Injury Prevention and Control for Children and Youth

■□■□■□■□■□■□■□■□■□■□■□■□■□■□■□■

Third Edition

Author: Committee on Injury and Poison Prevention
American Academy of Pediatrics

Editor: Mark D. Widome, MD, MPH

American Academy of Pediatrics
PO Box 927, 141 Northwest Point Blvd
Elk Grove Village, IL 60009-0927

Library of Congress Catalog No. 97-073556

ISBN 0-910761-90-6

MA 0024

Quantity prices on request.
Address all inquiries to:
American Academy of Pediatrics
PO Box 927, 141 Northwest Point Blvd
Elk Grove Village, IL 60009-0927

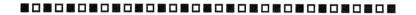

Acknowledgments

Many persons, mostly pediatricians, contributed to this manual. Although I am greatly indebted to my colleagues who contributed to the manuscript, the reader must assume that any deficiencies are the editor's. The Committee on Injury and Poison Prevention and the Section on Injury and Poison Prevention were always supportive, and special thanks go to Bill Boyle, MD, and Joel Bass, MD, the respective chairpersons at the time this project was begun, for their much-appreciated encouragement. I continue to gather encouragement and inspiration from the current committee under the able chairmanship of Murray Katcher.

I wish to acknowledge the following individuals whose contributions form the basis for the text:

Phyllis Agran, MD, MPH, University of California – Irvine, Irvine, CA

Jerold M. Aronson, MD, St Christopher's Primary Pediatrics, Philadelphia, PA

Jean Athey, MSW, PhD, Maternal and Child Health Bureau, Rockville, MD

M. Douglas Baker, MD, Children's Hospital of Philadelphia, Philadelphia, PA

Joel L. Bass, MD, MetroWest Medical Center, Framingham Union Campus, Framingham, MA

Roberta K. Beach, MD, MPH, Denver Health and Hospitals, Denver, CO

William E. Boyle, Jr, MD, Dartmouth Hitchcock Medical Center, Lebanon, NH

Bradley J. Bradford, MD, Mercy Children's Medical Center, Pittsburgh, PA

Marilyn J. Bull, MD, James Whitcomb Riley Hospital for Children, Indianapolis, IN

David L. Chadwick, MD, Children's Hospital and Health Center, Center for Child Protection, San Diego, CA

Ed Christophersen, PhD, Children's Mercy Hospital, Kansas City, MO

M. Denise Dowd, MD, MPH, Harborview Injury Prevention Research Center, Seattle, WA

Everett Dulit, MD, Albert Einstein College of Medicine, Bronx, NY

Lois A. Fingerhut, MA, National Center for Health Statistics, Hyattsville, MD

Jordan W. Finklestein, MD, The Pennsylvania State University, University Park, PA

Susan Gorcowski, MA, National Highway Traffic Safety Administration, Washington, DC

Joseph Greensher, MD, Winthrop-University Hospital, Mineola, NY

Marjorie Joan Hogan, MD, Hennepin County Medical Center, Minneapolis, MN

Murray L. Katcher, MD, PhD, University of Wisconsin Medical School, Madison, WI

Phillip J. Landrigan, MD, MSc, Mt Sinai School of Medicine, New York, NY

Gregory L. Landry, MD, University of Wisconsin Hospital and Clinics, Madison, WI

Barbara Lee, RN, PhD, National Farm Medicine Center, Marshfield, WI

Gerry Madden, MVB, MRCVS, Ambler, PA

Angela Mickalide, PhD, National SAFE Kids Campaign, Washington, DC

S. Donald Palmer, MD, Sylacauga Pediatric Clinic, Sylacauga, AL

Patricia Cresswell Parkin, MD, Hospital for Sick Children, Toronto, Ontario, Canada

Jerome Paulson, MD, George Washington University School of Medicine and Health Sciences, Washington, DC

Susan H. Pollack, MD, University of Kentucky, Lexington, KY

James Morrison Poole, MD, Capitol Pediatrics, Raleigh, NC

James S. Reilly, MD, Alfred I. DuPont Institute, Wilmington, DE

Frederick P. Rivara, MD, MPH, Harborview Injury Prevention Research Center, Seattle, WA

George C. Rodgers, Jr, MD, PhD, University of Louisville, Louisville, KY

Richard A. Schieber, MD, MPH, Centers for Disease Control and Prevention, Atlanta, GA

S. Kenneth Schonberg, MD, Albert Einstein College of Medicine, Bronx, NY

Donald F. Schwartz, MD, MPH, Children's Hospital of Philadelphia, Philadelphia, PA

Judy Sheese, PhD, James Whitcomb Riley Hospital for Children, Indianapolis, IN

Barbara L. Smith, MD, Tucson, AZ

Richard S. Stanwick, MD, MSc, The City of Winnipeg Health Department, Winnipeg, Manitoba, Canada

Victor C. Strasburger, MD, University of New Mexico School of Medicine, Albuquerque, NM

Robert R. Tanz, MD, Children's Memorial Hospital, Chicago, IL

Deborah Tinsworth, US Consumer Products Safety Commission, Washington DC

Susan B. Tully, MD, Los Angeles County Olive View Medical Center, Sylmar, CA

Lorrie Walker, Pennsylvania Traffic Injury Prevention Project, Bryn Mawr, PA

Flaura K. Winston, MD, PhD, Children's Hospital of Philadelphia, Philadelphia, PA

Carol L. Wright, Early Childcare Initiatives, Raleigh, NC

Joseph R. Zanga, MD, Children's Medical Center, Medical College of Virginia, Richmond, VA

The following contributed by reviewing chapters and helping polish various aspects of the book:

Judith Ann Bays, MD, CARES Program, Emanuel Hospital, Portland, OR

Stephanie Bryn, MPH, Maternal and Child Health Bureau, Rockville, MD

Mary Ellen Fise, JD, Consumer Federation of America, Washington, DC

Susan J. Gallagher, MPH, Children's Safety Network National Injury and Violence Prevention Resource Center, Newton, MA

Philip L. Graitcer, DMD, MPH, The Rollins School of Public Health of Emory University, Atlanta, GA

Donald E. Greydanus, MD, Michigan State University, Kalamazoo, MI

Allen H. Hanford, MD, The Milton S. Hershey Medical Center of The
Pennsylvania State University, Hershey, PA

Robert M. Reece, MD, Massachusetts Society for the Prevention of
Cruelty to Children, Boston, MA

Howard Spivak, MD, New England Medical Center, Tufts University
School of Medicine, Boston, MA

Deborah Davis Stewart, Editor, *Safe Ride News*, Seattle, WA

Thomas L. Young, MD, University of Kentucky, Lexington, KY

In each of the chapters, the contributors and the editor have tried to provide the reader with a selected list of references that we felt would be most useful to the reader. These lists may have, at times, failed to fully acknowledge other authors and sources whose ideas are incorporated into the manual. In particular, I have on my bookshelf (and wish to acknowledge) a few general references on injury prevention that I refer to on an almost daily basis. These books have shaped my thinking on the subject over the years, and therefore, many of the ideas of those authors are indirectly reflected in this manual. I recommend these books to the serious student of pediatric injury control. Each provides a unique perspective. The *Injury Fact Book* by Baker and colleagues is the best single source of general epidemiologic information and specific mortality data.[1] Good mortality and morbidity data on unintentional injuries are also available in the time-honored annual editions of the National Safety Council's *Accident Facts*.[2] Thought-provoking discussions of intervention strategies that go far beyond the scope of pediatrics can be found in *Saving Children* by Wilson and colleagues.[3] More general discussions of injury prevention epidemiology and public policy may be found in the extensive 1989 report by The National Committee for Injury Prevention and Control and in two excellent texts by Leon Robertson.[4-6] Julian Waller's *Injury Control* is a an excellent detailed text that emphasizes scientific rigor in the development of injury control strategies.[7] The best general reference on consumer products, for physicians and parents alike, is *The Childwise Catalog* by Jack Gillis and Mary Ellen Fise.[8] And finally, probably no recent work has been more influential in shaping national policy and the research agenda on injury control than *Injury in America*, the 1985 report to Congress by the Committee on Trauma Research of the National Research Council and the Institute of Medicine.[9] This short but powerful text is "must reading" for all modern students of injury prevention.

Special thanks are due to Michelle Esquivel, MPH, and Allison Rand, MPH, the AAP project managers for the manual, who assisted in all phases of this project; Barb Scotese, AAP senior medical copy editor; and Natalie Arndt, AAP word processor. Also, special thanks are due to Deborah Tinsworth of the Consumer Product Safety Commission who provided data, product reports, advice, and assistance to many of the authors, and good advice to the editor. Likewise, Lois Fingerhut of the National Center for Health Statistics provided recent mortality and morbidity data that were incorporated into various chapters and provide the basis for the Data Appendix.

Thanks are due for all I learned from the many members of the Committee on Injury and Poison Prevention with whom I had the pleasure of serving between the years of 1979 and 1991. I especially wish to acknowledge a debt to Jim Holroyd, MD, and Joe Greensher, MD, past chairpersons of the AAP Committee on Injury and Poison Prevention who preceded me in that post in the early 1980s.

My interest in injury control was originally sparked during my stay at the Johns Hopkins School of Hygiene and Public Health in 1976–1977. For her many insights, I owe thanks to Professor Susan Baker, who first showed me the vast unrealized potential in primary prevention.

Mark D. Widome, MD, MPH, Editor
Professor of Pediatrics
The Pennsylvania State University
College of Medicine
PO Box 850
Hershey, Pennsylvania 17033
717/531-8006 office
717/531-8985 fax

1. Baker SP, O'Neill B, Ginsburg M, Li G. *The Injury Fact Book*. 2nd ed. New York, NY: Oxford University Press; 1992

2. *Accident Facts*. Chicago, IL: National Safety Council; 1994

3. Wilson MH, Baker SP, Teret SP, Shock S, Garbarino J. *Saving Children: A Guide to Injury Prevention*. New York, NY: Oxford University Press; 1991

4. National Committee for Injury Prevention and Control. *Injury Prevention: Meeting the Challenge*. New York, NY: Oxford University Press; 1989

5. Robertson L. *Injuries: Causes, Control Strategies, and Public Policy*. Lexington, MA: Lexington Books; 1983

6. Robertson L. *Injury Epidemiology*. New York, NY: Oxford University Press; 1992

7. Waller J. *Injury Control: A Guide to the Causes and Prevention of Trauma*. Lexington, MA: Lexington Books; 1985

8. Gillis J, Fise MER. *The Childwise Catalog*. 3rd ed. New York, NY: HarperCollins; 1993

9. Committee on Trauma Research, National Research Council, and the Institute of Medicine. *Injury in America: A Continuing Public Health Problem*. Washington, DC: National Academy Press; 1985

4/26/96

■□■□■□■□■□■□■□■□■□■□■□■□■□■□■□■

Foreword: An Overview

This manual was assembled for pediatricians and others who are interested in the control of pediatric injuries. The focus of the chapters is meant to be practical, containing the kind of information that is useful in the office, but that is also useful to one preparing a talk or seminar for colleagues or for a community group. In all cases, I have exercised an editor's prerogative to cut and paste the work of the contributors to make the book seem whole.

The manual is divided into three sections: The Field of Pediatric Injury Prevention and Control, Injury Control in Specific Settings, and Specific Topics. The first section is meant to provide the reader with a broad overview of the field and to highlight the roles of the pediatrician in the control of injuries. Although a developmental perspective should be evident throughout the manual, the specific developmental concerns related to the prevention of adolescent injuries are surveyed in this section.

The second section looks at injury prevention at home, at school, in the workplace, and on the farm—the places where young people live, play, learn, and work. There is some overlap with the specific topics of the third section, but I have tried to provide cross references and an adequate index to efficiently guide the reader. Roadway and sports injuries are arbitrarily saved for the third section.

The final section covers specific injury topics related to mechanism of injury (fires, drownings, suffocation, etc.) or to specific products (toys, consumer products) or vectors (animals).

The Appendices provide mortality data, a guide to federal government involvement in injury control, and an introduction to available AAP materials.

As work progressed on this project, it became evident how much could not be covered. We gave priority to those topics and issues that appeared to have the greatest impact on child health. This is another book for the bookshelf, not *the* book for the bookshelf. The Committee on Injury and Poison Prevention and the Section on Injury and Poison Prevention hope that this manual will help you in your work in the control and prevention of pediatric trauma.

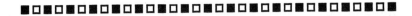

Contents

The Field of Pediatric Injury Prevention and Control

Injury Control in Specific Settings

Specific Topics

Appendices

■□■□■□■□■□■□■□■□■□■□■□■□■□■□■

CHAPTER 1

The Science of Injury Prevention

The practice of clinical pediatrics is based on the traditional basic sciences that include physiology, pharmacology, genetics, and pathology, among others. As pediatrics has evolved, newer basic sciences have assumed greater importance. Today's clinician must also have a firm foundation in behavioral sciences, epidemiology, and developmental biology. Likewise, as the science and practice of injury prevention has emerged into the mainstream of pediatric practice — both in the clinical setting and in community pediatrics — it has been built on three pillars of scientific investigation and understanding: epidemiology, biomechanics, and behavioral science. Epidemiology provides an understanding of the nonrandom distribution of injury risk among populations of children so that targeted interventions can be designed. Biomechanics gives an understanding of human vulnerability and resilience to energy transfers, so those energy transfers can be limited to tolerable amounts. Behavioral science provides knowledge about effective and ineffective ways of changing risk by changing behaviors not only of children and adolescents, but also of parents, decision makers, and entire communities. This chapter introduces the reader to these areas of basic knowledge. Further readings are suggested for the interested clinician.

1.1 Injury Epidemiology

1.1.1 Introduction

Injuries are understandable, predictable, and preventable. They are not, as we used to think, "accidents," ie, random, uncontrollable acts of fate or the result of a child being "accident prone." This is the central theme of injury epidemiology and has been the key to the development of injury prevention and control as a sophisticated science. Specific injuries share similar characteristics of person, place, and time. It is by understanding injuries that interventions can be developed and implemented to prevent or limit the extent of a given injury.

1.1.2 History

For the first half of this century the focus of injury prevention began with the premise that people who were injured were careless, stupid, or indifferent.[1, pp4-18] Movements in the 1920s (traffic safety) and 1950s (home safety) focused on the implementation of educational measures and the eradication of careless behavior. However, a landmark paper in 1942 by Hugh DeHaven, a pilot and physiology researcher, pointed out the great importance of injury thresholds and biomechanics and that damage in an injury event was not inevitable. He concluded that, "Structural provisions to reduce impact and distribute pressures can enhance survival and modify injury within wide limits in aircraft and automobile accidents."[2] In 1949, a seminal paper by Dr John Gordon introduced the concept of injury epidemiology.[3] Dr Gordon patterned the epidemiologic behavior of injury on a paradigm used in understanding infectious diseases. Thus, injuries could be characterized by episodic and seasonal variation, long-term trends, and demographic distribution. In addition, the occurrence of an injury could be thought of as the interaction of a host, an agent (or vector), and the environment. James J. Gibson modified this understanding by introducing the concept of energy transfer as the direct cause of injury.[4] Dr William Haddon, Jr, further developed this concept and summarized it in his phase-factor-matrix.[5]

The application of epidemiologic methods and other injury prevention strategies has met with substantial success in recent years. Motor vehicle injuries, as the most important cause of injury death for children and adolescents in the United States, have been the subject of a wide variety of injury prevention efforts. Efforts to reduce poisoning deaths among children have occurred at numerous levels. Reduction in the number of aspirin and iron tablets in one bottle to sublethal doses, the use of child-resistant packaging,[6] the development of poison center networks and poison information lines,[7] the use of syrup of ipecac in the home, and the development of effective protocols for the management of poisoning[8] have all contributed to a remarkable reduction in these deaths among preschool children.

Successful injury prevention campaigns have also been initiated and realized by individual efforts at the local level. Community pediatricians using concepts and interventions based on application of sound principles of injury prevention and control have made significant differences in childhood injury morbidity. A Tennessee pediatrician, Robert S. Sanders, MD, using a variety of approaches and considerable persistence, was responsible for the passage of the first US child safety seat law in 1977. In 1978, Kenneth Feldman, MD, a Seattle pediatrician, became concerned about the scald burns he saw in his practice.[9] Armed with a thermometer and the knowledge that serious burns will occur in less than 1 minute at water temperatures over 127°F (52.8°C), he visited households in his practice, where he measured the water temperature and routinely found temperatures of 150°F (65.6°C). With a combined strategy of community awareness, collaboration with the water company, and legislative action, all water heaters sold in Washington state eventually were set at a temperature of 125°F (51.7°C), thus greatly reducing the potential for scald injuries among children throughout the state as well as in his practice.

1.1.3 The Epidemiologic View of Injury

As William Haddon first outlined in his *phase-factor matrix* (Table 1.1, p 4), injuries can be studied in an organized fashion in much the same way as infectious diseases. Much like infectious disease, there is a "host" (the person with pneumonia or who has experienced blunt trauma), the "vector" (the bacterium or the vehicle), and the physical and socioeconomic environment (crowded living environment). However, unlike other diseases, the occurrence of an event leading to an injury (pre-event phase) can and should be distinguished from the actual injury-producing event (event phase). Finally, the ultimate morbidity and mortality from trauma are also affected by what happens after the injury occurs (postevent phase). Haddon's matrix allows one to consider an injury along all epidemiologic dimensions and at each phase in time. This generates further specific risk-factor hypotheses and determines points of intervention in the causal sequence.

Epidemiologic studies that investigate risk factors commonly concentrate on pre-event host factors, such as age or sex. However, injury prevention depends more on examining *modifiable* risk factors: pre-event factors such as separation of bicyclists from traffic, event factors such as

TABLE 1.1.
Matrix and Conceptual Framework for Injury Cause and Prevention: Example of Application to Bicycle Injuries*

Phases	Epidemiologic Dimension			
	Human Factor (Host)	Agent or Vehicle	Physical Environment	Socioeconomic Environment
Pre-event	Age Bicycle riding skill Judgment	Brakes, tires Reflectors	Separation from traffic Weather conditions	Funding for bike lanes Urban crowding Traffic
Event	Helmet wearing	Ease of control Protective covers on ends of handlebars	Riding surface Fixed objects in riding path	Affordability of helmets Helmet laws Attitudes about wearing helmets
Postevent	Age Physical condition		EMS systems Trauma centers	Support for trauma care Training of EMS personnel

*After Haddon.[5]

head protection offered by helmets, and postevent factors such as availability of emergency medical services and trauma center care. The field of injury control, then, attempts to reduce mortality and morbidity from trauma through primary prevention of the injury event, secondary prevention through better acute care, and tertiary prevention through improved and more accessible long-term rehabilitation.

Exposure measurement

A key element of any epidemiologic study design is the proper measurement of risk. Risk of a given injury is, in turn, related to exposure to a given environment, product, or activity. The risk of childhood drowning is clearly related to exposure to water. However, it is also related to the type of exposure (swimming vs wading), the length of the exposure, the duration of exposure per episode, and the number of episodes per year. The apparent increased risk of some types of injuries, ie, injuries to children in child care, may disappear when the number of hours of exposure are taken into account. If possible, calculation of rates of injuries should take these exposure measurements into consideration. For instance, motor vehicle fatalities are reported as both number of deaths per 100 000 population and as number of deaths per 100 million miles driven. Unfortunately, calculation of rates based on hours of exposure is difficult for most activities because of the lack of availability of such data.

Risk factor analysis

Risk factors are identified in order to apply epidemiologic methods to the study of injury. These risk factors become crucial to the planning of interventions directed at those persons at increased risk of a given injury. The questions "Who? What? Where? and How?" must be answered. The science of injury prevention and control seeks to determine *modifiable* risk factors through analytic epidemiologic studies. Study designs are chosen to minimize the probability of confounding factors biasing the estimate of risk.

The *case-control* and the *cohort* studies are two mainstays of analytic epidemiology that have been applied successfully in injury prevention research. The case-control design is ideal for the study of relatively rare problems, such as head injuries from bicycle crashes or suicides from home ownership of guns. It allows the researcher to measure the strength and direction of association between an injury and multiple risk or protective factors. Often, existing records and data sources are used, making these studies more economically feasible than cohort studies. Case-control studies do not require long-term follow-up. It was just such a study design that demonstrated that the risk of serious head injury increases dramatically if a bicycle helmet is not worn.[10] Challenges in the conduct of valid case-control studies include the proper selection of control subjects and accurate measure of the exposure of interest.

Cohort studies can be conducted either prospectively or retrospectively and are often more difficult and more expensive to conduct. Individuals are selected for the study based on the presence or absence of a particular potential risk factor. The subsequent occurrence of a specific injury is measured. Cohort designs can better show causality because the time sequence of exposure to risk factors and the injury event can be better determined. The major drawback of this design is that it may take a long time to gather a significant number of cases because specific injuries of a given mechanism are relatively rare events. By using both case-control and cohort methods, one can identify high-risk individuals, high-risk activities, or high-risk products (or combinations) to target interventions.

1.1.4 Data Sources

Readily available and accurate injury data are the foundation of the study of injury. Without them we have no valid way to quantify the problem, no basis with which to make informed decisions about prevention, and great difficulty in evaluating control measures. These data are also essential for educating the public and policy makers about the magnitude of injuries and the usefulness of prevention and control efforts. Population-based injury statistics are the ideal, although often difficult to come by (except for mortality statistics).

Although needs for accurate and adequate data are great, a number of data sources are available to the injury researcher or those interested in a descriptive or analytic evaluation of a local injury problem. In general, mortality data are much more readily obtained and more complete than are morbidity data. Mortality statistics are available from both national (National Center for Health Statistics at the Centers for Disease Control and Prevention) and state vital statistics offices.

Unfortunately, deaths due to injury are the "tip of the iceberg" and thus do not give a complete picture of the injury problem. Nonfatal injury data are much more difficult to obtain and may be less accurate. Most states have hospitalization discharges abstracted in a central database and coded by a diagnosis code (ICD-9 N Codes). Unfortunately, relatively few states code injury admissions by mechanism of injury using the available ICD-9 external cause of injury codes, or E-codes. Other local sources of injury data include the county or city medical examiner's office for injury fatalities, state or local trauma registries, and EMS databases, among others. All databases have limitations that must be understood and taken into account in the interpretation of the data (Table 1.2, p 7).

1.1.5 Interventions

Once causal factors are identified, appropriate preventive interventions should be devised. They should aim at preventing the injury from occurring in the first place, diminishing the damage caused by the injury event once it occurs, or limiting the long-term sequelae of the injury. As

TABLE 1.2.
Local and State Sources for Injury Morbidity and Mortality Data

	Level	Type of Data	Limitations
Vital statistics	State County	Deaths — demographics on person, cause of death, location (death certificates)	Often a considerable delay in reporting, death certificate not filled out in a standardized manner, may be completed before autopsy
Medical examiner data	County Local	Detailed data about injuries ending in death	Often not computerized, education of person completing report varies, may be difficult to obtain
Hospital discharge data	State (Uniform Hospital Discharge Data Sets) Local	All hospitalizations	May not contain E-coding, considerable lag time with state data
Trauma registries data	State Local	Hospitalizations due to trauma	Reflect regionalization of trauma care, may include only those hospitalized ≥ 24–48 h
EMS and prehospital reporting systems	State	All cases transported by EMS	A minority of injuries arrive via EMS
Criminal justice agencies	Local State	Assaults, homicides known to police	Ease of accessibility varies
Physicians of ces, HMOs	Local	All injuries presenting to offices	Data may not be computerized

shown in Table 1.1, a researcher could devise a number of strategies for all three phases: bike paths to separate riders from traffic, helmets on riders to limit injury should a crash occur, and further development of EMS systems and trauma centers.

Traditionally, interventions or countermeasures are considered either passive or active, depending on requirements for behavior change on the part of the host. Active interventions rely on actions taken by the host individual (the child or someone acting on behalf of the child, eg, the parent). For example, poisoning can be prevented by storing medications away from children's reach. Passive interventions, on the other hand, do not rely on the effort of the host to be successful. An effective passive strategy has been the packaging of medications in non-lethal amounts.

Many interventions cannot be classified as strictly active or passive but are somewhere between the two or use both active and passive strategies. For example, a helmet will help protect from head injury if someone falls off a bicycle, but the helmet must be properly worn in the first place. The likelihood that an intervention will be successful at preventing injury is inversely related to the amount of individual effort required.

Interventions — targeting

The first step in planning an injury control or prevention countermeasure is to define a target group or population in which to implement the intervention. Targeting is important because the intervention can be designed with a particular population in mind and population-specific goals can be set. A target group may be chosen because the injury occurs relatively frequently in that group (eg, age group), the intervention is most likely to be successful in the group, or a combination of the two. The Seattle Bicycle Helmet Campaign was targeted to school-age children because bicycle-related head injuries are common in this population and the behavior of 5- to 9-year-olds was perceived to be more open to change (as opposed to teenagers, for instance).[11]

Interventions — implementing

After the countermeasure is chosen and a target group is identified, the countermeasure must be implemented. This may involve several activities and may be carried out at a variety of levels: among patients in a given practice, among students at a given school, or in an entire community. Implementing an injury prevention effort is often a collaborative affair — the joint effort of health care educators, public relations specialists, community leaders, and other concerned groups.

Interventions — evaluating

One of the most important uses of epidemiology in injury research is the evaluation of interventions. The traditional evaluation of disease prevention programs has been based on examining subsequent reductions in disease and deaths. Injuries, however, are relatively rare, and reduction in the number of deaths or hospitalizations for a specific injury, particularly in a local study, may not be statistically feasible. Emergency departments remain a potential source of data, but many emergency departments do not routinely code injury data by mechanism. Ongoing emergency department–based surveillance systems, such as those that exist in children's hospitals in Canada and many hospitals in Australia, are clearly helpful.

At the other end of the outcome spectrum are surveys that measure changes in knowledge and attitudes. Although often used to measure the effectiveness of injury prevention programs, the evidence argues against them as valid measures in injury research since they correlate poorly with changes in behaviors. Likewise, self-reporting of behaviors can be misleading. Comparison of self-report data on safety belt use and observed use shows that safety belt use is substantially over-reported.[12,13]

One method that avoids those limitations and has proven useful in the evaluation of injury prevention programs is the use of proxies, or changes in behavior that lead directly to prevention. A proxy evaluation was used to measure the effectiveness of community bicycle helmet programs in Seattle, Wash. Bicycle helmet use among school-age children increased from 5% to 16% after 1 year of intervention. The control community, Portland, Ore, showed no such increase. Determining the effectiveness of a particular intervention is critical to use limited resources most effectively.[14]

1.1.6 Conclusion

Epidemiology is the cornerstone science upon which the field of injury prevention and control is built. It provides the direction for intervention efforts by helping to choose important injury problems and high-risk groups and to create strategies to decrease the most serious injuries. Epidemiology also plays a key role in evaluating interventions and directing scarce resources to programs that have the greatest impact. The greatest advances in injury control over the last decade have come from applying the science of epidemiology to our efforts and moving from programs that "seem to make sense" to those that are evidence-based. While large case-control studies and manipulation of computer databases are beyond the reach of many practicing pediatricians, the ability to understand the patterns of injury in a community is available to us all.

The pediatrician is referred to several basic texts on the epidemiology of injury.[1,12,15,16] A national directory of injury prevention professionals is available from the National Center for Education in Maternal and Child Health, 38th and R Streets, NW, Washington, DC 20057 (202-625-8400).[17]

1.2 Biomechanics

Effective injury control involves strategies for avoiding injury-producing events and minimizing the injuries that may result if these events should occur. While epidemiologists have identified risk factors for the child and the environment, bioengineers study injury events to design safety technologies that will reduce the risk of injury and the severity of injury. The key to understanding the use of specific safety devices is in understanding the biomechanical principles that led to their design.

1.2.1 Injury and Energy

All prevention strategies work by minimizing the burden of various harmful agents on the body. Just as viruses and bacteria are among the agents of infectious disease, energy is the agent of injury. And, in the same way that infectious diseases are prevented by minimizing the burden of pathogenic viruses and bacteria on the body, injury is prevented by minimizing harmful forms of energy. Injury results when a body is exposed to energy that surpasses the body's ability to absorb or dissipate that energy without structural or functional damage.

Energy may be mechanical, thermal, chemical, electrical, or ionizing radiation. When the human body is exposed to significant quantities of energy of any form, the body must somehow manage this excess energy or be damaged. For example, when the body is exposed to excess thermal energy or heat, blood vessels dilate to manage the excess energy. If the temperature is beyond the thermoregulatory capacities of the body, a burn or heat stroke may result.

Mechanical energy is of special importance in any general discussion of pediatric injury prevention. It is the energy of motion and the agent that can break bones and cause head injuries in falls, automobile crashes, and gunshot wounds. This form of energy is responsible for the majority of injury hospitalizations and fatalities. Mechanical trauma can occur without impact (eg, whiplash after rapid flexion-extension of the neck or avulsion fracture after twisting an ankle), but most of the severe mechanical traumas occur following impact. At low levels of excess mechanical energy, bodies manage the energy locally by bending and stretching; at higher levels, bones will break, often preserving the more vital internal organs.

1.2.2 Energy and Safety Technologies

The goal of many safety technologies is to aid the body in managing excess mechanical energy. An energy-absorbing surface beneath playground equipment can prevent serious injuries from falls. Seat belts can allow a child to survive what would otherwise be a fatal motor vehicle crash. A polystyrene-lined helmet can prevent brain damage in a fall from a bicycle.

These examples illustrate some of the most important principles in the management of energy by safety technologies. Safety technologies serve to reduce the severity of injury by minimizing the energy delivered to the child and by altering the *manner* in which energy is delivered. The severity of injury is related to the *amount* of energy the body must manage, the *direction* of impact, the *mechanical properties of the tissue* impacted, the *suddenness* of the impact, and the *localization* of the impact.

The relationship between *magnitude* of energy delivered and degree of injury is the most obvious. Magnitude of energy varies directly with the distance of a free fall and varies with the *square* of the velocity of impact. A child falling 6 ft onto a playground surface will suffer more severe injuries than a child falling 3 ft. The energy delivered is *twice* the magnitude because the distance of the fall is *twice* the distance. However, a car crashing into a tree at 30 miles per hour will *not* deliver twice the energy to occupants of one crashing at 15 miles per hour; it will deliver *four* times the energy, because energy varies as the *square* of speed. From the above, it can be concluded that limiting the height of playground equipment and enforcing speed limits are important injury prevention strategies based on biomechanical principles. It can also be concluded that limiting speed plays an especially important role in limiting energy transfers.[12]

Another important determinant of injury severity is the *direction* of impact. The body is not symmetrical. Impacts to the left side of the body will result in different injuries from impacts to the right side, the front, or the back. In particular, lateral impacts to the head are more closely associated with diffuse axonal injury and coma than impacts in other directions. This biomechanical principle of injury may partly explain the continued high prevalence of morbidity and mortality associated with side-impact motor vehicle collisions. To minimize the energy delivered to the body with lateral collisions, a side-impact air bag for automobiles has been developed.

Mechanical properties of biological tissues vary considerably with respect to medical condition and age. In particular, infants have relatively large head-to-body mass ratios and weak neck musculature. As a result, infants would be subject to severe whiplash injuries in frontal motor vehicle collisions. Because the majority of severe motor vehicle collisions are frontal, engineers have designed infant safety seats that face backward.

The *suddenness* of impact is another determinant of injury severity. Biological tissues have a property known as *viscoelasticity*; the faster they are struck, the more easily they are injured. Many safety technologies work to reduce the suddenness of impact to ease the blow. In other words, they are designed to deliver the energy over a long enough period of time that the tissues can manage it. Helmet liners crush on impact and seat belts stretch. These technologies all serve to increase the time (a larger fraction of a second) over which energy of an impact is delivered to the body.

The degree of *localization* of the impact is related to the amount of surface area exposed to the impact. For a given force, the larger the area over which an impact is distributed, the less severe the injury. (This is often measured in pounds per square inch.) As an extreme example, sitting on a sharp tack will result in injury while sitting on a chair will not. In both situations the force is the same but the area over which the force is distributed is different. When used properly, seat belts distribute an impact over the bones of the pelvis and thorax, thereby spreading the load and minimizing injuries. If seat belts are not worn, a properly shaped dashboard will cause less injury than one with edges and protrusions, though both may deliver the same total energy in a crash.

Some of the principles of biomechanical reasoning can be appreciated in the following examples: vehicle crashes and bicycle head injuries.

What happens to an unrestrained passenger during a motor vehicle collision?

During an impact, the vehicle decelerates suddenly and comes to a complete stop over a distance related to the amount the vehicle is crushed.[18] For a 30-mph frontal impact with a rigid barrier, this deceleration to a stop occurs over about 2 ft.

As the collision develops, the vehicle begins to stop but the unrestrained passenger continues to move at the original speed of the vehicle. Because the knees contact the instrument panel early in the crash phase, before the vehicle has come to a complete stop, the knees benefit from the deceleration, or impact ride-down, of the vehicle. Before impact, the head is approximately 2 ft from the windshield and will hit after the vehicle has come to a complete stop. Therefore, the head of an unrestrained occupant will be exposed to a sudden, short-duration stop and will not benefit from ride-down.

Unrestrained infants are at particular risk during motor vehicle crashes, especially if a passenger holds the infant in his or her lap. During the collision, the infant will not only experience a violent impact when thrown against the vehicle interior, but will also be crushed by the passenger. In effect, the infant will serve to cushion the blow of the passenger holding him. Older unrestrained children may be thrown against the interior of the vehicle or ejected through windows.[19]

Prevention technologies are created to increase the time and the surface area over which the energy of the crash is delivered to the body. The crushing of the front of the automobile absorbs some of the energy in addition to distributing the remaining energy over time. Restraint systems such as seat belts or child-restraint systems provide some additional ride-down time when they stretch. Additionally, they deliver forces over additional area given the width of the webbing. Most importantly, they deliver the energy load to parts of the body that can tolerate it better (eg, the pelvis) rather than parts that can poorly tolerate it (eg, the head).

As discussed in chapter 9, restraints must be used properly to achieve maximum benefit and to prevent injuries induced by the restraint system itself. The mechanical properties of tissues impacted are considerations in the recommendation that infants not face forward in the automobile. Large head, weak neck muscles, and small pelvis all make it imperative that the infant be rear-facing and allow the crash forces to be distributed along the long axis of the infant's body, thus avoiding spinal flexion injuries or abdominal injuries.

Prevention of bicycle-related head injuries

In a bicycle crash, the head is often the first body part to hit an object or the ground. The mechanical energy involved in the impact is transmitted directly to the skull and then to the brain and dural blood vessels. Helmets are designed to decrease energy transmitted to the head during impact.

During a crash, the head crushes the foam liner in the helmet. As the foam liner is crushed, it absorbs sufficient force to slow the head to a relatively gentle stop. This protects the head from the potentially lethal levels of energy it would otherwise sustain. In other words, helmets are designed to protect the head by absorbing and dissipating the energy of impact. Helmets are designed to spread a concentrated load over a larger portion of the head, protect against penetration, and remain on the wearer's head during an impact.

Until recently, all helmets protected against a single impact. Once the foam was crushed, the helmet was no longer protective for future impacts and needed to be replaced. However, a new generation of multi-impact helmets is emerging. These helmets are made of new foams that crush during impact, but then recover after crushing. The foam is able to crush multiple times, making these helmets ideal for sports involving multiple falls such as rollerblading.[20]

Helmets must be worn properly to give their greatest protective effect. Four key points should be considered when purchasing and fitting a helmet — the four S's: Sticker, Size, Straight, and Straps. A *sticker* indicating conformity with a recognized voluntary performance standard should be affixed to the inside of the helmet. (A sticker from The Snell Memorial Foundation on the inside of the helmet assures the buyer that the helmet has passed the most rigorous premarket and postmarket testing currently [1996] available for helmets.) The helmet should be *sized* to fit the child comfortably when placed on the head horizontally *straight* across the midforehead. Foam pads should be added to ensure a tight fit. Finally, the retention *straps* should be adjusted according to the manufacturer's instructions so that the helmet will not come off during an impact. Like safety seats, helmets are complicated to use and are often used incorrectly.

1.2.3 Conclusion

Safety technologies are designed to minimize the energy delivered to the child during impact and to deliver this energy to the child in a manner that will result in the least severe injuries. The pediatrician can serve as information resource for injury prevention strategies in the same way that he or she educates about disease. The frustration that accompanies using complicated safety devices can be lessened by counseling from a pediatrician who has an understanding of the biomechanical principles employed in the design of these technologies.

1.3 Behavioral Sciences and Pediatric Injury Control

Of all of the major mandates in health care today, injury control is perhaps the one to which behavioral scientists have the most to contribute. The complexity of the task provides a compelling rationale for professionals with a wide range of backgrounds to contribute to injury control efforts. Within the behavioral sciences alone, many productive professionals have died or had their productivity diminished or compromised by injuries. In the landmark 1985 document, *Injury in America*, several major approaches were identified to prevent injuries.[21] These include:

1. Persuading persons at risk of injury to alter their behavior to increase their self-protection — for example, to use seat belts or install smoke detectors.
2. Requiring individual behavior change by law or administrative rule — for example, by passing laws that require the use of seat belts or the installation of smoke detectors in all new buildings.
3. Providing automatic protection by product and environmental engineering — for example, installation of built-in sprinkler systems that automatically extinguish fires.

Each of these fundamental approaches to injury control can benefit from the behavioral sciences. Not only can behavioral scientists provide guidance in the design of strategies to modify personal behaviors, they can also suggest how to best influence demand for and acceptance of public policy to reduce injury (legislation and regulation). Even passive (engineering) strategies can greatly benefit from the behavioral sciences since all technologies require human motivation and acceptance in their design and implementation. Tragically, thousands of lives were needlessly lost on our nation's highways in the several decades that passed between the development of air bag technology and its final acceptance into automobile design.

This section will emphasize the application of the behavioral sciences to the first fundamental approach: persuasion. To that end, a review of the areas of health education and behavior management are of particular pertinence to the work of pediatricians.

1.3.1 Active and Passive Strategies

All injury control strategies can be placed on an active-passive continuum depending on how dependent each strategy is on modifying human behavior. Automobile air bags that automatically inflate in a crash are considered passive. The traditional seat belt that an individual uses every time he or she enters an automobile is considered active. There is a broad consensus in the injury control literature that active approaches are more difficult to implement and less effective than passive approaches.[22]

While passive ("nonbehavioral") strategies to injury control are preferred, such strategies are not possible in many instances. For example, parents can turn down their hot water heater temperature to protect their children from scald burns, but there is no practical way to remove all potential sources of drowning in a home (toilets, buckets, and bathtubs). In those instances where a totally passive strategy is not feasible, a combination of active and passive strategies is desirable.

Despite the preference for injury control solutions that depend minimally on behavior, there is little chance that injury control can be realized without the contributions of both active and passive strategies. Effective injury control will always depend, in part, on an understanding of what motivates safe and unsafe behaviors and how those behaviors might be reinforced or modified.

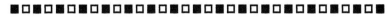
1.3.2 Health Education

Most of the early efforts at injury control involved some form of health education. Health care providers often informed patients of the potential benefits and dangers of particular behaviors that their patient engaged in and would, typically, make alternative recommendations.

It is unfortunate that so much early (and current) effort in health education has been conducted without adequate evaluation. Often, even intensive safety education efforts, when subject to scrutiny, have been shown to have little or no benefit.[23,24] It is therefore imperative that health education interventions be subject to the same objective scrutiny demanded for other kinds of injury control interventions.

Both Reisinger and Dershewitz tried brief (less than 2 minutes in duration) educational "pep-talks" for restraint-seat usage and smoke detector installation, respectively.[25,26] Both studies reported minor improvements in parents' implementation of injury control measures. Later studies have shown that when health care providers took more time and effort to give the health education messages, more promising results emerged. Christophersen and his colleagues reported high rates of compliance with infant automobile restraint-seat use when a multidimensional educational program was used.[27] Their program included the passage of state legislation, a hospital loaner program for provision of the restraint seats, nurses and physicians who encouraged and educated new parents about the need to use restraint seats, and a community-wide educational program about the advantages of restraint-seat use. The parents in the study correctly used restraint seats more than 85% of the time at hospital discharge and at 3-month, 6-month, and 12-month follow-up observations. It is unclear, however, how important a role the educational component played.

In an extension of this study, Treiber reported that similar health education approaches were effective in encouraging parents to use automobile-restraint devices for young children correctly.[28] Treiber demonstrated parents had the highest compliance rates when they were informed about both the dangers of automobile travel and the advantages inherent in using child-restraint devices. Discussions of only the dangers of automobile travel or of only the advantages of restraint-seat use produced lower rates than the two strategies combined.

In another study, Thomas and her colleagues demonstrated the potential effectiveness of an alternative health education format — called group well-child care — in encouraging parents to lower the temperature of hot water heaters in their homes.[29]

Future health education research should concentrate on identifying those components of multidimensional programs that may be critical to their effectiveness.

1.3.3 Behavioral Approaches

While health education efforts frequently have been used to encourage individuals to implement changes that will reduce the risk of injury that they face each day, a variety of behavior modification approaches also have been used in recent studies of injury control.

Behavioral researchers frequently have viewed problematic behavior as falling into one of two categories:

- Behaviors that need to be learned initially or increased in frequency, such as using seat belts and conscientiously monitoring children
- Behaviors that need to be eliminated or reduced in frequency, such as playing in the street, playing with matches, exceeding highway speed limits, and driving while intoxicated

Many standard behavioral interventions, including the use of tangible rewards and incentives, have been widely used in past research. Several researchers have applied these or similar interventions to injury control research.

Roberts and Turner used behavioral techniques to encourage parents and children to use automobile safety belts or child-restraint devices by rewarding parents for correct use.[30] The parents were given lottery tokens redeemable for prizes if their children were appropriately secured with an automobile seat belt when they arrived at the child's day care center. When the parents began receiving rewards based upon their seat belt use, there was an increase in their own use of seat belts. After the rewards were removed, seat belt use gradually declined.

Sowers-Hoag et al used behavioral strategies, assertiveness training, and social and contrived reinforcers to successfully establish and maintain automobile safety belt use in young children.[31] Geller and his colleagues

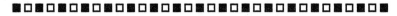

also showed the effectiveness of rewards on increasing the use of child safety devices.[32] These studies demonstrate that behavior modification strategies can be applied to injury prevention.

Mathews and colleagues reported on a program for teaching mothers to use standard child behavior management techniques to reduce the number of dangerous behaviors in their young children.[33] They showed that the use of techniques originally developed to reduce other undesirable behaviors in young children was also effective in reducing dangerous behavior. In this study, teenage mothers were taught through modeling and demonstration how to reward their infants with brief physical contact for age-appropriate behaviors. They were also taught to dissuade dangerous behaviors by placing their child in a playpen for a brief time-out. The infants in the study engaged in potentially dangerous behaviors approximately 55% of the time prior to training. After the mothers were trained in the use of these behavioral techniques, the children's potentially dangerous behaviors occurred less than 10% of the time. These results were maintained at a 6-month follow-up.

In the future, researchers should continue to study and refine promising techniques of behavioral modification to injury prevention problems. In the study by Mathews et al,[33] the mothers were trained using in-home demonstrations by behavior therapists. Future research can examine whether the same procedures might work if used in an office setting. Future studies must also examine whether behavior changes can be sustained over extended periods of time.

In 1985, Gallagher et al reported encouraging results from a program that utilized a three-part injury prevention strategy.[34] The three strategies were regulatory (identification and abatement of violations of existing housing codes), educational (counseling on potential safety hazards in the home), and technological (installation and/or distribution of inexpensive safety devices at no cost to the family). Gallagher et al showed that the homes in the intervention group had fewer household hazards — including fewer hazardous items and lower hot water heater temperatures. Future investigators should evaluate similar comprehensive programs that incorporate behavioral and nonbehavioral strategies.

1.3.4 Conclusion

The behavioral sciences play a complementary role to epidemiology and biomechanics in the development of focused injury control strategies. Pediatricians have traditionally relied on their behavioral science backgrounds to educate parents and patients to ensure compliance with recommendations. The application of behavioral sciences to injury control has the potential to extend the pediatrician's effectiveness in the office and in community-based endeavors.

References

1. National Committee for Injury Prevention and Control. Injury prevention: meeting the challenge. *Am J Prevent Med.* 1989;5(suppl 3):1–303

2. DeHaven H. Mechanical analysis of survival in falls from heights of fifty to one hundred and fifty feet. *War Med.* 1942;2:586–596

3. Gordon JE. The epidemiology of accidents. *Am J Public Health.* 1949;39:504–515

4. Gibson JJ. The contribution of experimental psychology to the formulation of the problem of safety: a brief for basic research. In: Jacobs HH et al, eds. *Behavioral Approaches to Accident Research.* New York, NY: Association for the Aid of Crippled Children; 1961:77–89

5. Haddon W Jr. A logical framework for categorizing highway safety phenomena and activity. *J Trauma.* 1972;12:193–207

6. Walton WW. An evaluation of the poison prevention packaging act. *Pediatrics.* 1982; 69:363–370

7. McIntire MS, Angle CR. Regional poison control centers improve patient care. *N Engl J Med.* 1983;308:219

8. Done AK. Aspirin overdosage: incidence, diagnosis and management. *Pediatrics.* 1978;62:890–897

9. Feldman KW, Schaller RT, Feldman JA, McMillon M. Tap water scald burns in children. *Pediatrics.* 1978;62:1–7

10. Thompson RS, Rivara FP, Thompson DC. A case-control study of the effectiveness of bicycle safety helmets. *N Engl J Med.* 1989;320:1361–1367

11. Bergman AB, Rivara FP, Richards DD, Rogers LW. The Seattle children's bicycle helmet campaign. *Am J Dis Child.* 1990;144:727–731

12. Robertson LS. *Injury Epidemiology.* New York, NY: Oxford University Press; 1992

13. Mawson AR, Biundo JJ Jr. Contrasting beliefs and actions of drivers regarding seatbelts: a study in New Orleans. *J Trauma.* 1985;25:433–437

14. DiGuiseppi CG, Rivara FP, Koepsell TD, Polissar L. Bicycle helmet use by children: evaluation of a community-wide helmet campaign. *JAMA*. 1989;262:2256–2261

15. Wilson MH, Baker SP, Teret SP, Shock S, Garbarino J. *Saving Children: A Guide to Injury Prevention*. New York, NY: Oxford University Press; 1991

16. Baker SP, O' Neill B, Ginsburg M, Li G. *The Injury Fact Book*. 2nd ed. New York, NY: Oxford University Press; 1992

17. *Injury Prevention Professionals: A National Directory*. Washington, DC: National Center for Education in Maternal and Child Health; 1992

18. Mackay M. Mechanisms of injury and biomechanics: vehicle design and crash performance. *World J Surg*. 1992;16:420–427

19. The Insurance Institute for Highway Safety. *Protecting Child Passengers: Crash Tests by the IIHS*. Arlington, VA: Insurance Institute for Highway Safety; 1990

20. Snell Memorial Foundation. *1994 Standard for Protective Headgear for Use in Non-Motorized Sports*. St James, NY: Snell Memorial Foundation Inc; 1994

21. Committee on Trauma Research, Commission on Life Sciences, National Research Council, and the Institute of Medicine. *Injury in America: A Continuing Public Health Problem*. Washington, DC: National Academy Press; 1985

22. Williams AF. Passive and active measures for controlling disease and injury: the role of health psychologists. *Health Psychol*. 1982;1:399–409

23. Derschewitz RA, Williamson JA. Prevention of childhood household injuries: a controlled clinical trial. *Am J Public Health*. 1977;67:1148–1153

24. Robertson L, Zador PL. Driver education and fatal crash involvement of teen-aged drivers. *Am J Public Health*. 1978;68:959–965

25. Reisinger KS, Bires JA. Anticipatory guidance in pediatric practice. *Pediatrics*. 1980; 66:889–892

26. Dershewitz RA. Will mothers use free household safety devices? *Am J Dis Child*. 1979;133:61–64

27. Christophersen ER, Sosland-Edelman D, LeClaire S. Evaluation of two comprehensive infant car seat loaner programs with 1-year follow-up. *Pediatrics*. 1985;76:36–42

28. Treiber FA. A comparison of the positive and negative consequences approaches upon car restraint usage. *J Pediatr Psychol*. 1986;11:15–24

29. Thomas KA, Hassanein RS, Christophersen ER. Evaluation of group well-child care for improving burn prevention practices in the home. *Pediatrics*. 1984;74:879–882

30. Roberts MC, Turner DS. Rewarding parents for their children's use of safety seats. *J Pediatr Psychol*. 1986;11:25–36

31. Sowers-Hoag KM, Thyer BA, Bailey JS. Promoting automobile safety belt use by young children. *J Appl Behav Anal*. 1987;20:133–138

32. Geller ES, Bruff CD, Nimmer JG. 'Flash for life': community-based prompting for safety belt promotion. *J Appl Behav Anal*. 1985;18:309–314

33. Mathews JR, Friman PC, Barone VJ, Ross LV, Christophersen ER. Decreasing dangerous infant behaviors through parent instruction. *J Appl Behav Anal.* 1987;20: 165–169

34. Gallagher SS, Hunter P, Guyer B. A home injury prevention program for children. *Pediatr Clin North Am.* 1985;32:95–112

■□■□■□■□■□■□■□■□■□■□■□■□■□■□■□■□■□■

CHAPTER 2

An Office-Based Approach to Injury Counseling

The pediatrician has a key role in educating parents and children about injury prevention strategies. As the professional who regularly sees parents of young children, and as the professional who establishes and maintains a continuing relationship based on concern for the child's health, growth, and development, the pediatrician is key in influencing parental behavior to reduce risk of injury.

An effective office-based injury prevention program for children is developmentally focused and cogent, emphasizes the most important injuries, and actively engages the parent in a dialogue regarding injury prevention. Such a program engenders a sense of responsibility and urgency to adopt and follow safe practices. Any such program must take into account the parent's own viewpoint on injury prevention. In addition, an effective program is adaptable to office practice and works efficiently with other health supervision activities.

2.1 TIPP

Although a wide variety of materials are available for injury prevention and many pediatricians have developed their own system of injury prevention counseling, the American Academy of Pediatrics (AAP) TIPP (The Injury Prevention Program) is the most comprehensive system that is readily available for practicing pediatricians. TIPP consists of three major elements:

- A policy statement on injury prevention by the American Academy of Pediatrics Committee on Injury and Poison Prevention
- Childhood Safety Counseling Schedules
- Safety information sheets and safety surveys for use in providing anticipatory guidance to parents

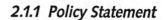
2.1.1 Policy Statement

The Academy's first policy statement on injury prevention was published in 1982. The most recent version of the statement (October 1994) reflects the Academy's attempts to address the most significant issues of the 1990s (see Appendix C).[1] The policy focuses on common injuries with known effective intervention strategies, such as child safety seats and smoke detectors, and addresses those issues of greatest significance to parents of children by age group. The policy has made injury prevention counseling a standard of care in pediatrics and provides an important benchmark defining comprehensive pediatric practice.

2.1.2 The Childhood Counseling Schedules

TIPP injury counseling schedules have been designed to correspond intentionally to the AAP Periodicity Schedule for children. An Early Childhood Safety Counseling Schedule and a Middle Childhood Safety Counseling Schedule are included in the program. Both schedules explain when to introduce concepts related to injury prevention, when they should be reinforced, and what materials are available to accomplish the goal.

2.1.3 Materials

Materials in TIPP include age-specific and topic-specific Safety Sheets (see Appendix E). Also included are the Framingham Safety Surveys, a series of developmentally oriented questionnaires that highlight specific risk areas for individual parents. TIPP sheets help focus the pediatrician's counseling at each visit on selected important injuries, ensuring compliance with the TIPP counseling schedules. The Safety Surveys highlight the education issues concerning injury that are most germane to the parent being counseled.

The Safety Surveys are a series of developmentally appropriate two-part forms on which only at-risk answers appear on the duplicate copy. The reading levels (fifth and sixth grade) of the surveys have made them adaptable to a wide range of clinical settings, and studies have shown them to be both well accepted and effective. TIPP sheets, Framingham Safety Surveys, and counseling schedules are color coded to allow for ease of use. In addition, TIPP includes a *Guide to Safety Counseling in Office Practice* that explains all the details of TIPP, as well as specific counseling guidelines for every question on each of the Framingham Safety Surveys.[2]

2.2 Additional Strategies

In addition to TIPP, other strategies are available to strengthen injury prevention counseling. The physician's office should be a model of safety in the waiting room, reception areas, and examining rooms. Posters promoting and demonstrating safety are available from many sources. In particular, announcements of hazardous products from the Consumer Product Safety Commission can be prominently displayed in the office. Use of such strategies creates an atmosphere in which parents can readily learn to appreciate the importance that the physician places on injury control.

2.3 Effectiveness of Physician Counseling

Although the AAP has recommended injury prevention counseling for more than a decade, the question of the validity of counseling has been raised in the literature over the years. At least three questions need to be addressed:

• Is there a need for the counseling?
• Is the counseling process effective?
• Can the results be documented?

2.3.1 Educational Needs

The need for injury prevention counseling is perhaps the easiest of these three questions to address. Several studies have demonstrated that parents do have varied and significant educational needs about injury prevention.

A 1980 study in Framingham, Mass, demonstrated the educational needs of parents regarding a wide range of injury prevention activities. This study included parents from suburban and clinic practices.[3] Extraordinary deficiencies were identified in parental awareness and reported practice of basic injury prevention techniques for parents of children of all age groups and among all social and ethnic groups studied. Knowledge deficiencies were noted in the areas of fire and burn prevention, poison prevention, and vehicular safety. Similar deficiencies were noted in a statewide survey that included nearly 1500 Massachusetts parents from urban, suburban, and rural communities.[4] In addition, a study of clinic patients in Tennessee documented the educational needs of parents regarding the developmental aspects of injury prevention.[5]

Although the three studies previously described date from the early 1980s and most closely reflect educational programs available to parents through the mid- to late 1970s, a more recent study using a nationwide telephone survey demonstrated that parents had significant educational needs concerning pedestrian and bicycle injuries, burns, and drowning.[6] An interesting aspect of this study was that parents thought they would be most likely to obtain information on child safety from the physician's office and physicians were cited as the parents' first choice for information on injury control and child safety.

2.3.2 Effectiveness of the Counseling Process

An effective injury prevention counseling program must:
• Be easy to administer
• Be readily comprehensible to parents
• Make efficient use of the physician's time
• Address relevant issues that concern parents

A recent study performed by the AAP Department of Research showed that different groups of parents each adopt injury prevention strategies that reflect their own concepts of good parenting.[7] Urban parents tend to believe that their children are safer indoors and are more concerned about hazards outside the home. They also think that keeping an eye on their children is most important for good parenting and that safety equipment is unnecessary provided supervision is available. Suburban parents, in contrast, tend to believe that good parents use safety equipment and supplies. Appreciation of such patterns of parental attitudes enables effective counseling to motivate compliance and overcome resistance to counseling suggestions.

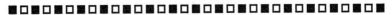
2.3.3 Outcomes of Counseling

When the effectiveness of injury prevention counseling is reviewed, three types of outcomes can be examined: educational change, behavioral change, and change in the occurrence of injury. A recent review of the literature on the effectiveness of pediatric counseling has shown that of 20 studies reviewed, 18 demonstrated positive effects.[8] The results and types of effects both for motor vehicle–related and non–motor vehicle–related injuries are summarized in Tables 2.1 and 2.2, p 28. This review included 11 randomized controlled reports. In view of these results, it is evident that physician counseling to prevent injury is an important component of pediatric primary care.

As a final point, the economic impact of injury prevention counseling may also be significant. A recently published analysis based on the AAP literature review estimated if the parents of all 19 million children from birth to 4 years of age received the TIPP counseling, approximately $230 million would be saved annually in medical spending due to injury and that injury costs overall would decline by $3.4 billion.[9] Each dollar spent on TIPP was estimated to return nearly $13 in economic value.

Considering both the efficacy studies and the economic analysis based on those studies, ample evidence exists that pediatric injury preven-

TABLE 2.1.
Outcomes of Pediatric Injury Prevention Counseling (1964–1991): Motor Vehicle*

	Outcome Measures		
Study Design	Educational	Behavioral	Injury Occurrence
Controlled/ randomized	Increased reported car seat use	Increased sales of car seats	
Controlled/ not randomized	Increased reported seat belt use Increased reported car seat use	Increased car seat use	Decreased auto passenger injuries
Multiple time series			Decreased traffic accidents

*From Bass et al.[8]

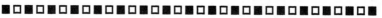

TABLE 2.2.
Outcomes of Pediatric Injury Prevention Counseling (1964–1991):
Non–Motor Vehicle*

| | Outcome Measures | | |
Study Design	Educational	Behavioral	Injury Occurrence
Controlled/ randomized	Increased recognition of household injuries Decreased reported hot water temperature at tap	Increased home safety Increased use of outlet covers Decreased hot water temperature at tap	
Controlled/ not randomized	Increased reported ipecac possession	Increased home safety Increased installation of smoke detectors	Decreased falls Decreased injury rates and relative risk for injury
Multiple time series	Increased knowledge of ipecac use		Decreased home accidents
Descriptive	Increased knowledge of poisoning prevention strategies		

*From Bass et al.[8]

tion counseling is an important effort of significant benefit to children and families.

References

1. American Academy of Pediatrics, Committee on Injury and Poison Prevention. Office-based counseling for injury prevention. *Pediatrics.* 1994;94:566–567

2. American Academy of Pediatrics TIPP Revision Subcommittee. *TIPP: A Guide to Implementing Safety Counseling in Office Practice.* Elk Grove Village, IL: American Academy of Pediatrics; 1994

3. Bass JL, Mehta KA. Developmentally-oriented safety surveys: reported parental and adolescent practices. *Clin Pediatr (Phila).* 1980;19:350–356

4. Halperin SF, Bass JL, Mehta KA. Knowledge of accident prevention among parents of young children in nine Massachusetts towns. *Public Health Rep.* 1983;98:548–552

5. Rivara FP, Howard D. Parental knowledge of child development and injury risks. *J Dev Behav Pediatr.* 1982;3:103–105

6. Eichelberger MR, Gotschall CS, Feely HB, Harstad P, Bowman LM. Parental attitudes and knowledge of child safety. *Am J Dis Child*. 1990;144:714–720

7. LeBailly SA, Fleming GV, Freel K, et al. *The Children's Safety Research Project*. Elk Grove Village, IL: American Academy of Pediatrics; 1990

8. Bass JL, Christoffel KK, Widome M, et al. Childhood injury prevention counseling in primary care settings: a critical review of the literature. *Pediatrics*. 1993;92:544–550

9. Miller TR, Galbraith M. Injury prevention counseling by pediatricians: a benefit-cost comparison. *Pediatrics*. 1995;96:1–4

■□■□■□■□■□■□■□■□■□■□■□■□■□■□■□■□■□■□■

Adolescent Injury Control: A Developmental Approach

The greatest challenges in the control of injuries occur during adolescence. Unintentional and intentional injuries account for 75% of deaths in youths 10 to 19 years of age. Motor vehicle crashes, homicides, suicides, and drowning are the major causes of adolescent injury death, yet their relative importance varies significantly with age, gender, and race (Table 3.1). Adolescent injuries have a greater impact — in human suffering, years of life lost, and financial cost to society — than any other

TABLE 3.1.
Leading Causes of Injury-Related Adolescent Deaths by Age, Gender, and Race: Number of Deaths per 100 000 Adolescents, 1992*

Age Group	Cause of Death			
	Motor Vehicle Crashes	Homicide	Suicide	Drowning
10-14 y				
White				
M	7.0	1.2	2.6	1.1
F	4.1	1.0	1.1	0.4
Black				
M	7.8	9.6	2.0	4.8
F	3.6	5.1	†	1.6
15-19 y				
White				
M	39.6	15.2	18.4	3.8
F	21.0	3.6	3.7	†
Black				
M	26.2	128.5	14.8	11.0
F	9.1	14.2	1.9	†

*Data from the National Center for Health Statistics, courtesy of Lois Fingerhut. The following are the standard ICD-9 E-codes that are included in each injury category: motor vehicle crashes, E810-825; drowning, E830, 832, 910; suicide, E950-959; and homicide, E960–978.
†Fewer than 20 deaths.

adolescent health problem.[1] Fortunately, several specific protective behaviors have been identified that significantly reduce the incidence of adolescent injury. Unfortunately, the risk-taking behaviors that result in injury often stem from inherent aspects of adolescent development, creating a major challenge to effective prevention. Understanding adolescent development is essential in counseling teenagers and parents about injury prevention and in planning community and public health programs.

3.1 Risk Behaviors

Risk taking can be defined as "the participation in potentially health compromising activities with little understanding of, or in spite of an understanding of, the potential negative consequences."[2] Some amount of risk is inherent in daily living. For example, anyone who travels in an automobile, goes swimming, walks a city street at night, or plays competitive sports is at risk of injury. Society distinguishes between "acceptable risk" and unnecessary risk-taking behavior. Prevention efforts are aimed at reducing unnecessary risk.

Four specific risk behaviors have been identified as causing the majority of preventable injuries during adolescence.[1]

3.1.1 Alcohol and Other Drug Use

Alcohol is directly involved in many adolescent injuries. Other drugs (eg, marijuana) are involved to a lesser extent. Half of adolescent deaths from motor vehicle crashes are alcohol related.[3] Alcohol is similarly involved in many drownings and bicycle and boating injuries. Studies show that 51% of teenagers who suffered brain injuries had measurable alcohol levels at the time of injury. Half of adolescent injury deaths could be prevented if adolescents did not drink alcohol.

3.1.2 Failure to Use Safety Devices

Despite widespread education and legislation, most teenagers are not in the habit of using the simple protective devices that prevent many injuries. Surveys show that 19% of teenagers do not wear seat belts, 40% do not wear motorcycle helmets, and 93% do not wear bicycle helmets consistently.[4] It is estimated that approximately 30% of deaths and 60% of injuries would be prevented by use of these safety devices.

3.1.3 Firearms

Firearms are responsible for 20% of deaths of youths 15 to 19 years of age (48% African-American, 18% white).[5] Mortality and morbidity from intentional injury are significantly associated with firearms. In 1993 guns, primarily handguns, were involved in 86% of adolescent homicides and 66% of suicides in the second decade of life (see Appendix A)

3.1.4 Sports and Recreation

Sports and recreational activities are the leading cause of nonfatal adolescent injury, representing 40% of all injuries in this age group.[6,7] They constitute the second leading cause of emergency department visits and hospital admissions in 13- to 19-year-olds. Sports with the highest risk include football, wrestling, and gymnastics. Swimming is the recreational activity with the highest risk.

3.2 Risk Reduction

Risk reduction through health education activities is an essential component of adolescent health care. Pediatricians have a significant role in educating teenagers to make wise choices and decisions to prevent injury. Understanding the previously described risk factors allows the formulation of very specific behavioral objectives that are achievable and realistic and have the greatest benefit in reducing mortality and morbidity from injury. The following messages about injury prevention are important to emphasize with adolescents[1]:

- Do not drink alcohol or use drugs. Specifically, do not drink (or use drugs) and drive or ride in a motor vehicle with those who do.
- Always use safety belts in motor vehicles.
- Always wear bicycle and motorcycle helmets.
- Avoid the misuse of firearms and people who illegally carry handguns.
- Learn and practice nonviolent methods of conflict resolution.

- Practice sports safety. Use protective sports gear: helmets, mouth guards, shin guards, and face protectors.
- Learn to swim.
- Use life preservers during boating and water sports.
- Use sunscreen.
- Learn first aid and basic life support (CPR).

Many other protective health behaviors have been identified for reducing injuries from the entire spectrum of causes discussed in this manual. The pediatric caregiver needs to target and individualize anticipatory guidance to the specific risk factors involved in the adolescent's environment and activities. However, the challenge remains to find effective ways of influencing adolescent behavior. For a useful guide to anticipatory guidance in the adolescent years, the reader is referred to *Guidelines for Health Supervision III* [8] and *Bright Futures.* [9]

3.3 Developmental Context of Risk Behavior

Adolescent risk-taking behavior is a complex topic that has been elegantly addressed by many authors. [2,10] At the risk of great simplification, essential concepts for the caregiver are summarized here.

3.3.1 Comorbidity

Accumulating data confirm that risk behaviors rarely occur in isolation, but tend to cluster as interrelated behaviors. For example, fighting and violence are related to substance abuse and subsequently to injury. Social problems become medical problems. Interventions designed to reduce injury, therefore, must also address coexisting health risk behaviors and target high-risk groups. [11]

3.3.2 Who Is at Greatest Risk?

Risk-taking behavior is an inherent part of adolescent development. Increasing amounts of data indicate there may be two subsets of risk takers: those who engage in risk behaviors throughout their lifetime and those who engage in unnecessary risks primarily during adolescence. [12,13] Although the research has been directed at substance abuse, delinquency, and criminal behavior, the findings are applicable to injury prevention because many injuries are associated with alcohol use and violence.

Individuals who are inclined to engage in high-risk behavior throughout their lifetime have the following characteristics:

- Show neuropsychologic vulnerability from birth, often recognized as "difficult" infants who have poor impulse control and attention-deficit/hyperactivity disorder–type behaviors
- Are poorly parented, with poor bonding and weak family connections, including dysfunctional or highly stressed family circumstances with parents who themselves model risk-taking behaviors and habits
- Live in high-risk environments that may be complicated by poverty, mobility, and endogenous criminal activity
- Early puberty in males, probably related to the influence of testosterone on aggressive behavior

These children at risk are often identifiable as early as first grade, with a behavioral profile during ages 7 to 11 that includes rebellious aggressive conduct, fighting, ignoring rules, and antisocial behaviors.

The recognition that some individuals are prone to risk throughout life emphasizes a need for early identification of problem behaviors in children, increasing social support for parents and families, teaching parenting skills, and preschool and early elementary school interventions. Intervention with young children becomes even more important given the relative ineffectiveness in the research literature of interventions with adolescents.[12]

Individuals with high-risk behavior primarily during adolescence are characterized by the absence of one or more protective factors: close family ties, parental skills in supervision and limit setting, wholesome adult role models, and early school achievement and success. Delayed puberty also seems to be protective. The reasons why these adolescents engage in typical risk-taking behaviors are subject to many hypotheses. Puberty as a biological and social event is clearly implicated because the timing of puberty is directly related to risk behaviors.[14] The prolonged 5- to 10-year gap between biological and social maturity creates a void in meaningful social roles. The adolescent may compensate for this void by seeking peer status through attention-getting risky behavior. Several studies indicate that adolescents perceive more benefit than risk from many dangerous behaviors.[12] The adolescent's search for identity, typified by hero worship and mimicry of adult behavior, is influenced by the modern glamorization of violent and antisocial role models. From these perspectives, risk-taking behavior limited to adolescence may be seen as part of normative adolescent adjustment.[13]

3.3.3 Developmental Stages and Changes

One of the most helpful concepts for office counseling is an understanding of the three stages of adolescent development. Psychosocial development is a dynamic process that continues throughout the life span. The transition phase between childhood and adulthood lasts for more than a decade, beginning around age 11 and extending through age 21 or later. Adolescence is commonly divided into three developmental stages: early (11 to 14 years), middle (15 to 17 years), and late (18 to 21 years). Age ranges are approximate and females tend to progress through the stages earlier than males. At each stage, characteristic changes in cognitive thinking, behaviors, and associated health concerns occur. The most effective approaches for health counseling are different at each stage. The full spectrum of adolescent developmental issues include four major task areas: emancipation from family, development of peer relationships, determination of educational and vocational goals, and establishment of identity and self-responsibility. Only aspects of development that relate specifically to injury prevention are discussed here (Table 3.2, pp 37–38).

Cognitive changes

During adolescence, youths progress from concrete operational thinking ("here and now") to abstract operational thinking, with a maturing ability to engage in deductive reasoning, to understand risk and benefit, and to appreciate future consequences of current choices and decisions. The level of cognitive development is believed to affect the ways adolescents understand their world and make decisions. Adolescents at lower levels of cognitive complexity (concrete thinkers) are at greater risk for participation in health risk behaviors because they are less capable of planning ahead or understanding the longer term consequences of behaviors.[14]

TABLE 3.2.
Adolescent Developmental Issues Related to Injury Control

	Early Adolescence, 11-14 y	Middle Adolescence, 15-17 y	Late Adolescence, 18-21 y
Cognitive changes	Concrete thinking: here and now; understands immediate results of behavior but has no or limited sense of future consequences	Early abstract thinking: inductive/deductive reasoning; starts to connect separate events; understands concepts but not reality of later consequences	Abstract thinking: adult ability to understand risk and benefit, but limited experience; philosophical; idealistic about societal issues
Physical changes	Puberty, rapid growth, hormonal surges, volatile moods; accident prone	Growth spurt finishes; physically awkward, lacks coordination, has poor reaction time; aggressive behavior (in males)	Peak health, physical strength, endurance; overconfidence in physical ability
Psychological changes	Transition from being obedient to rebellious	Insistence on independence	Emancipation (leaves home)
		Adult conflict increases	Requires little adult supervision
Independence — emancipation	Challenges rules but ambivalent (wants adult protection)	Resists parental supervision	Becomes legally responsible for action
	Hero worship is common	Often tests limits	Gains experience rapidly
	Lacks experience, has poor judgment	Learns from experience	
Peers-social development	Wants friends desperately	Strong need to please significant peers	Selects close friends, partners
	Makes constant comparisons ("Am I normal" concerns)	Highly vulnerable to peer pressure; will do whatever gives status with peers	Increasingly able to reject peer pressure if not in self-interest ("enlightened self-interest")
	Intensely curious	Risk-taking behaviors predominate	
	Experiments with risk behaviors		

TABLE 3.2.

Adolescent Developmental Issues Related to Injury Control, continued

	Early Adolescence, 11-14 y	Middle Adolescence, 15-17 y	Late Adolescence, 18-21 y
Identity	Has poor self-image Losing role as child but does not identify as an adult Tends to use denial ("It can't happen to me") Shows adolescent bravado, reckless behaviors	Confused about self-image Seeks group identity (conformity) Very narcissistic Impulsive, impatient Belief in invincibility ("I'll live forever")	Has a more positive self-image Begins to consider other's needs; is more protective Emerges as a leader or follower Seeks adult identity (rites of passage)
Values	Negotiable: good behavior in exchange for rewards	Conformity: behavior that peer group values	Social responsibility: behavior more consistent with laws and duty
Highest injury risks	Motor vehicle injury (unbelted passenger) Unintentional injury from firearm use Water sports injuries Sports injury from bicycles, skateboards, running sports, baseball	Motor vehicle injury (driving late at night, on weekends) Homicide (impulsive) Suicide (impulsive) Drowning Sports injuries from contact sports, football, basketball	Motor vehicle injury (drunk driving) Homicide (cultural risks) Suicide (depression) Work injuries (power equipment)

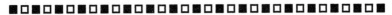
Physical changes

The onset of puberty, with rapid growth and dramatic physical and hormonal changes, heralds an increase in risk-taking behavior and number of injuries, especially for boys. The *early adolescent* is curious, confused, and anxious about early pubertal changes, and often at the mercy of volatile mood changes. Intense curiosity and daredevil behavior typify young teenagers.[15] The *middle adolescent* is coping with the effects of the rapid growth spurt, including poor physical coordination, awkwardness, and lack of confidence that predisposes to injury. The *late adolescent* begins to enjoy peak physical strength and agility, leading to a sense of invincibility in the face of danger.

Independence and autonomy

The developmental drive for emancipation starts in early adolescence with a transition from obedient to rebellious behavior. Young teenagers begin to argue about limits, but still desire adult supervision and protection. Middle adolescents have increasing amounts of freedom, privacy, and time unsupervised by adults, as well as a desire to challenge adult rules, leading to the risk behaviors and experimentation associated with injury (alcohol and driving).[16] Late adolescents become legally autonomous but lack the experience necessary for consistent sound judgment. They leave home to live alone or with peers and face the challenge of independent decision-making in new social contexts.

Peer group influences

Adult influence is replaced by that of the peer group as youths progress through adolescence. Although early adolescents may be intensely focused on "friends," they still respond to firm adult supervision. In middle adolescence the need for group conformity becomes paramount, influencing the teenager to engage in the behaviors valued by the peer group. Pressures exerted by friends struggling with their own insecurities may prompt late adolescents to engage in risky behaviors they may otherwise resist. The power of peers to influence adolescent behavior (both positively and negatively) must not be underestimated.

Identity and rites of passage

Early adolescents, caught between the role of a child and adult, may experience poor self-image and low self-esteem. In defense of emerging fears of inadequacy and fallibility, they tend to respond with denial ("it can't happen to me"). Middle adolescents cope with their uncertainty by seeking group identity, while internally becoming very self-absorbed, egocentric, and impulsive. Late adolescents begin to develop a realistic and positive self-image that allows them to consider other's needs and to reject group pressure if not in their own interest ("enlightened self-interest"). Insecure adolescents may search for an instant adult identity by mimicking unsafe adult behaviors (drinking, reckless driving, carrying guns).

Immaturity

Safety often is learned from experience. A lack of experience and judgment predisposes teenagers to dangerous experimentation and subsequent injury. Throughout the stages of adolescent transition, countless situations are "learning opportunities" that facilitate the development of mature decision-making skills.

Each stage of adolescent development contains intrinsic psychosocial needs that influence adolescents to take risks that can result in injury. However, risk taking may also be viewed as an inevitable component of healthy adolescent development to the extent that certain risk behaviors may enhance self-esteem, build experience and competence, help develop an understanding of natural consequences, and eventually lead to sound judgment.[2,17]

3.4 Intervention Strategies Based on Developmental Stages

To be most effective, professional approaches to office counseling should be matched to the current developmental stage of the adolescent (Table 3.3, pp 41–42). It is equally important to understand the context of the teenager's life, including the family situation, cultural background, socioeconomic status, peer group influences, and daily environment.[18]

3.4.1 Early Adolescence

Young teenagers respond to firm, direct adult support and supervision. Because they are concrete thinkers, expectations and behavioral goals should be conveyed as simple concrete choices. The young adolescent's

TABLE 3.3.

Injury Intervention Strategies Based on Adolescent Developmental Stages

	Early Adolescence, 11-14 y	Middle Adolescence, 15-17 y	Late Adolescence, 18-21 y
Of ce counseling	Utilize visual, graphic information; correct peer misinformation	Utilize interactive teaching methods (role play, rehearsal of scenarios)	Utilize adult-to-adult participation in decisions
	Provide firm, direct expectations for safe behaviors	Be an objective sounding board (but let them solve their own problems)	Act as a resource
	Convey simple concrete choices	Seek teenager's perception of risk/benefit	Idealistic stage, so convey "professional" (not parental) image
	Emphasize immediate "here and now" rewards of safe behaviors	Negotiate safer behaviors that also give status with peers	Obtain commitment to personal safety goals
	Do not ally with parents, but be an objective, caring adult	Stress immediate (not long-term) consequences of behaviors	Begin to discuss future consequences (on health, career, life plans)
		Modify perceptions of invulnerability	
Key community approach	Family support: encourage close parental supervision, limit setting	School support: strengthen school health and safety programs	Laws: support protective social legislation
Examples: • Drinking	Young teenagers are curious about alcohol, so provide graphic information (about liver damage, auto crash victims, peer disapproval of people "acting stupid"); advise parental supervision, curfews	Experimentation with alcohol is normal but dangerous: negotiate safe ride, designated driver contracts, rehearse the unexpected ("what if...")	Drinking is still illegal; identify those at-risk of alcoholism and refer them to support groups

TABLE 3.3.

Injury Intervention Strategies Based on Adolescent Developmental Stages, continued

	Early Adolescence, 11-14 y	Middle Adolescence, 15-17 y	Late Adolescence, 18-21 y
• Peer refusal	"I can't. My parents will ground me."	"I want to be your friend, but I don't need to drink to prove it. See you tomorrow."	"I am your friend, and I won't let you drive drunk. I'm taking the keys."
• Safety devices	Encourage parental role modeling and expectations of seat belt and helmet use to ingrain habits early	Legal driving age: teach driving safety, support graduated privileges, role play getting friends to use seat belts	Support seat belt/helmet legislation. Discuss work injury (eg, risk of using power equipment)
• Firearms	Because of intense curiosity, parents are encouraged to remove hand-guns from the home or lock them up separately from the ammunition; reinforce the dangers of firearms; teach conflict resolu-tion skills ("We could fight, but I'd rather be friends")	Because of pressure to join gangs, gang "wannabes," discuss alternatives to accomplish peer status (eg, become a peer counselor); role play nonviolent conflict resolution	Carrying weapons seen as "rite of passage" into adulthood: provide accurate informa-tion on personal risk, legal consequences
• Sports	Baseball, soccer, and running injuries are common (affecting the eyes and limbs): recommend use of protective safety gear ("no eye guard – no soccer")	Competitive sports injuries are common (football, wrestling, and gymnastics): support school/coach safety require-ments for sports participation	Unsupervised recreational injuries are common: emphasize physical conditioning, use of "spotters" and guards, discuss the impact of injury on job performance, finances

tendency toward hero worship of adults (other than their parents) can result in a healthy transference to good role models, including respect for their teachers and physician. Encourage parents to be present during the office visit, and counsel families on appropriate adult supervision and limit setting. Also interview the teenager alone in order to be seen as an objective, caring adult, rather than an extension of the parents. The intense curiosity of early adolescence represents an ideal time for appropriate information, especially to correct the misinformation teenagers may encounter. Visual, graphic, and interactive educational materials, including computer-assisted activities, are appealing to young teenagers. Stress the immediate (not long-term) consequences of risk-taking behavior. The most important community effort to reduce early adolescent injury involves family support programs to increase family skills in parenting young adolescents.

3.4.2 Middle Adolescence

Interactive teaching becomes very important during middle adolescence. Caregivers should become an objective sounding board, posing questions to assess the teenagers' perceptions of risks but allowing them to formulate their own goals and solve their own problems. The discovery of abstract thinking and the ability to begin inductive-deductive reasoning make middle adolescents great debaters. They will challenge authority, which encourages analysis and negotiation. Skills to deal with peer pressure are essential for teenagers at this stage. Role playing and rehearsing likely scenarios are useful techniques to develop these skills. Middle adolescents respond best to positive visualizations ("dos, not don'ts") and need help to identify healthy behaviors that the peer group values. Continue to stress immediate consequences of risk-taking behavior, but from the perspective of peer group status. For middle adolescents, the most important community focus for professionals is to support school and peer programs (peer education, peer *leadership* education).

3.4.3 Late Adolescence

Older adolescents are leaving home for college or jobs and respond best to an adult-to-adult approach. Because of the intense idealism of late adolescence, the caregiver should convey a professional, mature image. Older teenagers often seek information and resources as they become interested in personal protective and health-promoting behaviors. Discussing the long-term consequences of injury and obtaining the adolescent's commitment to personal goals for safe behavior are appropriate for this age. Outside the clinical setting, the most significant measures to protect older adolescents relate to social legislation (seat belt laws, drinking age, gun control).

3.5 Recommendations

A number of general recommendations emerge from understanding the developmental issues related to injury prevention in adolescents.[19]

1. Identify youth prone to risk in early childhood to facilitate family and educational support systems that foster social competency, impulse control, and effective parenting.

2. Individualize health risk counseling toward the teenager's specific risks, considering developmental stage, age, gender, and environment.

3. Express genuine concern for the adolescent from the perspective of a caring professional adult.

4. Emphasize personal vulnerability to counter bravado by adolescents and their belief in invincibility.

5. Address the perceived benefits of risk-taking behavior, which are more important to teenagers than the perceived risks. Empower teenagers to recognize their ability to choose either safe or risky behaviors. Encourage safer behaviors that also meet the adolescent's perceived needs.

6. Refer adolescents at serious risk (for violence or substance abuse) to professionals or support groups for active intervention.

7. Recognize that the most significant approaches to injury control involve social legislation, community campaigns, school programs, and family support systems.

8. Collaborate with school and youth programs in the community.

Risk-taking behavior is an intrinsic aspect of adolescent development. The reduction and prevention of adolescent injury ultimately depends on collaborative, comprehensive, and continuous community action.

References

1. Elster AB, Kuznets NJ, eds. Rationale and recommendations: intentional and unintentional injuries. In: *AMA Guidelines for Adolescent Preventive Services (GAPS): Recommendations and Rationale.* Baltimore, MD: Williams & Wilkins; 1994:29–39

2. Ryan SA, Irwin CE Jr. Risk behaviors. In: Friedman SB, Fisher M, Schonberg SK, eds. *Comprehensive Adolescent Health Care.* St. Louis, MO: Quality Medical Publishing; 1992

3. American Academy of Pediatrics, Committee on Injury and Poison Prevention and Committee on Adolescence. The teenage driver. *Pediatrics.* 1996;98:987–990

4. Centers for Disease Control and Prevention. CDC Surveillance Summaries. Youth risk behavior surveillance – United States, 1993. *MMWR Morb Mortal Wkly Rep.* 1995;44(SS-1)

5. American Academy of Pediatrics, Committee on Adolescence. Firearms and adolescents. *Pediatrics.* 1992;89:784–787

6. Rome ES. Sports-related injuries among adolescents: when do they occur, and how can we prevent them? *Pediatr Rev.* 1995;16:184–187

7. Bijur PE, Trumble A, Harel Y, Overpeck MD, Jones D, Scheidt PC. Sports and recreation injuries in US children and adolescents. *Arch Pediatr Adolesc Med.* 1995;149:1009–1016

8. American Academy of Pediatrics, Committee on Psychosocial Aspects of Child and Family Health. *Guidelines for Health Supervision III.* Elk Grove Village, IL: American Academy of Pediatrics; 1997

9. Green M, ed. *Bright Futures: Guidelines for Health Supervision of Infants, Children, and Adolescents.* Arlington, VA: National Center for Education in Maternal and Child Health; 1994

10. Jessor R. Risk behavior in adolescence: a psychosocial framework for understanding and action. In: Rogers DE, Ginzberg E, eds. *Adolescents at Risk: Medical and Social Perspectives.* Boulder, CO: Westview Press; 1992:19–34

11. Orpinas PK, Basen-Engquist K, Grunbaum JA, Parcel GS. The co-morbidity of violence-related behaviors with health-risk behaviors in a population of high school students. *J Adolesc Health Care.* 1995;16:216–255

12. Rivara FP, Farrington DP. Prevention of violence: role of the pediatrician. *Arch Pediatr Adolesc Med.* 1995;149:421–429

13. Moffitt TE. Adolescence-limited and life-course-persistent antisocial behavior: a developmental taxonomy. *Psychol Rev.* 1993;100:674–701

14. Orr DP, Ingersoll GM. The contribution of level of cognitive complexity and pubertal timing to behavioral risk in young adolescents. *Pediatrics.* 1995;95:528–533

15. Arnett J. Reckless behavior in adolescence: a developmental perspective. *Dev Rev.* 1992;12:339–373

16. Brooks-Gunn J. Why do adolescents have difficulty adhering to health regimens? In: Krasnegor NA, Epstein L, Johnson SB, Yaffe SJ, eds. *Developmental Aspects of Health Compliance Behavior.* Hillsdale, NJ: Erlbaum; 1993:125–152

17. Irwin CE Jr. The theoretical concept of at-risk adolescents. *Adolesc Med.* 1990;1:1–14

18. Hoffman AE. Clinical assessment and management of health risk behaviors in adolescents. *Adolesc Med.* 1990;1:33–44

19. Cavanaugh RM Jr. Anticipatory guidance for the adolescent: has it come of age? *Pediatr Rev.* 1994;15:485–489

■□■□■□■□■□■□■□■□■□■□■□■□■□■□■□■

CHAPTER 4

Injury Prevention in and Around the Home

The home is the most frequent place that fatal and nonfatal injuries occur in children younger than 15 years, and especially in preschool-age children.[1] The most common mechanisms of death related to injury in the home among infants and young children are suffocation, fires and burns, and drowning.[2] During early adolescence, deaths caused by unintentional discharge of firearms account for one third of all fatalities in the home.[1]

Falls are the leading cause of nonfatal injuries in the home.[3] Home injury prevention programs have proved effective at increasing injury prevention behavior and decreasing injuries that occur in the home.[4]

This chapter provides comprehensive room-by-room safety tips for parents, highlighting many of the injury booby traps found in typical homes. The chapter also reviews falls and ingestion of poisons, two causes of nonfatal injury that occur most frequently at home. Burns, product-related injuries, and animal bites, the other classes of injury that are most closely associated with the home environment, are discussed in chapters 11, 14, and 18, respectively.

4.1 General Safety Tips

- Never leave children home alone.
- Keep the doors locked at all times, whether you are at home or away.
- Keep all doors and screens secured with toddler-proof locks.
- Mark glass doors with decals to enhance their visibility.
- The following areas should be off-limits: garage, basement, greenhouse, workshop, and exercise room.
- Guns in the home are a danger to the family. If a gun is kept in the home, keep it locked up, inaccessible, and unloaded, and store the bullets in a separate, locked location. Use a trigger lock.

- Install a fire extinguisher.
- Install smoke alarms throughout the house, test them monthly, and replace batteries annually.
- Install a carbon monoxide detector.
- Install child-guard latches on drawers and cabinets that contain dangerous items.
- Ensure that furniture is stable.
- Ensure that cabinet and furniture knobs are secure and large enough that they do not present a choking hazard.
- Cover sharp edges of furniture, for example, coffee tables, with corner guards.
- Keep heavy and fragile objects out of reach.
- Install wall-to-wall carpeting, or ensure that area rugs have nonskid backing.
- Keep window blinds or drapery cords out of reach by attaching the cord to a blind with a clamping device, wrapping the cord around a cleat near the top of the blind, tying the cord to itself, or installing a tie-down device on the window sill. Cut all looped cords and attach tassels to each end.
- Avoid falls from above-ground windows by installing window guards or installing a locking device that will not allow a window opening of more than 4 in.
- Keep furniture away from unprotected windows (so that children cannot climb out).
- Keep ash trays, matches, and cigarettes and lighters out of reach.
- Minimize the use of electrical cords and move them behind furniture so the child cannot chew or tug them.
- Avoid the use of extension cords.
- Cover electrical outlets with shields, and place heavy furniture in front of them.
- Do not leave light bulb sockets empty in lamps or other fixtures.
- The use of infant walkers is strongly discouraged.
- If an infant walker is used, block off stairways and exit doorways; avoid uneven floors, carpets or thresholds; clear objects off tables; keep a child in a walker away from ovens, space heaters, and fireplaces; keep hot liquids away from children in walkers.

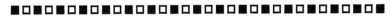
- Never leave a child unattended in a walker.
- Do not use infant walkers near stairs because they may tip over when going through doorways or down stairs.

4.2 Room-by-Room Home Safety Tips

4.2.1 Kitchen

General

- Keep preschool children out of the kitchen, especially during meal preparation when hazards are greatest, unless supervision is close.
- If necessary, provide a safe zone, for example, a playpen.
- Place an appliance latch on the refrigerator.
- Do not use small refrigerator magnets that could cause choking.
- Do not place infants on the kitchen counter.
- Do not place infants in an infant seat on the kitchen counter or other elevated area.
- Keep garbage secured behind a latched door.
- Rearrange storage areas so dangerous items, cleaning compounds, and foods are kept in the upper, out-of-reach cabinets and drawers, and safe items are kept in the lower cabinets and drawers.
- Set aside one cabinet for safe items that the child may use to explore.
- Clean up spills immediately to avoid slipping and falling.

Scalds and burns

- Playpens should be located well away from the stove.
- Do not carry hot liquids when you are carrying a child.
- Do not place hot items at the edge of the counter or table.
- Use back burners of the stove when possible.
- Turn pot handles inward on the stove.
- Use knob covers as barriers to burner controls.
- Keep the child out of reach of the outside of ovens or other appliances that may be hot.
- Never leave an appliance cord plugged into an outlet when the cord is disconnected from the appliance.

- Keep appliances, electrical cords, and knives out of the child's reach and away from the edges of counters.
- If a microwave oven is used, use a low setting in a microwave-safe dish for a brief time. Mix food thoroughly after heating, and test it before serving the child.

4.2.2 Living Room and Family Room

General

- Avoid the use of glass-topped tables.
- Keep heavy objects, for example, bookends, out of reach.
- Keep electronic equipment, for example, VCRs, CD players, and televisions, out of reach.
- Install a VCR guard on the cassette loader.
- Avoid falls from above-ground windows by installing window guards or installing a locking device that will not allow a window opening of more than 4 in.

Burns and electrical hazards

- Keep hot light bulbs out of the child's reach.
- Install protective barriers to fireplaces, heaters, stoves, and radiators.
- Avoid the use of space heaters.
- If a space heater is used, ensure that it turns off automatically if toppled and that it is turned off when adults are out of the room or asleep; keep it out of the reach of children.

Playpen

- A playpen may be used as a safe area.
- The playpen should have fine mesh sides with openings smaller than $1/4$ in or vertical slats less than $2^3/8$ in apart.
- The playpen should always be fully open so it does not collapse or allow creation of a space between the mattress and mesh side.

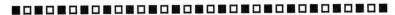

4.2.3 Dining Room

General

- Do not use tablecloths that overhang the table.

High chairs

- The high chair should have a wide base to ensure that it will not topple over easily.
- Always use the safety strap when the child is in the high chair.
- Do not leave the child unattended in the high chair.

4.2.4 Bedroom

General

- Destroy all bean bag infant cushions.
- Do not put infants to sleep on an adult bed.
- Do not place an infant on a water bed.
- Do not leave an infant unattended on a changing table.
- Use a covered wastebasket in the bedroom, or do not place hazardous items in an open wastebasket (eg, plastic bags, small or sharp items, rubber bands, batteries, or latex balloons).
- Avoid using toy chests, or install a spring-loaded lid-support device that keeps the lid open at any angle to which it is lifted and will not automatically snap shut; air holes should be drilled in the body of the box. Open bins, baskets, and shelves are safer for toy storage.

Cribs

- Cribs should have slats that are not more than 2⅜ in apart.
- The crib should be free of splinters and cracks and be painted with lead-free paint.
- Do not use cribs with corner posts because the posts can catch clothing.
- Do not use cribs with decorative cutouts in the headboard that could allow entrapment of the child's head, leg, or arm.
- There should be no cross bars on the sides of the crib.
- The sides, when lowered, should be at least 9 in above the mattress.
- Never leave the crib rails down when a baby is in the crib.

- The sides should be operated with a locking, hand-operated latch that is secure from accidental release.
- The mattress should be the same size as the crib so no gaps will be created that could cause entrapment.
- The minimum rail height should be 26 in from the top of the railing to the mattress set at the lowest level.
- Cribs should meet all current federal and voluntary industry standards. Older cribs should be discarded and replaced.
- Bumper pads should be used around the entire crib until the infant begins to stand, and then the bumper pads should be removed.
- Begin to lower the crib mattress before the baby can sit unassisted; have it at its lowest point before the baby can stand.
- No hanging crib toys should be within reach.
- When the child is beginning to push up on hands and knees or is 5 months of age, remove all crib toys that are strung across the crib. In general, it is best if toys are not strung across the crib.
- Do not leave large toys in the crib because the baby may use them as steps to climb out.
- Place a rug or carpet beneath the crib to cushion a fall.
- Begin using a bed instead of the crib by the time the child is 35 in tall.

Toddler's bed

- Install safety rails on the bed.
- Place the bed at least 2 ft from windows, heating vents, radiators, wall lamps, drapery, or window-blind cords.

Bunk beds

- Children younger than 6 years should not sleep in the top bunk.
- Attach additional boards to the bunk bed to close any space more than $3\frac{1}{2}$ in between the lower edge of the guard rails and the upper edge of the bed frame to prevent entrapment of the child's head, leg, or arm.
- The upper and lower bunks should have guard rails next to the wall and at both ends, and the upper bunk should have a guard rail on the outer side as well.
- Guard rails should extend at least 5 in above the mattress.

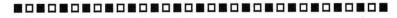

- Mattresses should be supported by well-secured cross supports of wood slats, metal straps, or sturdy wires.
- Children should not play roughly on bunk beds.

4.2.5 Bathroom

General

- The bathroom should be inaccessible when not in use by keeping the door closed and installing a hook-and-eye latch or doorknob cover on the outside.
- Ensure that the door lock can be opened from the outside if locked from the inside.
- Keep the toilet lid closed with a safety latch.
- Use nonskid bath rugs.
- Use a covered wastebasket.
- Keep medications and cleaning products in a latched cabinet.
- Keep other products and harmful items out of reach.

Bathtub

- Never leave an infant or child unattended in the water, even in a special tub or seat, until the child is at least 5 years old.
- When bathing an infant or child, ignore all other interruptions, such as answering the telephone.
- Use an infant tub for younger infants.
- Ensure that the tub bottom is slip-proof, or add nonskid decals.
- Lower the household water heater thermostat to 120°F.
- Use an antiscald device to keep water temperature at the tap less than 120°F.
- Turn on the cold water before the hot water, and turn off the hot water before turning off the cold. Single faucets are safer than separate hot and cold water faucets.
- Install a protective cover for the tub spout to prevent bumps and burns.
- Test the water temperature before placing the child in the tub.
- Never leave water in the tub when the tub is not in use.

- Do not leave soap bars or containers, shampoo containers, or other bath products on the edge of the tub.

Electrical hazards

- Keep hair dryers away from children.
- Do not leave electrical appliances plugged in.
- Keep electrical appliances away from water.
- Install ground fault circuit interrupters.

4.2.6 Halls and Stairways

General

- Keep stairs clear of objects.
- Keep plants out of reach.
- Install carpet with nonskid backing on the stairs, at the foot of each staircase, and in hallways.
- Banisters should be secure, and the distance between the upright posts should be no more than 4 in.
- Keep hallways clear of clutter, and keep floors in good repair.
- Do not overwax floors.
- Clean up spills immediately to avoid slipping.
- Ensure that halls and stairways are well lit at night.
- Install and secure gates at the top and bottom of the stairs.
- Gates at the top of the stairs should be permanently installed; gates at the bottom of the stairs may be portable.
- Gates should have vertical slats no more than $2\frac{3}{8}$ in apart or be made with fine mesh or acrylic plastic sheets (ie, Plexiglas).
- If the gate has small diamond-shaped openings, these should be no greater than $1\frac{1}{2}$ in wide. Do not use accordion-style gates with large diamond-shaped openings.

Laundry room

- Keep the laundry room off-limits.
- Keep the dryer door closed at all times.
- Keep detergents, bleach, and other products in a cabinet out of reach.
- Keep children away from standing water in buckets, diaper pails, and other containers.

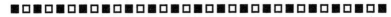
4.3 Home Injuries: Falls

4.3.1 Scope of the Problem

Falls are the most common cause of nonfatal injury, accounting for approximately 783 000 hospitalizations annually and more than 11 million visits to emergency departments.[5] Falls are also the second leading cause of death by injury, after motor vehicle injury, for the population as a whole.[6] Two and a half million children and adolescents receive medical attention for falls each year. Half of these falls occur at home, and a quarter occur at school.[3] Fortunately, falls are an infrequent cause of death during childhood, with the National Center for Health Statistics recording 233 deaths in 1992 in children and youth aged 19 years or younger. There is, however, considerable morbidity and expense associated with falls in children and teenagers. Falls account for about one third of emergency department visits for injury.[7] In Washington State alone, falls accounted for almost one third of hospital admissions for trauma; the annual cost of these injuries was $4.5 million.[8]

The home is the site of most childhood falls, especially in children younger than 4 years. Falls from one level to another, such as from stairs and furniture, predominate; windows are the primary site of falls from heights of more than 10 m. In older children, falls on the same level, from slipping or colliding with another person, are increasingly important. Bicycles, playground equipment, and sports-related injuries play a larger part, as discussed in chapters 5, 16, and 17.

Lacerations are the most commonly treated injuries resulting from falls, and other soft tissue injuries occur frequently. In falls from *heights,* fractures are the most common injuries treated.[9] Children who have fallen are most often hospitalized for fractures or dislocations and for head injuries.[8] Head injuries account for most of the deaths.[8]

4.3.2 Risk Factors

Injuries from falls are caused by an abrupt dissipation of mechanical energy; the intensity of this energy (and the resultant severity of injury) increases with the velocity of the fall which, in turn, is related to the height from which the fall occurred and whether the fall was interrupted. Severity of the injury is also determined by the surface with which the impact occurred, the size of the contact area (energy applied over a wider area is less likely to cause serious injury), and by complex biomechanical factors, such as the position in which the victim fell and the resistance of the tissues to injury.

Age is an important variable; the high-risk groups are young children and the elderly. The death rate is highest in the first year of life.[7] In childhood, the rate of injury from falls declines with age, with toddlers not surprisingly having the highest rates.[10] Boys fall more than girls do. This difference is not noticeable in children younger than 4 years, but becomes substantial in school-age children, especially those in urban areas. Several studies have indicated that poor children are at higher risk, as are those who are not white. This is most likely related to deficiencies in the environment, as is the substantially higher rate of injuries from falls in urban, as compared with suburban and rural children. Falls are not distributed evenly in time: the frequency varies by month (most occur in spring and early summer) and by hour of the day (most occur from noon to 6 pm).[10]

The contact surface is also related to the severity of injury. Injuries are much more likely to occur with falls onto unforgiving surfaces, such as concrete or asphalt, than with falls onto grass or carpet.[10] Falls on stairways are highly associated with the use of infant walkers.

4.3.3 Intervention Strategies

Enforcement

Building codes that modify the environment have substantial potential to prevent falls, especially those in the home. Because stairways are the site of many falls, enforcement of building safety codes dealing with construction, maintenance, and illumination of stairways may prove fruitful. Building codes also contain requirements for the construction of balconies and the spacing of the slats in railings.[11] When local building codes require window guards in multistory buildings, falls from windows are substantially reduced.[12,13] Because of the association between walkers and stairway falls, mobile walkers should be banned.[14,15]

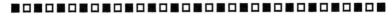
Equipment or environmental modification

Stairway gates do prevent falls, although they must be used conscientiously and consistently to be effective. Gates with accordion tops should not be used because of their documented risk as a cause of strangulation. Modification of equipment known to be dangerous, such as replacement of mobile baby walkers with "stationary walkers," has promise in prevention. Modification of surfaces in areas where falls frequently occur, such as bathrooms, so they are less slippery, helps to avoid such falls, as does removal or modification with nonskid backing of throw rugs and rounding of contact points, such as table edges and cabinet corners. Devices exist that can be used to soften corners of furniture in homes where toddlers live. Product regulations that specify the design of nursery furniture, such as changing tables and cribs, can reduce the incidence of falls from them.

An association has been described between a child's footwear and the incidence of falls because of loss of footing. Low-top sneakers have the lowest injury rate; rough soles and rubber (as opposed to other sole materials) are more protective.[16]

Education

Counseling of parents of young children by pediatricians has been proven effective in reducing the incidence of falls.[17] Such counseling should be geared to the child's stage of development, with information about the likely hazards at each age and developmental level. The mainstay of counseling regarding infant and toddler falls is that young children should never be left unattended in situations where they could fall. Education about the use of the aforementioned equipment should also be part of anticipatory guidance, as should compliance with laws and regulations dealing with home safety.

Prevention of falls and injury while using playground equipment and while engaged in sports and recreation, both common causes of injury, is discussed in chapters 5, 16, and 17.

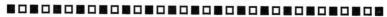
4.3.4 Recommendations for Pediatricians

Anticipatory guidance

Counseling about the risks for and prevention of falls in the home should be a routine part of anticipatory guidance, especially for the infants and toddlers who are most likely to fall at home and not in sports or recreation. Suggested content for counseling of parents of infants includes the following:

- Never leave an infant unattended on any furniture, even if the infant has never rolled over before. Place the infant on the floor or in a crib.

- Purchase nursery equipment that meets current safety standards (beware of buying used cribs or other baby furniture) and use the equipment as it was intended (eg, use the straps on high chairs, strollers, and changing tables). Infant seats do not protect infants from falls.

- Lower the mattress in cribs as the infant gets older and develops the ability to sit and stand. Avoid using toys or pillows that the child could use to stand on to crawl out of the crib.

- Infant walkers do not enhance development and they are dangerous, especially in houses with stairs. Their use is strongly discouraged.

For toddlers and preschoolers, the following points should be emphasized:

- Install and use stairway gates for all stairs. Teach all household members, including older children, to latch the gate whenever they use it.

- Install padding on sharp corners, especially coffee tables.

- Install window guards in dwellings in multistory buildings, especially from the second floor up. Do not place furniture near open windows; children may climb to the window and fall out.

- Examine home floor surfaces, and, whenever possible, modify slippery surfaces. For example, use a rubber mat in the tub, put nonskid backing on throw rugs, and consider installing nonskid stair runners. Soft flooring around cribs can minimize the severity of injury should children fall out. Electrical cords and floor clutter are common environmental hazards that lead to falls; route cords behind furniture or near the wall, and keep clutter away from major walkways in the home.

- Think about fall prevention when buying shoes for children. Low-cut sneakers with rough, rubber soles are optimal to prevent falls.

In school-age and older children, falls in the home are much less frequent than those occurring during sports and recreational activities. Prevention of those injuries is discussed in chapters 5, 16, and 17. Emphasis of the following points may help prevent falls in the home by older children:

• Parents should discourage active physical play on decks, balconies, and roofs because most serious falls in school-age and older children occur from these areas. If possible, remove climbing aids in yards or balconies (eg, furniture near the balcony or deck railings and storage areas and woodpiles next to the backyard fence or a tree).

4.4 Poison Prevention

See also chapters 3, 6, 7, and 8.

4.4.1 Scope of the Problem

Exposure to toxic substances is common in the pediatric population, particularly in the first few years of life. Of the almost 2 million exposures to poison compiled by the 65 participating regional poison centers that constituted the Toxic Exposure Surveillance System in 1994, more than half were to children younger than 6 years of age and 40% were to children younger than 3 years.[18] Another 120 000 exposures to poison occurred to children aged 6 to 12 years and almost 140 000 to teenagers. Considering that many exposures to poison are handled by nonparticipating poison centers, by other providers of health care, or without medical advice, the actual number of poisonings for the whole US population may be double the number reported.

Common categories of substances reported to poison centers include cleaning products, analgesics, cosmetics, plants, and cough and cold preparations. Categories that cause the largest number of deaths include analgesics; antidepressants; sedatives, hypnotics, and psychotics; stimulants and illicit drugs; cardiovascular drugs; and alcohol.[18]

Although exposure of children to poisons commonly causes minor symptoms, major health effects and fatalities are uncommon. In 1994, of the 1.3 million reported toxic exposures in the pediatric age group, there were only 26 deaths of preschoolers, 5 deaths in the 6- to 12-year-old age group, and 44 deaths in the teenage group.[19]

The pattern of poisoning varies with gender and age. In all preadolescent age groups, exposure to poison is slightly more common in boys than in girls. Among adolescents, 58% of cases are female. With increasing age, the likelihood increases that exposure to poison is intentional. Among preschoolers, virtually all exposures to poison are classified as *unintentional*. Among grade school age children, more than 90% of exposures are unintentional. Among teenagers, intentional and unintentional exposures to poison are almost equally divided.[18] This reflects the large percentage of exposures to poison in the older age groups associated with suicide attempts or gestures and substance abuse. Fatalities in teenagers almost exclusively fall into one of those two categories.

4.4.2 Risk Factors

In addition to the gender and age factors, consideration of developmental and environmental factors may be useful.

Developmental factors

Risk factors for poisoning reflect normal child and family development. Young infants have a limited ability to acquire and ingest poisons because of their limited motor abilities and the close supervision they receive from their parents. However, toward the end of the first year of life, dramatic changes occur. Children become mobile enough to open the cabinet under the sink or reach objects on the countertop. They have developed the fine motor skills required to remove unsecured caps, empty containers or bring them to their mouths, and grasp and ingest small objects, such as pills. The older infant and toddler have the curiosity and oral instincts to assure that almost any novel object or substance will be brought to the mouth, tasted, and occasionally swallowed.

Preschoolers become increasingly capable and resourceful in their ability to acquire and ingest poisons. They lack the ability to comprehend the danger of poisoning, and they spend increasing amounts of time out of their parents' direct line of sight and supervision. Children of a given age vary in their abilities to obtain potentially poisonous substances, based on motor skills and cognitive ability. Likewise, it seems reasonable that temperament varies from child to child (ie, in impulsiveness, activity level, and risk taking), placing some young children at greater risk than others.

School-age children are at lower risk of unintentional self-poisoning as they begin to develop the ability to understand rules, comprehend danger, and develop self-control. Yet, inadequate supervision when the child must take medications can lead to an inadvertent overdose by the well-meaning child.

Adolescence brings a new set of risks. The first is the problem of intentionally taking an overdose of medication to cause self-harm or to cry for help. Girls are more likely to intentionally take an overdose of pills, whereas boys are more likely to cause self-injury by other mechanisms (see chapter 8.2 for a full discussion). Carbon monoxide from automobile exhaust is one example that can easily result in death. Such events are sometimes related to an immediate crisis in the young person's life, but more often are a reflection of long-standing personal or family problems. Adolescents of both sexes are exposed to "recreational" drugs, that may be illicit (eg, cocaine or heroin) or illicitly obtained legitimate drugs (eg, amphetamines). Peer pressure, easy availability, and the natural propensity for taking risks all contribute to substance abuse and the resultant toxic effects in early and midadolescence.

Environmental factors

The American home typically contains dozens of potentially toxic substances. Many families have little idea of the products that have accumulated in the medicine cabinet, among the cleaning supplies, in the garage, and in kitchen cabinets. Prescription drugs are kept on hand long after they are no longer needed. Highly promoted over-the-counter cough and cold preparations and analgesics are kept on hand in sufficient varieties and numbers that they create substantial risk to the curious young child. And because some household products are not clearly labeled for their toxicity, highly poisonous substances (eg, furniture polish, drain cleaners, and solvents) are stored side-by-side with the nontoxic substances (eg, soaps, shampoos, and toothpaste). To children and parents, poisonous plants are indistinguishable from nontoxic plants.

Safe storage of potentially toxic substances varies from household to household. Even when families choose to store products out of reach or in locked cabinets, they often present a risk when they are being used and there is a lapse in supervision.

The adolescent's environment may also be more or less conducive to poisoning, in this case, intentional poisoning. Communities, schools, and neighborhoods where illicit and recreational drugs are available put all young people at risk. Lack of vigilance for children at risk for substance abuse or suicide denies these children the early intervention and counseling that may be lifesaving.

4.4.3 Intervention Strategies

Intervention strategies are divided into primary, secondary, and tertiary prevention.

Primary prevention

Primary prevention consists of strategies to make poisons unavailable for ingestion. Because at least 80% of poisonings during childhood occur in the home, this is logically the central focus for education and intervention.[3] Prevention may be accomplished by keeping toxins out of the household, ensuring that they are unavailable to children in the home, or formulating them in ways that they will not be ingested or will not be ingested in toxic amounts. Within the purview of primary prevention, there are roles for education, enforcement, and engineering.

Education

Parent education has been a key component of many prevention programs designed by physicians and local and regional poison control centers. The Injury Prevention Program (TIPP), initiated by the American Academy of Pediatrics, is, in part, a nationally recognized *poison prevention* program. Many poison control centers have designed and used individually tailored programs. None of these programs, including TIPP, have been rigorously evaluated for their ability to prevent poisoning during childhood. Where evaluations have been done, generally over a few weeks to a few months, minimal changes have been noted in parental behavior as the result of active education programs. Programs have generally focused on activities such as "poison proofing" the home, acquiring syrup of ipecac for use at home, and distributing stickers to place on the phone. These activities are designed to improve the awareness of parents and children about the risk of poisoning. Access to parents has often been through school and community organizations, social groups, and preschool programs. Public service announcements in the mass media are also used, but they are usually brief, and no data support their influence on long-term parental behavior. There is a need for a nationally adopted, rigorously tested, and effectual program to educate parents and other caregivers about the prevention of childhood poisoning.

Many programs focus on the direct education of the child. They are geared toward preschool children and use various activities, including audiovisual and arts and crafts projects designed make the child aware of the poisoning hazards in the environment. Unfortunately, most unintentional incidents of poisoning occur in the early years (2 years old and younger), and it is unlikely that education for children this young will be effective in prevention. Again, no validation exists about the effectiveness of these programs, particularly in changing medium- to long-range behavior patterns.

Several programs are geared to school-age children, particularly at the elementary level. While these programs work for children who are more amenable to the education process, they are unlikely to substantially influence the incidence of poisoning because accidental poisonings in the school-age population are uncommon. Some of these programs use the child as a conduit to younger siblings and the family in general with take-home materials that can be used in the home. While this may be a productive approach, no national program exists, and there is little to no validation of the effectiveness of such programs at the local and regional levels.

Office-based parent education should be focused and guided by specific objectives. Of central importance should be increasing awareness that poisoning is a developmental and situational risk. Parents can be educated to keep all potential poisons inaccessible to the toddler by using child-resistant cabinet latches and high cabinets. Parents must recognize the need for duplication in protective strategies (ie, layers of protection), so they should also use child-resistant closures on medication containers and toxic household products. Products and medications should be stored in their original containers and never in food or drink containers that could confuse children as they learn to distinguish between edible and nonedible items.

Parents should be urged to purchase the least toxic products that will do the job, to purchase those products in reasonable quantities, and to dispose of potential toxins when they are no longer needed. Old prescription medications should be disposed of so they are inaccessible to toddlers (ie, flushed down the toilet). Bleach for use at home is of lower concentration and toxicity than bleach manufactured for commercial and industrial use. Certain products are of such high and irreversible toxicity, such as crystal drain cleaners, that parents of young children should avoid purchasing them for use at home.

The toxic effects of medications should be considered when they are prescribed for families with children. Tricyclic antidepressants and theophylline preparations may have safer and equally effective therapeutic alternatives, or at least they can be dispensed in small quantities.

Another approach to primary prevention that has been aggressively promulgated, particularly in the United States, is the use of warning labels on packaging. These warning labels may be placed by the manufacturer, using the skull and crossbones poison symbol, or by parents using stickers such as the "Mr. Yuk" sticker designed to warn children about the hazardous contents of the container. While conflicting data exist about the efficacy of such symbols, the consensus is that this approach to prevention has limited value and, in fact, may attract the child to the container.[20,21] A major risk of using these labels is that the parent will assume that adequate preventive measures have been taken and will not supervise the child sufficiently when toxic materials are in use or will not effectively prevent the child's access to potentially toxic materials.

Enforcement

Legislative and regulatory measures have been and are being used to prevent unintentional poisonings of children. The Child Protection Act of 1966 and the Poison Prevention Act of 1970 recognized the risk of childhood injury from unintended ingestion of medications and other common household products and the potential for reducing such risks with the appropriate use of safety closure packaging. Since then we have had a major shift in the use of such packaging for toxic products commonly found in the home. Currently, legislation and regulations require that most prescription medications, some over-the-counter medications, and many toxic, corrosive, and irritant household products be dispensed or sold with child-resistant closures (CRCs).[22,23] A result of these laws has been a dramatic fall in the incidence of fatal poisonings of children, although the data about reduction of overall poisoning episodes are less clear.[24] A more recent move at the federal level is the effort to limit the quantity of a potentially toxic material in a unit package, particularly for over-the-counter products, to minimize the potential for substantial injury should the child gain access to the product. Such packaging restrictions are now being applied to analgesic products and will probably be extended to iron preparations.

Child resistant closures do not provide absolute protection against unintended ingestion of toxic substances, and the parent should not rely on them as foolproof methods of prevention. The regulations governing CRCs state only that no more than a certain percentage of children will be able to gain access to the contents within a specified time and that at least a certain percentage of adults will be able to open the containers with relative ease. Furthermore, the regulations allow consumers to request the pharmacist to substitute standard closures for CRCs. Physicians and pharmacists should discourage such requests. Regulations published in July 1995 require that the child-resistant containers be easier for *older* adults to open, which discourages leaving difficult-to-open containers open.

Engineering

(See the discussion about CRCs in preceding section, Enforcement.)

During the last decade, many storage and locking devices that are specifically designed to prevent access of children to toxic materials have become available for use in the home. These devices generally take two forms: specific containers, such as buckets or boxes that allow easy access by parents through a locking device but prevent most children from gaining access, and devices that secure cabinet or door locks to allow easy access by parents but make entry by children difficult. Many of these latter devices are available in forms that do not damage the woodwork when they are installed and are convenient and inexpensive. The use of such devices should be actively encouraged in pediatric preventive health counseling.

In addition to child-resistant packaging and safe storage, the product itself may be formulated in such a way that ingestion is either encouraged or discouraged. Overdoses of iron supplements produce toxic effects. Iron pills that are small, round, smooth, and colorful (like candy) are attractive and easy to swallow. Some household detergents contain an artificial "bittering" agent (denatonium benzoate [Bitrex]) to discourage a second or third swallow.[25] The approach is logical, but strong evidence for its effectiveness is lacking.

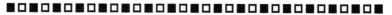
Secondary prevention

Secondary prevention includes strategies that prevent illness or injury once the exposure or ingestion has occurred. These strategies include familiarity with first aid and life support, use of poison information centers, and use of detoxifying measures such as emesis, charcoal, specific antidotes, and catharsis.[26–28]

Poison control and information centers

Since they were first envisioned in the 1950s, a successful system of poison control centers has been established in the United States.[19,29] The centers are staffed 7 days a week, 24 hours a day by trained and certified information specialists. They use extensive computerized databases to provide parents, physicians, and hospitals with current information about toxicity and management of exposure to poisons. While most areas of the United States are served by regional poison centers, coverage is not yet universal. Also, awareness of poison centers is far from universal, particularly among some cultural and socioeconomic groups. The 1990 National Health Interview Survey revealed that among households with children younger than 10 years, only three fourths had heard of the poison control center, only half knew the phone number, and only one fourth had syrup of ipecac on hand.[30] Awareness increases with education and income, and it is greater in white and non-Hispanic families and in those living outside of the inner city.

Gastric decontamination

Keeping syrup of ipecac in the home has been a traditional recommendation to parents. Because the use of syrup of ipecac has decreased dramatically recently as a result of more realistic assessments of many common poisoning episodes and the awareness that more effective means of gastric decontamination exist, the value of having syrup of ipecac in the home may be questioned. However, many physicians believe that purchasing and storing syrup of ipecac in the home represent a sentinel event that increases parental awareness of the risk of poisoning and the measures needed to prevent injuries. In this sense, the emphasis on syrup of ipecac, particularly in parental counseling in the pediatric office, is probably of some value. Clearly, along with the emphasis on syrup of ipecac must come parental education about a variety of other techniques that can be used in the home to prevent poisonings.

Except in extraordinary circumstances, syrup of ipecac should be used only on the specific advice of a poison information specialist or knowledgeable health professional. Emesis is hazardous and contra-indicated in certain ingestions (caustic agents and hydrocarbons) and situations (compromised airway or decreased level of consciousness).

Activated charcoal, with or without cathartics, is the method of choice for gastric decontamination in the emergency department. It may also become the treatment of choice for home use when a more palatable, smaller dose preparation becomes available.[28]

Tertiary prevention

Tertiary prevention includes interventions that minimize injury or toxic effects once symptoms have appeared.[19] Poison centers, emergency medical services, emergency departments, and pediatric inpatient ser-vices have played a role in minimizing toxic effects. The specific inter-ventions used to treat poisoning are beyond the scope of this chapter but are covered in detail in a companion volume.[31]

4.4.4 Recommendations for Pediatricians

Pediatricians can intervene to lessen the impact of poisoning on child-hood morbidity and mortality through two major avenues: clinical inter-vention and community intervention.

Clinical intervention

General counseling themes

Through anticipatory guidance, pediatricians can educate parents about the interaction of child development and risk of poisoning. This can begin toward the middle of the first year of the child's life as parents begin to appreciate how the development of fine and gross motor skills and the persistence of oral behavior necessitates poison proofing the home. Pediatricians should specifically recommend a home survey at or before the 6-month visit and periodically thereafter (see section 4.2). Parents should survey specific areas of the home for well-recognized risks, assuring that household products, prescription and nonprescription medications, household plants, and lawn and garden chemicals are safely stored. Strategies include safe (and original) packaging and use of inaccessible cabinets or cabinets with safety latches. Parents should also be asked, as part of the home survey, to consider whether some toxic or poisonous substances in the home are unessential; those should be removed. Table 4.1, p 69, provides a general walk-through of the home from the viewpoint of preventing poisoning, identifying the specific risk areas and substances, and suggesting approaches to removing these materials effectively from the child's access.

Parents should be counseled to store medications in containers with CRCs, and those containers should be stored in a locked medicine cabinet or special container or box. Many parents have found a box such as a fishing tackle box or tool box with an external latch and lock to be an appropriate place to store medication. This box can be placed conveniently in a closet or cabinet. Child-resistant closures should not be left off when medication is being used over a period of time because children may then gain access to it.

It is also important that medication not be confused with candy. A common technique to entice children to take medication is telling them that it is candy. The child may then be unable to distinguish medication from candy. Medication should always be labeled as medication, and it should be continually emphasized to the child that medication is only taken in the presence of the parent and is only used to treat illness. All medication intended for young children should be given under the direct supervision of the parent or the designated caregiver.

Parents should be encouraged to keep a 1-oz bottle of syrup of ipecac at home and to post the telephone number of the poison control center near the telephone. A second bottle of syrup of ipecac could be kept in the glove compartment of the car or packed for family trips. Parents should be informed that the regional poison control center should be the first source for information about poisons in an emergency, rather than the physician or the local hospital emergency department.

Cardiovascular medications, iron supplements, antidepressants, hydrocarbons, pesticides, and caustic agents are particularly hazardous and require special caution. Parents should be made aware of these substances and their inherent risks.

Parents should be told that a substantial percentage of ingestions of toxic medication — perhaps as many as one third — occur with medications intended for someone other than an immediate family member, most often a grandparent.[32] Grandparents often take medications with

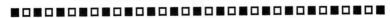

TABLE 4.1.
Poison Prevention: The Home Survey

Home Area	Risks	Preventive Approaches
Kitchen	Detergents (particularly dishwasher) Cleaners (particularly oven) Drain cleaners	Store on higher shelves, put food in lower cabinets Use locking devices on cabinet doors and drawers Do not store chemicals in the refrigerator
Bathroom	Medications (prescription and over the counter) Perfumes and colognes (contain alcohol) Cosmetics and hair care products	Store in locked cabinet, locked box, or locked closet Store on upper shelves, preferably locked
Bedrooms	Medications and contraceptives Perfumes and colognes (contain alcohol) Cosmetics and hair care products	Store out of sight or preferably in locked cabinet or box Store out of sight and reach
Living and dining rooms	Plants Cigarettes, cigarette butts, and tobacco products Alcohol Insecticides, traps, and baits	Identify and, if toxic, keep out of children's reach or remove the plant Keep out of sight and reach Keep in a locked cabinet; dispose of partially consumed drinks Do not use in locations to which children have access
Garage or basement	Paints and solvents Insecticides and herbicides Chemicals for use in hobbies	Store in locked cabinet Always store materials in original containers
Laundry	Cleaning supplies	Keep out of reach
Outside areas	Plants, berries, and bulbs	Identify plants in yard Do not leave unplanted bulbs in areas to which children have access

substantial intrinsic toxicity: cardiovascular medications, asthma medications, and antidepressants. They may not be accustomed to children being around, and failing eyesight or arthritis often discourage their use of CRCs. Therefore, the homes of grandparents should be surveyed by parents when families arrive for a visit.

Physicians should consider the risk of poisoning when they prescribe medications. Less toxic therapies should be prescribed when appropriate (eg, use of an alarm system for enuresis instead of imipramine). When medications — even those with low toxicity — are routinely prescribed or recommended (eg, fluoride supplements), it is instructive to mention the importance of keeping *all* medications out of reach of children.

Clinical interventions to prevent suicide and substance abuse are covered in chapters 3 and 8.

Seasonally appropriate counseling

Physicians, particularly in northern areas of the country and during cold weather, should discuss carbon monoxide poisoning. Carbon monoxide is a common killer of both children and adults. It is produced by the combustion of any carbon-based fuel, including gasoline, oil, coal, and natural gas. The production of carbon monoxide can and should be minimized by efficient maintenance of heating devices, assuring an adequate flow of oxygen, which minimizes the production of carbon monoxide, and assuring a safe venting system for combustion gases. Parents should be encouraged to have appropriate yearly maintenance of appliances that use such fuel and purchase carbon monoxide detectors that are readily available and inexpensive. Children are particularly susceptible to carbon monoxide because it tends to accumulate at low heights. Thus children, who spend more time closer to the floor, are more likely to be affected than are adults. Children will also show more pronounced symptoms at any given level of carbon monoxide than will adults.

Physicians should also counsel parents about insect repellents. A variety of materials are used as topical insect repellents on children. Most notably, deet (diethyltoluamide) has been associated with encephalopathy and seizures in young children when it is applied in high concentrations over large body surface areas and left on for extended periods of time. Care should be taken by parents to use all such materials as directed. Manufacturers' recommendations should be followed for all insecticides used in the home. Questions about the use of these materials should be referred by parents to the pediatrician or a poison control center.

Competent diagnosis of poisoning

Pediatricians should keep poisoning in mind as part of the differential diagnosis when examining a child for altered consciousness, vomiting, shock, new seizures, or altered cardiac rhythm. Toward that end, clinicians should be familiar with the "toxidromes" associated with the ingestion of classes of toxins such as anticholinergics, opiates, iron, phenothiazines, and tricyclic antidepressants.[33]

Community intervention

Pediatricians can promote poison prevention efforts in the community and nationally by speaking out for continued and better funding of regional poison information centers. Because prevention of poisoning is a public health issue, it is demanding and deserving of public funding.[19] Pediatricians are encouraged to participate in community efforts to raise awareness about poison prevention activities in schools, child care centers, parenting classes, and adult education programs.

References

1. Pollock DA, McGee DL, Rodriguez JG. Deaths due to injury in the home among persons under 15 years of age, 1970–1984. *MMWR Morb Mortal Wkly Rep.* 1988;37:13–20

2. Widome MD. Pediatric injury prevention for the practitioner. *Curr Probl Pediatr.* 1991; 21:428–468

3. Scheidt P, Harel Y, Trumble AC, Jones DH, Overpeck MD, Bijur PE. The epidemiology of nonfatal injuries among US children and youth. *Am J Public Health.* 1995; 85:932–938

4. Bass JL, Christoffel KK, Widome M, et al. Childhood injury prevention in primary care settings: a critical review of the literature. *Pediatrics.* 1993;92:544–550

5. Rice DP, Mackenzie EJ, and Associates. *Cost of Injury in the United States: A Report to Congress.* San Francisco, CA: Institute for Health & Aging, University of California and Injury Prevention Center, and Baltimore, MD: Injury Prevention Center, School of Hygiene and Public Health, The Johns Hopkins University; 1989

6. Baker SP, O'Neill B, Ginsburg M, Li G. *The Injury Fact Book.* 2nd ed. New York, NY: Oxford University Press; 1992

7. Wilson MH, Baker SP, Teret SP, Shock S, Garbarino J. *Saving Children: A Guide to Injury Prevention.* New York, NY: Oxford University Press; 1991

8. Rivara FP, Alexander B, Johnston B, Soderberg R. Population-based study of fall injuries in children and adolescents resulting in hospitalization or death. *Pediatrics.* 1993;92:61–63

9. Meller JL, Shermeta DW. Falls in urban children: a problem revisited. *Am J Dis Child.* 1987;141:1271–1275

10. Garrettson LK, Gallagher SS. Falls in children and youth. *Pediatr Clin North Am.* 1985; 32:153–162

11. Stephenson EO. The silent and inviting trap. *The Building Official and Code Administrator.* 1988;Nov/Dec:28–33

12. Spiegel CN, Lindaman FC. Children can't fly: a program to prevent childhood morbidity and mortality from window falls. *Am J Public Health.* 1977;67:1143–1147

13. Lehman D, Schonfeld N. Falls from heights: a problem not just in the northeast. *Pediatrics.* 1993;92:121–124

14. Chiaviello CT, Christoph RA, Bond GR. Infant walker–related injuries: a prospective study of severity and incidence. *Pediatrics.* 1994;93:974–976

15. American Academy of Pediatrics, Committee on Injury and Poison Prevention. Injuries associated with infant walkers. *Pediatrics.* 1995;95:778–780

16. Baker MD, Bell RE. The role of footwear in childhood injuries. *Pediatr Emerg Care.* 1991;7:353–355

17. Kravitz H, Driessen G, Gomberg R, Korach A. Accidental falls from elevated surfaces in infants from birth to one year of age. *Pediatrics.* 1969;44(suppl):869–876

18. Litovitz TL, Felberg L, Soloway RA, Ford M, Geller R. 1994 annual report of the American Association of Poison Control Centers Toxic Exposure Surveillance System. *Am J Emerg Med.* 1995;13:551–597

19. Lovejoy FH, Robertson WO, Woolf AD. Poison centers, poison prevention, and the pediatrician. *Pediatrics.* 1994;94:220–224

20. Vernberg K, Culver-Dickinson P, Spyker DA. The deterrent effect of poison-warning stickers. *Am J Dis Child.* 1984;138:1018–1020

21. Fergusson DM, Horwood LJ, Beautrais AL, Shannon FT. A controlled field trial of a poisoning prevention method. *Pediatrics.* 1982;69:515–520

22. Poison Prevention Packaging Act of 1970, 15 USC §1471–1475

23. Poison Prevention Packaging Act of 1970 Regulations. 1988, 16 CFR Part 1700

24. Walton WW. An evaluation of the poison prevention packaging act. *Pediatrics.* 1982; 69:363–370

25. Sibert JR, Frude N. Bittering agents in the prevention of accidental poisoning: children's reactions to denatonium benzoate (Bitrex). *Arch Emerg Med.* 1991;8:1–7

24. James LP, Nichols MH, King WD. A comparison of cathartics in pediatric ingestions. *Pediatrics.* 1995;96:235–238

27. Mandl KD, Lovejoy FH Jr. Common poisonings. *Pediatr Rev.* 1994;15:151–156

28. Lovejoy FH Jr. Childhood poisonings: what role for ipecac and charcoal? *Contemp Pediatr* 1992;9:99–108

29. Scherz RG, Robertson WO. The history of poison control centers in the United States. *Clin Toxicol.* 1978;12:291–296

30. Mayer M, LeClere F. *Injury Prevention Measures in Households With Children in the United States, 1990.* Hyattsville, MD: Centers for Disease Control and Prevention, National Center for Health Statistics; 1994. US Dept of Health and Human Services publication PHS 94–1250

31. American Academy of Pediatrics, Committee on Injury and Poison Prevention. *Handbook of Common Poisonings in Children.* 3rd ed. Elk Grove Village, IL: American Academy of Pediatrics; 1994

32. Jacobson BJ, Rock AR, Cohn MS, Litovitz T. Accidental ingestions of oral prescription drugs: a multicenter survey. *Am J Public Health.* 1989;79:853–856

33. Woolf AD. Poisoning in children and adolescents. *Pediatr Rev.* 1993;14:411–422

CHAPTER 5

■□■□■□■□■□■□■□■□■□■□■□■□■□■□■□■

Injury Control in Child Care, Preschool, School, and Camp Settings

While injuries that occur in and around the home receive emphasis in early preventive efforts, as children grow, they spend an increasing amount of their time away from home. Even infants and toddlers are likely to spend part of their days in child care settings because increasingly both parents work. This chapter addresses injuries that occur in child care settings, schools, and camps and during transportation to and from these settings.

5.1 Injury Prevention in Child Care, Preschool, and After-school Programs

5.1.1 Scope of the Problem

The family, the work force, and child care

In the last two decades, work and family life have changed dramatically. Some of the change is related to (1) the increased mobility of the work force, which has resulted in a decrease in contact with the extended family, (2) an increase in mothers entering the work force and in two-wage-earner families, (3) the high divorce rate, and (4) the increase in single parenting (by either the father or mother). In 1993, about 10 million children younger than 5 years — more than half of that age group — had mothers who were employed.[1] The mothers of more than 21 million children 5 to 15 years old are in the work force.

One result of these dramatic changes in the American family is that more children, including infants, toddlers, preschoolers, and school-age children, are spending their days or hours after school in out-of-home child care programs. Seventy percent of mothers in the work force with children younger than 6 years use child care. Of all children, 40% now receive full- or part-time child care.[2] More than 13 million children are estimated to be enrolled in some form of child care.

Increased demand for child care has led to a rapid increase in the numbers of child care facilities (centers and family child care homes) for infants, toddlers, and preschool children and after-school programs for school-age children. This expansion of programs has heightened concern about the quality and safety of out-of-home child care arrangements in general. For many school-age children, no after-school programs are available. More than 44% of school-age children with working parents have no adult supervision after school.[3]

Children enrolled in child care spend their days in a variety of settings—center-based care, family child care homes, special facilities, school-age child care facilities, and drop-in facilities.[4] Programs vary widely in organization, size, sponsorship, quality, and cost.

- Center-based care: This type of nonresidential child care may provide services for fewer than 25 children, while others provide services for several hundred children. *Full-day centers* provide care for more than 4 hours per day; *part-day centers* offer shorter day programs, such as Head Start, preschool, and after-school programs.

- Family child care homes: These facilities are in the homes of the caregiver, who employs assistants to meet requirements for staff-to-child ratios. *Small-family child care homes* provide care for one to six children; *large-family child care homes* provide care for seven to 12 children. *Family* child care homes may be *registered* or *unregistered.*

- Special facilities: *Special facilities for ill children* provide care only for children with illnesses. They are designed to meet the needs of working parents and their children when the children are unable to attend regular child care because of a minor illness. *Facilities for children with special needs* offer child care for children with developmental disabilities, chronic illness, or other impairments. These facilities may be residential or nonresidential.

- Facilities for school-age children: These facilities include before- and after-school programs.

- Drop-in facilities: These facilities, which may be residential or nonresidential, provide occasional care for children that is limited to less than 10 hours per day and no more than once a week.

Injury patterns

Because reporting of injuries is far from accurate, determining the scope of injuries in child care settings with any precision is difficult. Deficiencies in data result, in part, from concerns about increased liability and the state surveillance that may result from such reporting. Furthermore, much child care takes place in unlicensed child care homes, where reporting of injuries is unlikely. Also, the case definition of an injury, particularly if the injury is minor and does not require medical attention, is problematic. The injuries most commonly reported by child care professionals are listed in Table 5.1.

The epidemiologic aspects of injuries that occurred in out-of-home child care settings were reviewed in a series of presentations at a 1992 Centers for Disease Control and Prevention–sponsored international conference about child care.[5–9] Rivara and Sacks[5] noted that risk of injury may be less in child care settings than at home. (The injury rate in child care is about 2/100 000 child-hours compared with 3 to 5/100 000 child-hours at home.) About half of the injuries occur outdoors and 40% are due to falls that occur both indoors and outdoors. Falls from playground equipment are the most common cause and

---

TABLE 5.1.
**Injuries Most Commonly Seen and Reported
by Child Care Professionals**

Bites inflicted by other children

Choking on food

Fingers pinched in doors

Forehead lacerations from falls

Insect stings

Minor and superficial head trauma

Minor dental trauma from falls and collisions

Minor fractures

Minor trauma to the mouth and lips

Nose bleeds

Other minor lacerations

Scrapes and bruises from falls

Scratches from falling outside

Superficial injury from children colliding with each other

account for the largest numbers of serious injuries. Other injuries are associated with furniture, architectural elements (eg, doors and floors), or toys, or caused by interaction with other children (eg, biting and hitting).[8] A substantial proportion of injuries sustained in child care centers occurs as a result of interaction with other children.[5]

Alkon and colleagues,[9] who prospectively followed-up 141 children in four San Francisco child care centers, found that most children in child care sustained multiple minor injuries. The children in their study suffered a total of 886 injuries during a 1-year period; 18% sustained half of the injuries and only 10 children (7%) had no injuries. Nine of 10 injuries were mild, but those who sustained frequent minor injuries were also the most likely to sustain moderate or severe injuries.

Deaths in child care settings seem uncommon, but can result from strangulation, suffocation, pedestrian injury, and other causes that are common for the age group.[7]

5.1.2 Risk Factors

A variety of variables may influence the risk of injury in child care settings, including:
• Age and sex of the children
• Size of the center
• Adult-to-child ratio
• Specific program offerings, eg, swimming, field trips
• Overall quality of the center and its program
• Playground equipment and supervision
• Licensure and enforcement of regulations

Sacks and colleagues[10] reviewed the epidemiologic factors associated with medically attended injuries at 71 child care centers in Atlanta, Ga. They found that injury rates were low for infants and increased with the age of the child. Little difference in injury rates was noted by gender in the child care setting for preschoolers. At age 5 years, however, the rate of injuries indicated a male predominance. Injuries were more common in the summer, late in the morning, and late in the afternoon. The seasonal variation probably reflects outdoor play and particularly the use of playground equipment. The time-of-day pattern seems to reflect activity cycles, fatigue, and variations in the level of supervision throughout the day. The higher injury rates observed in the larger centers also may reflect the level of supervision.[10]

Rivara and Sacks[5] noted that poverty as a risk factor for child injury may be less a factor in the child care setting because protection from a hazardous home environment may be provided. However, hazardous conditions (such as unsafe playgrounds) at the child care setting increase the risk of injury.[11]

Alkon and colleagues[9] studied factors contributing to injuries and divided them between *child-related factors* (eg, falls or involvement with another child) and *environment-related factors* (eg, floors, equipment, and furniture). Environmental factors did not contribute to most minor injuries, but were implicated in most moderate-to-severe injuries.

A large study in Sweden[6] of the factors contributing to injuries in child care centers found the following percentages for each factor: playground equipment (eg, climbing frames and slides), 13.0; other child involved (eg, pushing, colliding, or throwing), 12.8; furniture (eg, chairs or bookshelves), 11.5; part of building (eg, doors or radiators), 10.7; vegetation (eg, trees or berries), 8.4; toys, 5.2; fixed equipment outdoors (eg, fence or gate), 3.1; bicycle, 2.5; sleds, 2.5; and other and unspecified factors, 30.5.

Hot tap water can contribute to injury. Many child care providers do not know the temperature of the tap water in the facility.[12] To meet the needs for both kitchen sanitation, which requires a water temperature above 120°F, and safety from scalding, which requires a water temperature of no more than 120°F, separate hot water heaters or safety valves are necessary. State regulations should mandate that the temperature of tap water in child care facilities be set to no greater than 120°F.

Playground safety is discussed in section 5.4. Several studies have revealed the playground to be the major site of injury in child care settings, accounting for 50% to 60% of all child care injuries.[6,10,13] Factors related to injuries on the playground include the ground surface material, safety gates, swings, children of different age groups playing on the playground at the same time, and permitting younger children to use equipment sized for older children. Injuries result from falls from the playground equipment and entrapment on equipment.

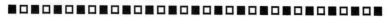
5.1.3 Intervention Strategies

Theoretically, interventions to control injuries in child care settings can be categorized as educational, enforcement, and environmental. In practice, much overlap exists.

Parents should be educated so they are informed purchasers of child care, paying attention to the safety features and supervision in various programs. Table 5.2 offers a sample safety survey that parents may use for general assessment during consideration of the child care programs. The same checklist may be used to make child care staff aware of potential safety hazards and problems.

TABLE 5.2.
Child Care Facility Safety Survey for Parents

This list is not all inclusive, but is intended to provide parents with a sample of items to screen for safe child care settings.

Are children greeted when they arrive and acknowledged when they depart?

Are the caregivers trained in pediatric first aid?

Are injuries recorded in a logbook?

Are emergency phone numbers posted by the telephone?

Are plastic bags stored out of sight and reach?

Is playground equipment secured on an energy-absorbing surface?

Are lists of allergies of the children readily available to staff in the classroom and the kitchen?

Is the hot water temperature at the tap 120°F or less?

Are barriers on stairs adequate to prevent children from falling?

Are there screens covering all heat sources?

Are there smoke detectors in each area of the center? Are they checked monthly?

Do high chairs have safety harnesses?

Are cribs sturdy with hardware in good condition?

Do changing tables have sides to prevent infants from rolling off?

Are the outdoor play areas adequately fenced?

Can the caregiver see the entire playground?

Is the playground free of hazardous litter (for example, rocks, cans, and bottles)?

Do children in an after-school program use the playground at the same time as do the younger children?

Are sand boxes covered?

Is sports equipment (such as balls) soft?

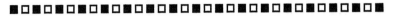
Child care providers should be educated about effective safety practices and procedures as outlined in simple checklists (Table 5.3), detailed in

---

TABLE 5.3.
Safety Checklist

Parking Lot
Maintained appropriately when snow and ice are present
Designed so pedestrians do not need to walk between cars
Cars are not left running unattended
Children are supervised by an adult and not allowed to run in the lot

Entrance
All steps have a handrail
Entrance and exit are at sidewalk level or onto same-level landing
All elevated areas (such as porches) are appropriately fenced (have vertical pickets with less than 4-in spacing)
Doors open outward and are never locked from the inside
Monitoring is done to prevent strangers from entering the facility

Hallways and Stairs
Areas are kept clean and unobstructed (to prevent physical injuries and fire hazards)
Lighting is adequate
Exits are well-marked, lighted, and unobstructed
No corners or counters have exposed sharp edges (they are covered)
Safety glass is used in doors and windows
Stairways are carpeted and have a child-height railing on the right side for descending
Smoke detectors are working
No peeling paint is visible; no lead-based paint is used

Rooms and Storage Units
Electrical sockets are high and out of reach or securely covered
No dangling or covered electrical extension cords are present
Cabinets or file boxes that contain medications and diluted cleaning

solutions (concentrated solutions are never kept in the classroom or playroom) must be locked
All hardware on cribs, tables, and bookcases is checked monthly (screws and bolts are tight)
Hot plates are not used (crock pots are allowed for warming bottles)
Chairs or tables are not used as ladders to hang items
No sharp corners are exposed on tables or other furniture
Toys are safe, with no sharp areas, pinch points, or small parts
Fire exit from room requires only one turn or pull-down action
Accessible above-ground-level windows are protected with adequate grills or screens
Hot surfaces, hot pipes, heaters, and vents cannot be reached by children; freestanding space heaters are not used
Temperature of tap water for hand washing is maintained at 120°F or less
Lighting is adequate in all rooms
Walkways are clear between sleeping cots for children and staff
Children are not left alone in high chairs or chairs
Infant walkers are not used
Pacifiers with strings longer than 6 in are not allowed
Emergency phone is accessible
Trash cans are covered and secured
No smoking is allowed
Floors are smooth, clean, and not slippery

Kitchen
Only authorized personnel are allowed in the kitchen
Sharp utensils are kept out of reach
All containers are clearly marked and have secure lids

TABLE 5.3.
Safety Checklist, continued

Kitchen, continued
Fire extinguishers are easily accessible
Items on shelving units, such as cans of
food, are neatly organized, secure, and
not piled high
Separate sinks are used for hand washing
and food preparation
Bathrooms
Cleaning supplies are not accessible
Toilets and sinks are appropriate for use
by children; step stools are provided
Water temperature for hand washing is
maintained at 120°F or less
Floors are nonskid

Outdoor Playground (section 5.4.)
Equipment is checked weekly for sharp
protrusions
Bolts are covered; swings have soft seats
Ground is covered with loose-fill surface
material (round gravel may be used
for children at least 3 years old)
Play area is fenced; gate has safety locks
Equipment is age-appropriate; slides are
enclosed or have hand rails; only one
child at a time uses the equipment; and
no spaces where a child's head, leg, or
arm could be trapped (3½ in to 9 in)
Constant supervision is provided
No poisonous plants, trash, or sharp
objects are in the area surrounding
the playground

Toxic Chemicals
Kitchen and cleaning supplies should have
their own locked storage unit
Cleaning solutions for use in classrooms
and playrooms are stored in a locked
cabinet

*Computers, Televisions, and Electrical
Equipment*
Ensure that the equipment is flush against
the wall so the electrical outlet is not
exposed
Only authorized people provide service
for equipment
Liquids are not allowed near equipment
Children are supervised while equipment
is in use

Vans and Other Vehicles
First aid kit is available
Child restraint devices are appropriate for
child's size and weight
Seat belts are used and maintained
Radio sound level is kept at a minimum,
and the program content is appropriate
for children
Vehicle tires, oil, and brakes are maintained
regularly
Driver has a current driver's license that
authorizes the driver to operate the
vehicle driven and is properly trained
Children are not allowed in the front seat
Vehicle is checked for sharp or rusty metal

Staff Training
Person certified in pediatric first aid that
includes rescue breathing and first aid
for choking on site at all times
Children are taught safety and emergency
procedures
Staff is fully trained in emergency procedures

Art Supplies
Nontoxic and natural materials such as
dyes and water-based products are used
Use of scissors is supervised
Aerosol sprays and solvent-based glues are
avoided

Field Trips
Adequate supervision is supplied by child
care center or camp personnel, not personnel at the location of the field trip
Identification is worn by each child
Young children hold hands in pairs or hold
onto a rope when walking in a group

Equipment
First aid kit is appropriately stocked
Sports equipment is safe and soft

Fire and Severe Weather Drills
All children are safely evacuated to a safe
area within 3 min
Monthly fire drills are held
Smoke detectors and the alarm system are
in place and working

guidelines published by the American Red Cross, or included in comprehensive health and safety standards such as those developed jointly by the American Academy of Pediatrics (AAP) and the American Public Health Association.[4,14,15] Pediatricians serving as consultants to child care facilities can provide up-to-date information about vehicle occupant safety, toy safety, and environmental hazards.

Personnel in child care facilities must document injuries, whether minor or major, to identify patterns and hazards in the facility and have a basis for corrective action where appropriate. A sample incident report form is shown in Fig 5.1, p 84.

State child care regulations provide incentives to providers to keep the environment safe and hazard free only to the extent that the regulations are known and enforced and technical support is provided. Unfortunately, child care regulation and inspection offer scant protection in the United States. Inspection varies greatly from state to state. Many inspectors lack special knowledge of child health and safety and are given little support or training for their roles. Furthermore, much of the child care provided in family child care homes is unlicensed and unregulated. The millions of children in these small home settings do not necessarily receive the benefits of centers or programs that have implemented child care health and safety standards. Some family child care homes may place children at risk for fire, burns, playground injuries, drowning, and exposure to toxic substances.

Environmental protection from injury that is *built into* the design of the child care center and its equipment does not require ongoing maintenance. Environmental, or "engineered" protection is usually more effective than that provided solely through education of staff or enforcement of regulations. For example, if the stairs are designed with wide steps and shallow risers, are well carpeted, have a landing, and have a child-height railing on both sides, considerable protection is built in, which eliminates the need for constant supervision of children as they climb and descend the stairs.

5.1.4 Recommendations for Pediatricians

Because most children seen by pediatricians are enrolled in some form of child care during childhood, pediatricians should become knowledge-

FIG 5.1.
Child care incident report form

NAME OF INJURED _____

SEX _____

AGE _____

DATE WHEN INJURY OCCURRED _____

TIME WHEN INJURY OCCURRED _____

DESCRIPTION OF HOW
INJURY OCCURRED _____

DESCRIPTION OF PART OF
BODY INVOLVED (IF ANY) _____

NAME OF CONSUMER PRODUCT
INVOLVED (IF ANY) _____

ACTION TAKEN ON BEHALF
OF THE INJURED _____

WAS PARENT/LEGAL GUARDIAN
SPECIFICALLY ADVISED OF INJURY? _____

WAS PARENT/LEGAL GUARDIAN
SPECIFICALLY ADVISED TO OBTAIN
MEDICAL ATTENTION? _____

NAME OF INDIVIDUAL(S) INVOLVED
IN SUPERVISION AT TIME OF INJURY _____

NAME OF PERSON COMPLETING
THIS REPORT FORM _____

DATE OF COMPLETION OF FORM _____

Reprinted from: Caring for Our Children: National Health and Safety Performance Standards: Guidelines for Out-of-Home Child Care Programs. Washington, DC: American Public Health Association (and) American Academy of Pediatrics; 1992.

able about child care issues. Pediatricians can assist in controlling injuries in child care settings by:

1. *Advising parents.* Pediatricians can provide parents with information, advice, and guidelines about safety when decisions are being made concerning child care for their children, just as pediatricians provide counseling for injury control in the home. Many of the issues involved in a home safety survey apply to the child care setting (see chapter 4.1).

2. *Advising child care facilities and their staff members.* Pediatricians are asked formally or informally to serve as consultants to child care facilities. Although often the initial interest of the facility is related to infection control, the pediatrician can extend the consultation to issues of injury control. Table 5.4, pp 86–87, lists useful discussion topics for the education of child care workers and parents.

3. *Advocating affordable, safe child care.* Standards in child care (as elsewhere) have been opposed on economic grounds. Some argue that the expense to comply with standards will make licensed child care unaffordable to many families, leaving them only with less safe unlicensed options. Pediatricians can use their influence to persuade government officials, employers, insurers, and consumers that children deserve a safe environment and knowledgeable caregivers at home and in out-of-home child care facilities. Safe child care must be a high priority; it cannot be left to chance. Childhood injuries are expensive for everyone in the community. Parents, government officials, employers, and members and staff of voluntary organizations must assume a share of the responsibility for assuring affordable and safe child care so the task does not fall on any one sector of the community. Pediatricians must advocate for consistent enforcement of reasonable child care health and safety standards.

5.2 School Safety

The school system in the United States is a monument to democracy and to social engineering. The public school system alone is monumental in scope and complexity. Yet its population of 48 million students and 2.1 million teachers, in 115 000 schools spread across 17 000 school districts, offers substantial heterogeneity.

TABLE 5.4.
Child Safety Points to Discuss With Caregivers

Birth to 3 mo

Child safety seats must be used correctly in an automobile or van

Crib safety: crib gyms should not be used, side rails must be up, dangling window cords must not be within the infant's reach, pillows should not be used, and the infant's sleeping position should be on the back or side

Infant's should be fed formula or breast milk, not water

Never leave infants unattended, especially with toddlers present

Never shake an infant (head trauma may result from shaking)

Necklaces or pacifiers on strings should not be worn (risk of strangulation)

Always check water temperature; set tap hot water temperature below 120°F

Never drink hot beverages while holding an infant

Do not suspend or rest an infant carrier above the floor

Avoid direct sunlight onto an infant

3 to 6 mo

Car safety seats must be used correctly

Ways to prevent falling, sunburn, choking, and poisoning (have poison control number) should be discussed

Stationary walkers only should be used

Toys should not have strings, sharp edges, or detachable parts

Purses must be inaccessible to crawling infants

Electrical outlets and extension cords must be inaccessible to children

Expanding gates should be sturdy, not accordion style

Infants should not have access to plastic bags or balloons

Use microwaves with extreme caution (risk of burns, container explosion, and uneven heating of food items)

6 to 12 mo

Sharp corners should be covered

Cabinets containing chemicals, medications, matches, or sharp objects should be locked

Purses must be inaccessible

Avoid foods that could cause choking (eg, peanuts, popcorn, chunks of meat, hot dogs, carrots, celery sticks)

Toys should not have small parts

Vehicle child restraint systems should be used correctly (children should face backward in a safety seat in the back car seat until they weigh 20 to 22 lb, and then face front until they weigh 40 lb)

Infants require constant supervision near water, including buckets, toilets, bathtubs, and pools

1 to 2 y

Constant supervision is necessary with increased mobility

Do not use collapsible gates within a classroom or playroom

Tap water temperature must not exceed 120°F

Poison and aspiration control, burn prevention, and climbing and falling precautions should be addressed

Children should not be allowed to walk in the street or parking lot; they should be carried

Avoid foods that can cause choking (eg, hot dogs, jelly beans, and peanuts)

2 to 4 y

Reinforce safety seat use, safety related to drowning, ingestion of small objects, falls, burns, and electrical injuries; and pedestrian safety

Alter window-blind loop cords to prevent strangulation

Most pets should not be present in child care settings (to avoid dog bites, cat bites and scratches, and *Salmonella* infections from turtles)

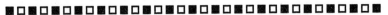
TABLE 5.4.
Child Safety Points to Discuss With Caregivers, continued

2 to 4 y, continued	*4 to 6 y*
Never leave a child unattended	Reinforce motor vehicle occupant safety
Use extreme caution at a swimming pool or natural body of water, using a 4:1 child to staff ratio	Reinforce pedestrian safety
	Discuss bike safety with use of helmets
	Children should avoid strangers
Small portable pools are prohibited, and built-in pools are to be covered when not in use	Teach children their home phone number and address
	No mechanical equipment or yard equipment should be within the child's reach
	Do not use a lawn mower when children are outside

Because children spend much of their waking lives in school, more than 1000 hours per year from the age of 5 years to about the age of 18 years, a safe school environment is paramount. Beyond the safety of the environment is the vast, largely unrealized potential for school personnel to teach and model safe behaviors and lifestyles. This section therefore addresses the topic of school safety broadly as it applies to primary, middle, and secondary education. School transportation safety is discussed in section 5.5.

5.2.1 Scope of the Problem

More than 2 million injuries requiring medical attention are sustained in schools each year.[16] An estimated 10% to 20% of the injuries sustained by school-age children occur at school.[17] In some schools, trauma is the most frequent reason for a visit to the health room.[18] More than one third of school injuries are related to sports and recreational activities, and nearly one third result from falls during other activities.[16] Reported rates of injury vary widely because of underreporting, lack of inclusion and exclusion criteria, and local factors, ie, some schools are safer. A Swedish study reported rates of 22 injuries per 1000 student-years[19]; Boyce et al[20] reported 49 injuries per 1000 student-years in Tucson; Lenaway et al[21] reported 92 injuries per 1000 student-years; and 15% of parents surveyed in Canada reported that their children had been injured at school during the previous month.[22]

Injuries occur nonrandomly in school populations. A prospective study of injury in nine Colorado schools found that rates for substantial injury peaked in the middle school years, injuries were most prevalent in the first 2 months of the school year (in part, because of football), and sports activities accounted for the largest percentage of injuries.[21] Elementary students are at particular risk on the playground, middle school students in the gym, and high school students on the playing field.[21] Injuries to elementary school students are much more likely to occur in unsupervised areas and activities than in areas and activities monitored by school personnel.[23]

5.2.2 Risk Factors

Studies of injuries at school show boys having at least a 50% greater risk than girls, with the injury rate for boys during midadolescence three times that for girls in the same age group.[20,21,24] A variety of behavioral characteristics, including aggressiveness and overactivity, have been reported to predict risk of injury during the school-age years (although not necessarily in the school setting).[25] The preponderance of hyperactivity disorders in school-age boys may help explain their higher injury rates. However, Davidson et al[26] found that hyperactivity in 6- to 8-year-olds was unlikely to be a significant risk factor for injury. Boyce and Sobolewski[27] studied children who experienced recurrent injuries during a 3-year period in Tucson, Ariz. They found that although a small group of children sustained more than their share of injuries in any given year, few children remained in that group for more than a year. Among other factors, they found recurrent injuries were more frequently related to athletics, occurred during early adolescence (12- to 13-year-olds in junior high school), and occurred in certain school settings (ie, schools with extended hours or open classrooms and in magnet schools). They concluded that students transiently become "accident repeaters" because of developmental, social, and environmental influences, rather than enduring personality traits or predispositions. This is promising for those seeking to prevent injuries in the school setting.

5.2.3 Intervention Strategies

The school setting offers barriers to and opportunities for injury control efforts. The responsibility for injury control in schools is typically ill-defined, delegated at times to administrative personnel, to school health personnel, to school transportation personnel, or to the athletics department. Furthermore, with increasingly limited funds, comprehensive injury control plans and programs in schools are rarely a priority. School personnel are often forced to address problems as they arise, rather than plan for their prevention. Systematic surveillance of injury patterns within school districts is not routinely done, which is particularly unfortunate given the seeming complexity of injuries — resulting from multiple mechanisms, occurring in multiple settings within the school framework, and affecting multiple age groups.[17]

The school setting offers some unique advantages for injury control efforts. The public *expectation* for school safety is high. Parents and others expect children to be safe at school, if nowhere else. The activities and curricula of schools are overseen by school boards that are accountable to the public. Schools, with their well-defined buildings, grounds, and personnel, should be subject to enforceable regulations and routine inspection. Also, in keeping with the educational mission, school curricula may integrate safety education with safety practice. In many schools where parental involvement is actively encouraged (eg, in parent-teacher organizations or as classroom aides), the safe practices learned by students in school may also have a positive influence on safety in the home. Finally, with a captive audience of school children, surveillance and epidemiologic analysis should be easily accomplished, thus facilitating development and implementation of targeted injury countermeasures.

Physical environment

Traditionally, the physical plant of the school has been considered a safe haven for children. For several reasons, this is less certain today, but pediatricians working with parents and school and community leaders can work together to make the school environment safe. The National Education Association has published a Hazard Survey Form (reprinted in the AAP manual, *School Health: Policy and Practice*), which can help identify hazards in the school environment.[28,29(p384)] Such a survey can help school faculty and staff assess such issues as the safety of chemicals available in schools (eg, for cleaning and use in science laboratories), ventilation of the building and classroom spaces (especially because many schools are air conditioned, with the windows sealed for all or most of the year), and the availability of unobstructed stairways and emergency exits. Smoke detectors and a regularly practiced plan for orderly evacuation of the building are of equal importance.

While these important concerns are being met, safety issues that are potentially broader in scope should be addressed. The "sick building syndrome" has recently emerged as a school problem as a consequence of materials used in construction and because of the lack of ventilation in the buildings.[30,31]

All persons responsible for school safety must be aware of asbestos used in construction. Approximately 10 000 schools built between 1946 and 1973 contain asbestos, although air contamination may be low.[32] Many experts recommend that the asbestos be contained rather than removed.[33] In either case, asbestos content in the ambient environment must be monitored and asbestos-containing materials inspected for deterioration at least every 3 years.

In certain parts of the country, radon is as much a concern in schools as in homes. Federal-, regional-, or state-designated environmental protection service offices can provide information about potential hazards and assist in decontamination.[34] Possible lead contamination of the water supplies in older schools has also come under scrutiny. All schools should have the water tested for lead content, and schools with metal piping should have the water tested at intervals recommended by the US Environmental Protection Agency. If the water supply contains 20 parts per billion or more of lead, decontamination of the system or filtering the water supply is mandatory.

Equipment in the schools is potentially hazardous, particularly to young children. Tall rolling carts used to transport audiovisual equipment are often top heavy and their contents may fall onto a child. Fatalities have been reported. Fatalities also have been associated with children moving or riding on heavy folding tables, such as those used in school cafeterias. Young children should not be permitted to participate in the moving of such heavy equipment in school.

Toxic, flammable, or explosive products may be used in science laboratories, art classes, or in industrial arts classes. Smoke detectors, fire extinguishers, and running water must be readily accessible; protective eye wear and aprons should be available and their use required where appropriate. In elementary schools, only nontoxic arts, crafts, and industrial arts materials should be used. In secondary schools, potentially toxic creative and industrial arts materials can be used safely only with proper student education and faculty guidance. In physical education programs, safe design of the physical plant includes appropriate padding on basketball goal posts, well-anchored (and padded) soccer goals, *nonanchored* softball bases, and playgrounds that meet the safety specifications outlined in chapter 16.

Over the years, the belief in the perimeter of the school as a safe haven has eroded, and schools have begun to use security fencing not to keep the children in, but to keep the neighborhood out. Walls, barbed wire, and locked gates have been installed in some areas. When more protection is necessary, students, faculty, and staff remain behind locked doors and barred windows. Although most of these security measures have been effective in keeping the occupants of the school safe, a new and more serious problem has recently emerged — an increasing number of students who are themselves armed with weapons in the schools.

Of high school students surveyed nationally by the Youth Risk Behavior Surveillance System of the Centers for Disease Control and Prevention, 12% have carried a potential weapon on school property — a knife, a gun, or a club — during the previous 30 days; 7% reported that they had been threatened or injured by a weapon on school property during the previous 30 days. One in six students had been in a physical fight on school property during the previous year.[35]

Installation of metal detectors for safety is often not a simple task because detectors are required at each building entrance, unless all the entrances are locked except those with detectors, which poses a hazard should a fire or other emergency occur. Successful safety programs have used a combination of metal detectors at selected school entrances and security personnel equipped with hand-held metal detectors to patrol the school corridors and randomly search students.[29]

Teaching

Age-appropriate safety education should be integrated into the curriculum for all school children and emphasize areas likely to reduce childhood morbidity and mortality; house fires, drowning, falls, and traffic safety are obvious examples. When possible, curricula that have been carefully designed and evaluated should be used, such as the National Highway and Transportation and Safety Administration Willie Whistle pedestrian safety program.[36] Traditional gun safety curricula have not been adequately evaluated and may potentially be counterproductive.[37,38] The worth of high school driver education is controversial (ie, its effectiveness as measured in reduced crash and injury experience); review of the published literature is discouraging.[39]

Many, if not most, schools lack adequate in-house expertise to teach a full safety curriculum. Schools, however, are in an ideal position to call upon community experts[37] — local police, fire officials, physicians, nurses, engineers, scientists, and others — to assist in the program. In many cases, injury prevention expertise and enthusiasm can be found among the families of students. Local colleges, industries, and medical centers are often willing to participate in the interest of community service. Guest speakers and appropriate field trips can make learning about injury prevention interesting as well.

In secondary schools, topics on safety can be integrated into the regular curriculum within several subject areas — much the same way writing has been incorporated across the curriculum. Subject areas may include physics (study of the biomechanics of an automobile crash), history or civics (study of a safer environment), health (study of primary prevention), and biology (study of the effects of substance abuse on human functioning, especially in the operation of a motor vehicle).[37]

To reduce violence in schools, programs that teach conflict avoidance and resolution are becoming increasingly popular.[40] These programs must be tailored to the age level of the child and to the environment and culture in which the child lives. Programs for rural areas are not necessarily applicable to the inner city. Introduction of conflict resolution skills and attitudes should begin in the primary grades and be continued (and intensified) in the secondary grades. Involvement of the community — and particularly parents — in this teaching and learning experience is especially important in the high schools. Because violence that erupts in school often results from conflict in the community, pediatricians and other health care professionals should participate in such curricula, along with teachers, school administrators, law enforcement personnel, and other community leaders.

Modeling

All adult school personnel must demonstrate safety practices. Classroom teaching can be positively reinforced by student observation of proper use of cleaning supplies and equipment and appropriate attire being worn by janitorial staff. Student observation of teachers and other staff using vehicle safety belts also may have a positive influence. A smoke-free environment in schools models health and safety behaviors for children and adolescents, as does faculty use of protective equipment in the laboratory, in the shop, and on the playing field.

5.2.4 Recommendations for Pediatricians

Because of the numbers of hours children and adolescents spend in schools, the educational mission of the schools, and the impact of adult role models in the school, pediatricians recognize the paramount importance of the school environment in influencing safe behaviors and practices. Many pediatricians are called on to speak to school groups (ie, students, parents, and faculty), to advise school boards, and to serve as school physicians and health consultants. Physicians can, in these capacities, help assure the safest school environment possible and the best use of the school's resources to educate and influence students and therefore reduce the number of unintentional injuries and control violence.[41]

5.3 Injury Control at Summer Camps

Camping has become an integral part of American life for many years. Each year, more than 5 million children attend summer camps. Camps for children and adolescents range from day camps to overnight camps, wilderness camps, and camps that are designed for children with special needs. The latter type of camp usually accommodates children with chronic illnesses such as cystic fibrosis, diabetes, or asthma. In recent years, with the advent of the Americans With Disabilities Act, many children who previously attended specialized camps have been assimilated into more traditional summer camps.

The following discussion highlights the features of camps that relate to injury prevention and control. The pediatrician's role as a consultant to individual families and camp personnel is emphasized.

5.3.1 The Pediatrician's Role in Advising Families

The child's physician can play a key role in helping parents choose a camp by providing a developmental perspective on the camping experience, offering advice pertinent to the child's special medical or emotional needs, and helping parents assess the adequacy and quality of a camp's health and safety program.[42] The pediatrician is in an ideal position to help parents match a camping experience with a child's individual characteristics, such as temperament.

Parents are generally well-attuned to the developmental, social, and health advantages of camping experiences for children. At the same time, parents are often concerned about their children's health and safety, especially when they are away from home for an extended period or in a remote location under the care of other adults. Parents may seek the pediatrician's advice about the advisability of summer camp and the selection of a specific camping experience. Likewise, the pediatrician may recommend a particular camping experience to meet specific patient and family needs. To help families assess risks and benefits of various camping opportunities, pediatricians should consider the following questions:

• What are the advantages of camps for children with special needs compared with those that are primarily for healthy children? Are there advantages for children with specific medical conditions attending camps that specialize in meeting their needs? These camps may be specially equipped and staffed to handle the injury risks associated with bleeding in the camper with cancer, hypoglycemia in participants with diabetes, or seizures in those with epilepsy.

• What are the concerns related to injury control in residential camps compared with day camps? In each setting, the physical environment, the program of activities, the quality of supervision, and the availability of trauma care should be considered.

• What are the concerns related to injury prevention that apply to so-called wilderness camp experiences? Children with medical conditions that require medication (eg, epilepsy or diabetes) may be at particular risk during rock climbing, rafting, or camping in an area that is remote from a nurse and health station.

• How competent is the camp staff in responding to the health problems, limitations, and special needs of each child to ensure a safe, rewarding experience? Can the staff accommodate unusually aggressive, inattentive, or clumsy children or sleepwalkers?

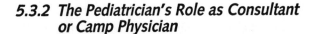
5.3.2 The Pediatrician's Role as Consultant or Camp Physician

Pediatricians have a valuable opportunity to use their public health, preventive medicine, and health promotion skills — including expertise in injury prevention — as either a pediatric consultant or camp physician.

Pediatric consultants must appreciate that the prevention of injuries is influenced by multiple aspects of the camp setting, including the following:

- Inherent risks in different camping activities (eg, backpacking vs music and art)
- Remoteness of the camp from emergency care facilities
- The ages, maturity, and training of the camp staff
- Access to parents in case of an emergency or where medical decision-making is necessary
- The population of campers (eg, age or special needs)
- The size of the camp and its physical location

Whether serving as camp consultant or camp physician, the pediatrician should consider the "epidemiologic triangle" — agent, host, and environment — when assessing the risk for injury and advising camp personnel about controlling and preventing injury (see also chapter 3).

Agent

As indicated in chapter 3, injury results from the transfer of energy (or energy deprivation) in rates and amounts that exceed human tolerance. Therefore, camping activities that involve rock climbing, white-water rafting, and archery are potentially hazardous. The pediatric consultant should ensure that such activities are adequately planned and supervised to prevent injury-producing energy transfer.

Host

The pediatric consultant must also consider the variability and vulnerability of the campers to injury. Campers must supply the camp staff with adequate health information so the staff can assess and reduce the likelihood of injury. This information includes the following:

- Chronic illnesses
- Medication requirements

- Immunization status
- Developmental and psychological problems (eg, sleepwalking, attention-deficit/hyperactivity disorder, fears, difficult temperament)
- Pertinent medical information needed in an emergency (eg, whether the child has asplenia or needs prophylaxis for subacute bacterial endocarditis)
- Allergies, food intolerances (eg, to bee stings or food items such as eggs)
- The need for special equipment or medications, ear plugs, orthodontia devices, orthopedic appliances, hearing aids, or syringes and insulin

Environment

Finally, prevention of injuries involves a survey of the camping environment. Specific attention must be paid to the buildings and housing facilities (eg, heating and repairs), the safety and quality of the water supply, food preparation, the potential for food-borne illnesses, and the physical setting and terrain of the camp.

The camp grounds may expose children to poisonous berries and vegetation or irritants such as poison ivy (eg, rhus dermatitis). Children may be exposed to excessive amounts of sun or heat; the animals and insects in the environment may carry the risk of trauma, infectious disease, or toxic reactions.

Other considerations

Pediatricians must also be certain that the camp implements policies and procedures for health and safety,[42] including the following:

- Adequate record keeping and staff to review the health information of the campers
- The role and responsibilities of the camp nurse[43]
- Administration of medications[44]
- Requirements for using appropriate protective equipment (eg, equestrian helmets, life jackets, and baseball batter helmets and face guards)
- Reporting, recording, treating, and following up on minor injuries
- Emergency trauma plans that include access to medical resources and notification of parents

- First-aid and basic life support administered by appropriately certified and trained camp staff

5.3.3 Health and Safety Concerns and Challenges Faced by Camps

The American Camping Association, the national organization that accredits camps, creates national standards for camping.[45] These standards encompass health care, sites and facilities, and special activities such as aquatics, trips and travel, and horseback riding. Despite these standards, there are many areas of ongoing concern about health and safety at children's camps, which include the following issues:

- Adequacy of training and supervision of camp staff
- The increasing number of children receiving medications or requiring specialized care
- Lack of full parental disclosure of the health and behavioral history of the child
- The complexity of integrating children with special needs into the camp
- Providing campers safe, valuable experiences while minimizing inherent risks (eg, during equestrian and aquatic activities)

The concerns listed pose challenges to camps and their medical advisors. Camping can be a rewarding, maturing, and educational experience for children. Pediatricians must help assure that health and safety concerns are addressed.

Prevention of injuries in camps requires that pediatricians understand the camp setting and program. The skills and expertise necessary are analogous to those used by pediatricians who participate in school health programs.

5.4 The Playground and Playground Equipment

5.4.1 Scope of the Problem

Each year, more than 170 000 children — perhaps as many as 250 000 — are treated in emergency departments for injuries sustained on outdoor playground equipment; about 70% of those injuries occur on public playgrounds; most of the rest occur on home playground equipment, some of which is homemade.[46,47] One third of the injuries occur to preschoolers and another 40% to children between the ages of 6 and 8 years, making those the highest risk years. Table 5.5 provides 1994 estimates of injuries from the Consumer Product Safety Commission.

Each year between 10 and 20 lives are lost as a result of injuries that occur on playgrounds. Half of the deaths are due to strangulation, typically entanglement of clothing in equipment. Another third of the deaths are due to falls, usually involving serious head injury.[46] Three out of four students are injured by falls from play equipment. Nine out of ten serious injuries result from falls.[37] Fifteen percent of head injuries are related to playground equipment. Slides, swings, and monkey bars account for eight of 10 of these injuries.[48]

Children can also become entrapped in playground equipment, be injured by sharp objects, or be injured because of inadequately designed or maintained equipment.[49] Inadequately supervised children playing on public playgrounds may have access to a roadway where they can be struck by traffic.

TABLE 5.5.

Estimated Injuries to Children From Birth to 19 Years of Age Treated in Emergency Departments in 1994: Playground Equipment*

Product	Total Estimated 1994 ED Visits	Percent Distribution by Age			
	0-19	0-4	Age, y 5-9	10-14	15-19
Climbing equipment	79 310	17.1	66.5	15.4	1.1
Seesaws	9 463	37.5	47.7	14.5	0.2
Slides	50 011	44.6	42.5	11.5	1.4
Swings	87 602	32.0	47.8	17.8	2.4
Other equipment	13 572	31.8	43.7	21.9	3.1
Unspecified equipment	12 437	26.3	55.4	17.2	1.1
Total	**252 395**				

*Data from a special product summary report, Consumer Product Safety Commission, courtesy of Joel Freedman. Numbers are estimates based on emergency department (ED) sampling. They are subject to sampling and nonsampling errors, which may be considerable.

5.4.2 Risk Factors

Surfaces beneath swings and climbing equipment, especially asphalt, constitute the most obvious risk factor for injuries related to falls.[50] The height of the climbing equipment and absence of barriers and guard rails also contribute to injuries from falls.[51] Poorly spaced equipment predisposes children to crashing into one another and into stationary objects such as trees, fences, and the equipment itself. Certain equipment configurations also make adult supervision more difficult. Lack of adult supervision is a particular problem when equipment is used by many children or by children of different ages and abilities.

Lack of proper routine maintenance of surfaces beneath swings and climbing equipment may cause loose, soft material to become packed and hard. The play equipment itself can become loose or worn, leading to sharp protrusions or collapse.

5.4.3 Intervention Strategies

Equipment design and layout

Proper layout and safe spacing must be observed. The "fall zone" is the area *under* and *around* play equipment in which protective surfacing must be installed. The fall zone beneath jump-off points must be of adequate diameter to protect the child. Generally, a 6-ft open radius around any stationary structure 6-ft high is adequate, with a 1-ft increase in the radius for each 1-ft increase in height. Thus, an 8-ft-high structure would need a minimum fall zone of 8 ft. Formulas for calculating adequate fall zones around moving equipment (such as swings) have been published by the Consumer Product Safety Commission.[49] The clear area between play zones and hazard points, such as buildings or asphalt walkways, should be adequate. Children exiting from playground equipment, such as slide chutes or moving swings, need sufficient space to exit without colliding with others.

The height of the equipment is of critical importance because it determines the distance of a fall. It is reasonable to design equipment so children cannot fall more than 6 ft (5 ft for equipment intended for preschoolers) and to provide a sufficient energy-absorbing surface under the equipment to prevent serious injury.[52] Detailed design recommendations are available to those who are contemplating design or purchase of equipment.[46,49]

Visibility

The entire playground should be visible to the teacher or supervisor if the playground is on school or child care property. On public playgrounds, despite the frequent lack of attendance by a supervisor, large equipment or natural barriers should not interfere with requisite visibility.

Surfaces

Falls are the most common cause of injury on playgrounds. Impacts from falls account for approximately 75% of all injuries on playgrounds. Fractures and head injuries account for the largest number of serious injuries. The height and orientation of the body during the fall and — crucially — the resilience of the surface on which the child falls determine the severity of the injury. Nothing is more critical in reducing the severity of injuries from falls than the choice of ground cover, and all too often this aspect of playground design and maintenance is overlooked or ignored.

Paved (asphalt or concrete) and natural (grass or dirt) surfaces absorb an insufficient amount of energy and are inappropriate for playgrounds. Although packed dirt is better than asphalt, it is far inferior to other ground cover, such as wood chips or mulch. Synthetic surfaces and loose fill are acceptable if they are sufficiently thick to absorb the energy from a fall. Synthetics are often expensive, however, and the loose-fill surface materials require more maintenance than synthetics.[46] Pine bark, wood mulch, and hardwood chips are readily available, relatively inexpensive, and energy absorbent. A 10-ft fall onto a bed of pine bark 1-ft deep has an impact equivalent to a fall of 16 in on to concrete.

The concept of *critical heights* is a useful way to think about the relative resilience of surfacing materials. The critical height is the minimum distance of a fall that is likely to result in life-threatening head injury. Table 5.6, p 101, shows typical critical heights for loose-fill surface materials. For example, 9 in of wood mulch should theoretically protect from life-threatening injury in a 10-ft fall. This, however, is based, in part, on preventing any impact greater than a $200g$ impact. However, the threshold for serious head injury is felt to be only $50g$.[37] Pediatricians should therefore recommend a substantial buffer zone of protection. A conser-

TABLE 5.6.
Critical Heights of Selected Loose-Fill Materials*

| Materials | Uncompressed Depth | | | Compressed Depth |
	6 in	9 in	12 in	9 in
Wood mulch	7	10	11	10
Double-shredded bark mulch	6	10	11	7
Uniform wood chips	6	7	>12	6
Fine sand	5	5	9	5
Course sand	5	5	6	4
Fine gravel	6	7	10	6
Medium gravel	5	5	6	5

*Critical heights are reported in feet. US Consumer Product Safety Commission.[49]

vative estimate of a 10- to 12-in-thick layer of loose-fill material (such as sand or wood chips) can be recommended when the height of the fall would be no greater than 6 ft for school-age children and 5 ft or less for younger children.[52] Lesser depths of fill material and greater distances of falling may be acceptable compromises with the understanding that the likelihood of serious injury is greater. Critical heights for manufactured synthetic surfaces must be obtained from the manufacturer.

The resiliency of the ground cover must be maintained by correcting worn or low spots and removing litter, such as rocks, glass, and cans. Tree roots must be eliminated or covered with at least 8 in of ground cover.

Barriers

Where possible, the playground should be enclosed with a fence at least 4-ft high. The fence must be at least 6 ft from the play equipment. Such a barrier will contain the children within the safe area and facilitate supervision. It also limits the number of children being supervised at a given time and facilitates housekeeping by reducing litter. Fences themselves should be inspected regularly for jagged or protruding areas or other defects. Gates should be located on the nonstreet side of the playground.

Climbing equipment

Climbing units account for almost one of three playground injuries. Energy-absorbing surfaces are necessary to reduce injuries from falls. Sharp edges and open holes that can entrap fingers, limbs, and heads (if the angles between adjacent surfaces are less than 55° or if openings are between 3½ in and 9 in in diameter) are hazards requiring monitoring. All units should be firmly mounted in concrete, which then must be covered by protective surfacing.

Swings

Swings account for one fourth of all playground injuries, which are chiefly caused by falling or jumping from the swing. Metal or wood seats can cause serious facial injury and should be replaced by softer material such as canvas, rubber, or plastic.

Shock-absorbing ground cover on the playground is important, especially in areas of high use, such as under swings or at exits from slides, where ground cover becomes attenuated and inadequate. A minimum of 24 in between swings and at least 30 in between the end swings and the frame is necessary.[49] The frame must be solidly mounted in concrete and covered by protective surfacing. Swing ropes or chains must be monitored for wear.

Slides

Slides are ubiquitous. Most injuries result from children falling off the ladder or the platform at the top of the slide. Occasionally, children fall over the side of the slide on the way down or while trying to ascend the slide by climbing up the chute. Children can also strangle if clothing is caught.

The maximum height of the platform above the protective ground surface should be 5 ft for preschoolers or 6 ft for school-age children.[46] A modification of the standard slide is to build a hill under the slide. Thus a child who falls would only fall a foot or so and then roll down the hill.

Deteriorated slides with jagged edges and corners, insecure footings or inadequate ground cover over footings, and platforms that are too small or unprotected by guard rails are also hazardous. The exit of the slide should be horizontal, the length of the horizontal area at the exit should approximate the thigh length of the largest users, and the height of the exit above the protective surface should approximate the tibial length of the users. Standards and recommended design characteristics are published.[46,49]

Metal slides become blisteringly hot in the sun and should be protected by shade or by facing them in the direction that receives the least direct sunlight. Plastic slides are less likely to become dangerously hot.

Merry-go-rounds, teeter totters, and spring rockers

This equipment should have adequate protective ground cover and be securely fastened to the ground. Sharp corners and areas of the equipment that may potentially pinch skin are hazardous. Are the handholds adequate? Handholds, seats, and footrests must be checked frequently.

Platform units and sliding poles

Adequate guard rails are necessary for this equipment. There should be no more than an 18 in drop from one platform to the next. Sliding poles require exit openings sized such that they require children to reach no more than 20 in to grab the pole, yet provide a minimum of 18 in clearance when sliding down the pole. Sliding poles are not recommended for preschool playground equipment. Wooden platform units may cause splinters.

Tire formations

If steel-belted tires are used in the formation, ensure that they have no projections. Are the suspension devices adequate and does accumulated water drain adequately? Are horizontally stacked tires secured to prevent slipping?

Supervision

Preschoolers require close supervision when using playground equipment. Older children benefit from supervision by teacher's aides or parents to assure that equipment is not misused (eg, several children on the slide at once or riding bicycles around the swings) and that rough play does not create hazardous conditions for children.

Routine inspection

Playgrounds, whether school, municipal, or private, must be regularly inspected for safety. The inspection should be detailed and meticulous. Sample inspection sheets are available and may be adapted for local use.[51]

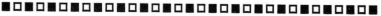
5.4.4 Recommendations for Pediatricians

Most playgrounds can be improved by putting an energy-absorbing surface underneath the playground equipment. Pediatricians can make parents aware of the need for proper surfacing and urge families to insist that schools and other public facilities upgrade their surfacing. Table 5.7, p 105, offers guidelines for parents wishing to check the safety of local playgrounds; more detailed lists are available.[46,51,53]

Playground safety is a logical topic for discussion at community group and parent-teacher organization meetings where pediatricians are asked to speak or attend. Educational brochures are available from the AAP and other organizations.[52,54]

5.5 School Bus Safety

5.5.1 Scope of the Problem

School bus safety, particularly the issue of safety belts, is currently one of the most controversial transportation topics. According to the Transportation Research Board of the National Research Council, approximately 400 000 school buses are used to transport 22 million children almost 4.3 billion miles to and from school and to school activities each year. Most of the children are transported in large type I school buses that are not usually equipped with safety belts.[55]

In 1993, approximately 9000 school bus occupants were injured and 13 persons died.[56] With a denominator of 94.2 billion annual passenger miles, school bus travel is exceedingly safe. A passenger in an automobile has a risk of fatality 30 to 70 times that of a passenger in a school bus.[57,58]

Despite this low rate of injury and death, many experts suggest that using safety belts on buses would further reduce school bus–related injuries and deaths. The AAP recommends installation of safety belts on all newly purchased school buses.[59] The AAP and other organizations believe that children are better protected on buses with safety belts, while still others believe that the current padded seats (compartmentalization) are adequate protection. Data about injuries that occur on the bus are incomplete.

TABLE 5.7.
Is Your Playground Safe?

Parents can use the following abbreviated checklist to assess the adequacy of public and school playgrounds used by their children.*

- Is there loose fill material maintained to a depth of 9 to 12 in (or adequate synthetic surfacing) beneath swings, slides, and climbing equipment?
- Does protective surfacing extend beyond the equipment at least 8 ft to provide an obstruction-free "fall zone" in all directions that a child might fall from the equipment?
- Are swing seats constructed of a soft, light material and at least 2-ft apart?
- Are platforms for climbing equipment and slides not more than 5-ft high for pre-schoolers and 6-ft high for school-age children, and do they have adequate guardrails to prevent falls?
- Are there any openings in equipment with dimensions of between 3½ and 9 in that could cause entrapment?
- Are there open "s" hooks or other protrusions where children could catch clothing and strangle?
- Is the equipment and hardware free of corrosion, rusting, bending, or excessive wear?
- Are the footings buried?
- Are there any environmental hazards such as rocks, tree roots, glass, trash, or collections of water that have not drained?

---

*If hazards are identified, inform the person or persons responsible for operating the playground about the hazards and request appropriate modification or repairs. (Adapted from Gillis and Fise.[53])

Three additional issues affect the safety of bus occupants. First, many school districts still use buses manufactured before 1977, when the current motor vehicle safety standards became effective. The need to remove these buses from service is urgent. They should not be sold or donated to camps and youth groups. Second, the buses in many school districts do not have enough seats for all passengers, requiring some passengers to stand, which is hazardous. Third, for reasons discussed in section 5.5.4, standard school buses transport large numbers of infants and preschool-age children. Buses are not designed to transport this age group safely.

The larger fatality problem in school bus–related crashes occurs *outside of the bus,* where about 40 pedestrians and 80 occupants of other vehicles are killed each year. Two thirds of the school-age pedestrians killed are struck by the school bus itself, and one third are struck by another vehicle.[60] Table 5.8, p 106, shows that during a bus crash children are typically injured as passengers, but are more likely to be killed as pedes-

TABLE 5.8.
Persons Killed or Injured in US School Bus Crashes, 1993

Person Type	Killed, n	Injured, n
School bus driver	1	2000
School bus passenger	12	7000
Pedestrian	40	1000
Pedal cyclist	2	< 500
Occupant of other vehicle	86	10 000
Total	**141**	20 000

Data From National Highway Traffic Safety Administration.[56]

trians.[56] Although the number of pedestrian injuries is far fewer than passenger injuries, they are more likely to be serious or fatal.

5.5.2 Risk Factors

School bus travel compares favorably with automobile travel because many of the risk factors associated with occupant fatalities in automobile crashes are absent in school bus transportation. School buses travel during the day, on familiar roads, at reasonable speeds, and with sober adult drivers under nonrecreational circumstances. The vehicles themselves are protective. While passenger ejection from an automobile is highly associated with fatality, ejection from a school bus is uncommon because of the location of the doors. During a crash, the large size and weight of the school bus are defensive.

Less fortunate are the pedestrians who find themselves near school buses. Young age and its accompanying immature judgment and lack of experience put early elementary school children who are waiting at the bus stop or getting off the bus at special risk. Since 1984, half of all school-age pedestrians killed in school bus crashes were between 5 and 7 years of age.[60] Young pedestrians are at risk because they move in directions and at speeds unanticipated by drivers. School buses, by virtue of their size and design, also inherently limit the visibility of the bus driver, and pedestrians near buses may be hidden from drivers of other vehicles. For pedestrians, the afternoon is more dangerous than the morning for being injured or killed. Between 1984 and 1994, 44% of school bus–related pedestrian fatalities occurred between 3:00 and 4:00 pm.[60]

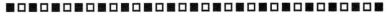
5.5.3 Intervention Strategies

Compartmentalization

School buses manufactured after April 1, 1977, with a gross vehicle weight rating of greater than 10 000 lb depend on strong, well-padded, energy-absorbing seats and high seat backs to protect passengers during a crash.[61] Compartmentalization on school buses is achieved by installing the seats close together, assuring that the seat backs are well padded, and assuring that the seat backs are high enough to provide head and neck support and to prevent a child from being thrown forward over the seat back. Current standards require that seat backs rise about 22 in above the seat, but the National Transportation Research Board recommends raising the seat back height another 4 in, thereby providing improved compartmentalization and better head support.[55,59]

Safety belts

Small school buses, those weighing less than 10 000 lb, must conform to the same Federal Motor Vehicle Safety Standards (FMVSS) for safety belt restraints and anchorages that apply to passenger automobiles (FMVSS 208, 209, and 210). Buses that weigh more than 10 000 lb are exempt from the above federal motor vehicle safety standards, in favor of compartmentalization (FMVSS 222). New Jersey and New York and some school districts elsewhere have enacted regulations that require safety belts on larger school buses. New Jersey law *requires* use of the belts, a key to the effectiveness of belt installation requirements.

The arguments for and against safety belts on large school buses are extremely controversial. Advocates for safety belts argue that children receive conflicting messages when they are required to wear safety belts in personal vehicles but not on buses, which causes confusion about their importance for safety. Proponents of safety belts also argue that safety belts, if installed and used properly on large buses, save lives and prevent at least several dozen serious injuries to occupants each year.

Opponents of safety belts on large school buses state that the cost outweighs the potential benefit and that compartmentalization is adequate to protect children. They point to the 1987 National Transportation Safety Board (NTSB) study of 43 crashes that concluded that injuries to occupants usually resulted from direct crash forces, making it unlikely that safety belts would have prevented the injuries.[62] The NTSB report also dispelled the concern that safety belts cause injuries. It recommended that limited funds would be better spent on other strategies to prevent school bus injuries.

Safety belts in new buses should only be installed at the factory. Buses manufactured before 1977 cannot be fitted with safety belts because the seats and floors may not be strong enough to support a child in a belt during a crash. Installation of safety belts on buses manufactured since 1977 usually requires reinforcement of the seats and may not be done properly because of a lack of adequate guidelines.

Although small school buses have seat belts, they are often not used. In 1993, eight unbelted children were ejected from a small bus in Oklahoma that was hit by a tractor-trailer; four of the passengers died and the others suffered minor to serious injuries.[63] An NTSB study found that lap belts may protect occupants outside of the impact area from injury.[64] Currently six states require use of safety belts on small school buses.

Bus drivers

Licensing requirements for bus drivers vary from state to state. Despite these variations, all transportation personnel should be trained in school bus operation, management of passengers, and dealing with various medical emergencies. Safety belt use by bus drivers should be enforced, not only to provide a good example to students, but to ensure that drivers can retain control of the bus in a crash.[62] Annual physical examinations and vision screening of drivers should be required.

Bus drivers and monitors for children with special needs should be familiar with necessary interventions for emergency care of children who have seizures, those with tracheostomies or feeding tubes, and those requiring ventilation.

Bus safety rules and equipment

Children *and parents* must know and follow bus safety rules. Children must be taught safe riding and pedestrian behavior. The following guidelines promote the safety of children when they board the school bus:

• Arrive early.
• Line up off the shoulder and road.

- Wait until the bus stops completely.
- Use the handrail when boarding the bus.
- Follow street-crossing rules (crossing the street on the way home from school is most hazardous).
- Eliminate or fix loose straps and ties on clothing or book bags that may catch on handrails and doorways (a number of children have been dragged to death in recent years).
- Contain papers and books in book bags so they will not be dropped and cause distraction.

Parents should monitor their children, particularly younger children, at bus stops until they are safely aboard or off the bus. Student monitors or school "safety patrol" students should be assigned at bus stops where older children and elementary grade children interact.

When riding in the school bus, children should sit quietly, one student to a seating position. Children should never stand while the school bus is moving. Parents should be supportive of discipline imposed by the driver.

When exiting the school bus, children should comply with the following guidelines:

- Allow passengers closest to the front to leave first.
- Move out of the danger zone before crossing the street. The *danger zone* is the space within 10 ft around the entire bus, within which the driver does not have a good view.
- Remain within the bus driver's view when exiting the bus.
- Look left-right-left before stepping into the street and beyond the side of the bus, keeping in mind that not all cars will stop when the bus stops.

School districts (usually) conduct emergency drills. Children should be instructed about how to behave in an emergency on a bus. They should know the location of emergency exits, and older children should be instructed to help younger children.

Given the epidemiologic factors associated with school bus–related injuries, pedestrian training should have high priority. Students must stay clear of the bus and never be close enough to touch it.

Crossing control arms on buses, new devices that are mounted to the front bumper, help keep children out of the danger zone. When the door of the bus opens, the arm swings out from the bumper, forcing children to walk well in front of the bus.

About 10 of the approximately 30 children killed as pedestrians at bus loading zones each year are killed by vehicles *other than* school buses.[60] Often, these vehicles are attempting to illegally pass a bus that has stopped to unload passengers. To minimize this problem, buses are required to have eight warning lights: two flashing red lights and two flashing amber lights on the front and on the rear of the bus. The amber lights indicate that the bus is preparing to stop, and the red lights indicate that the bus has stopped.

In addition, stop signal arms are required in most states, but are still optional in some states. Some experts have recommended installing strobe lights on buses for use during adverse weather conditions (eg, fog or darkness).

Whenever feasible, children should be picked up and dropped off on the same side of the road that they live on.

Additional recommendations for safety equipment designed to minimize the chance of the bus hitting a child include mirrors on the front corners of all school buses and the installation of at least one cross-view mirror. To allow for better detection of children or other objects around or under the bus, electronic systems have been developed to alert the driver of possible danger. Such systems sound an alarm if they detect any object near the bus when the driver begins to pull away from a stop.

Improving school bus safety requires a variety of interventions that address the epidemiologic peculiarities of this class of injuries. Selected recommendations from two government studies are summarized in Table 5.9,[55,62,63] p 111.

5.5.4 Children With Special Needs

The increasing numbers of children with physical or developmental disabilities being transported in school buses has piqued interest in providing them adequate crash protection.[65] Ninety percent of school districts transport preschool-age children to special programs. The provisions of the Individuals With Disabilities Education Act (PL 102-119), enable these children to receive developmental and rehabilitation services from the state department of education through local school districts. Head Start programs are transporting increasing numbers of

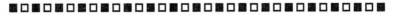
TABLE 5.9.
Selected Recommendations to Improve School Bus Safety

Recommendation	Rationale
Retire from service all school buses manufactured before April 1977.[62]	These "prestandard" buses lack "unibody" construction, have roofs that may not withstand rollover, and may not have shatterproof glass and protected gas tanks. Seat backs may be too low for adequate compartmentalization.
Improve drivers' safety belts and require that they be worn.[62]	This will help assure that drivers can maintain control of the bus in a crash or other emergency.
There should be a sufficient number of buses so every student has a seat.[55]	To assure that every student has the advantage of compartmentalization and so students are less likely to collide with and injure one another during a crash.
Seat backs should be 4 in higher than currently required.[55]	This would further improve compartmentalization in a crash.
Pedestrian training for students should receive higher priority, especially for 5- to 7-year-olds and their parents.[55]	Pedestrian fatalities outnumber fatalities of school bus occupants by more than two to one. Half of the student pedestrian fatalities are in this age group.
Equipment requirements on buses should be upgraded to include, for example, signal arms with flashing lights and better cross-view mirrors.[55]	This equipment is aimed at reducing pedestrian injuries by warning other motorists and making children more visible to bus drivers.
Where belts are installed, school districts should require their use.	Belts offer additional protection in a crash — but only if they are used.[64]

Adapted from Widome.[57]

3- and 4-year-olds, and many states have programs for even younger children of migrant workers. Furthermore, infants may attend school with their teenage mothers.

Two main issues concerning the transportation of children with special needs must be addressed — the transportation of children to school in wheelchairs and the transportation of infants and preschoolers. While there are federal safety standards for securing wheelchairs into school buses (1994 amendment to FMVSS 222), wheelchairs themselves are not primarily designed as occupant restraints and are not subject to crash tests. Safe transportation of infants and preschoolers requires special restraint devices attached to seats with safety belts. Most school buses do not have safety belts.

In a 1994 policy statement, the AAP[66] recommended the following:

- Any child who can be reasonably moved from a wheelchair to a standard seating position equipped with an appropriate safety belt (or a properly secured child safety seat, if appropriate) should be moved.
- Passenger seats that hold child safety seats or restraint systems should have reinforced frames and factory-installed belts that meet the same standards as automobiles for protection of occupants during a crash (FMVSS 208, 209, and 210). (Nonfactory installation of seat belts is fraught with hazards.)
- All restraint systems used for children who weigh less than 50 lb must meet federal crash protection standards for child safety seats (FMVSS 213).
- Children who weigh less than 20 lb must be transported rear-facing in devices that meet federal crash standards.
- Occupied wheelchairs must face forward and be secured to the wheelchair frame using four-point tie-down devices that can sustain a frontal crash at 30 mph. Wheelchair trays should be removed.
- Wheelchair occupants should be provided with upper and lower torso restraints that have been crash tested at 30 miles per hour (20g).

School officials and others should refer to the complete policy statement and subsequent revisions.

The National Coalition for School Bus Safety, in a November 1974 position paper, recommended the following additional criteria be met for transporting preschool children:

- Various restraint devices for preschool children, infants, and toddlers should be crash tested.
- The safety belts used to secure restraint devices must be installed at the factory on new buses only. Installation of lap belts on older model buses is prohibited.
- Passenger monitors must be provided in the same caregiver-to-child ratio required of licensed child care centers.
- Fire resistant, fire retardant, nontoxic upholstery material must be used on bus seats.

- For proper documentation of all injury and fatality statistics, age must be included in the school bus records.

Because travel by school bus plays such an important role in the daily lives of children from preschool through high school, pediatricians can help reduce the number of injuries by serving as resources, educators, consultants, and advocates for school bus transportation safety.

School bus safety for all children is an important issue, and with more preschoolers and children with special needs being transported by bus, concern for passenger safety and protection will continue. The most recent AAP policy statement provides further information.[59]

5.6 Resources

1. American Camping Association
Bradford Woods
5000 State Rd 67 North
Martinsville, IN 46151-7902

   The American Camping Association has accumulated descriptive data that are useful for pediatricians trying to understand the scope of the camping experience and publishes health history and examination forms for campers.

2. American Red Cross
2025 E St, NW
Washington, DC 20006
202-728-6531

   Through its local chapters, the American Red Cross sponsors an AAP-approved child care course for caregivers that includes modules on injury prevention and pediatric first aid. Sample checklists and injury report forms are provided.

3. Consumer Federation of America
1424 16th St, NW
Washington, DC 20036
202-387-6121

   The Consumer Federation of America has an extensive set of recommendations, including model legislation relating to playground safety.

4. Consumer Product Safety Commission
4330 East West Highway
Washington, DC 20207
301-504-0990
800-638-2772 (Consumer Hotline)

The Consumer Product Safety Commission publishes the *Handbook for Public Playground Safety* and has a number of reports on the same subject.

5. Educational Development Center, Inc
Children's Safety Network
55 Chapel St
Newton, MA 02158-1060
617-969-7100

With a grant from the Carnegie Corporation of New York, the Educational Development Center is preparing a book about school injuries entitled *Preventing Injuries in the School Environment*. The Educational Development Center is a good resource for statistics and background information about intervention strategies. The Children's Safety Network is partially funded by the Maternal and Child Health Bureau of the US Public Health Service.

6. National Association for the Education of Young Children
1509 16th St NW
Washington, DC 20036-1426
202-232-8777

The organization has manuals and guidelines available for child care programs.

7. National Center for Education in Maternal and Child Health
Children's Safety Network
2000 15th St North, Suite 701
Arlington, VA 22201-2617
703-524-7802
703-524-9335 (fax)

8. National Highway Traffic Safety Administration
National Center for Statistics and Analysis
400 Seventh St, NW
Washington, DC 20590
202-366-4198
202-366-7078 (fax)

The National Highway Traffic Safety Administration provides up-to-date and detailed information about school bus–related fatalities.

9. National Safety Council
1121 Spring Lake Dr
Itasca, IL 60143-3201
630-775-2276

The National Safety Council maintains data about school- and school bus–related injuries and deaths and is a source of educational materials and recommendations about these topics.

References

1. Casper LM. What does it cost to mind our preschoolers? *Curr Population Rep: Household Economic Studies.* 1995;52:70

2. Strauman-Raymond K, Lie L, Kempf-Berkseth J. Creating a safe environment for children in daycare. *J School Health.* 1993;63:254–257

3. *National Child Care Survey, 1990: A National Association for the Education of Young Children Study.* Washington, DC: Urban Institute Press; 1990

4. American Public Health Association, American Academy of Pediatrics. *Caring for Our Children: National Health and Safety Performance Standards: Guidelines for Out-of-Home Child Care Programs.* Washington, DC: American Public Health Association; 1992

5. Rivara FP, Sacks JJ. Injuries in child daycare: an overview. *Pediatrics.* 1994;94:1031–1033

6. Sellström E, Bremberg S, Chang A. Injuries in Swedish day-care centers. *Pediatrics.* 1994;94:1033–1036

7. Good SE, Parrish RG, Ing RT. Children's deaths at day-care facilities. *Pediatrics.* 1994;94:1039–1041

8. Mackenzie SG, Sherman GJ. Day-care injuries in the data base of the Canadian Hospitals Injury Reporting and Prevention Program. *Pediatrics.* 1994;94:1041–1043

9. Alkon A, Genevro JL, Kaiser PJ, Tschann JM, Chesney M, Boyce WT. Injuries in child-care centers: rates, severity, and etiology. *Pediatrics.* 1994;94:1043–1046

10. Sacks JJ, Smith JD, Kaplan KM, Lambert DA, Sattin RW, Sikes RK. The epidemiology of injuries in Atlanta day-care settings. *JAMA.* 1989;262:1641–1645

11. Sacks JJ, Holt KW, Holmgreen P, Colwell LS Jr, Brown JM Jr. Playground hazards in Atlanta child-care centers. *Am J Public Health.* 1990;80:986–988

12. O'Connor MA, Boyle WE Jr, O'Connor GT, Letellier R. Self-reported safety practices in child care facilities. *Am J Prev Med.* 1992;8:14–18

13. Briss PA, Sacks JJ, Addiss DG, Kresnow M, O'Neil J. A nationwide study of the risk of injury associated with day care center attendance. *Pediatrics.* 1994;93:364–368

14. Lie L, Runyan CW, Petridou E, Chang A. American Public Health Association/ American Academy of Pediatrics Injury Prevention Standards. *Pediatrics.* 1994; 94(suppl):1046–1048

15. *American Red Cross Child Care Course: Health and Safety Units.* Washington, DC: American National Red Cross; 1990

16. Scheidt P, Harel Y, Trumble AC, Jones DH, Overpeck MD, Bijur PE. The epidemiology of nonfatal injuries among US children and youth. *Am J Public Health.* 1995; 85:932–938

17. Children's Safety Network. *Injuries in the School Environment: A Resource Packet.* Newton, MA: Educational Development Center Inc; 1994

18. Nader PR, Brink SG. Does visiting the school health room teach appropriate or inappropriate use of health services? *Am J Public Health.* 1981;71:416–419

19. Bergström E, Björnstig U. School injuries: epidemiology and clinical features of 307 cases registered at hospital during one school year. *Scand J Primary Health Care.* 1991;9:209–216

20. Boyce WT, Sprunger LW, Sobolewski S, Schaefer C. Epidemiology of injuries in a large, urban school district. *Pediatrics.* 1984;74:342–349

21. Lenaway DD, Ambler AG, Beaudoin DE. The epidemiology of school-related injuries: new perspectives. *Am J Prev Med.* 1992;8:193–198

22. Hodgson C, Woodward CA, Feldman W. Parent report of school-related injuries. *Can J Public Health.* 1985;76:56–58

23. Sheps SB, Evans GD. Epidemiology of school injuries: a 2-year experience in a municipal health department. *Pediatrics.* 1987;79:69–75

24. Schelp L, Ekman R, Fahl I. School accidents during a three school-years period in a Swedish municipality. *Public Health.* 1991;105:113–120

25. Bijur P, Golding J, Haslum M, Kurzon M. Behavioral predictors of injury in school-age children. *Am J Dis Child.* 1988;142:1307–1312

26. Davidson LL, Taylor EA, Sandberg ST, Thorley G. Hyperactivity in school-age boys and subsequent risk of injury. *Pediatrics.* 1992;90:697–702

27. Boyce WT, Sobolewski S. Recurrent injuries in schoolchildren. *Am J Dis Child.* 1989; 143:338–342

28. National Education Association, Affiliate Services. *Health and Safety Handbook for Education Employees.* Washington, DC: National Education Association; 1988

29. American Academy of Pediatrics, Committee on School Health. *School Health: Policy and Practice.* 5th ed. Elk Grove Village, IL: American Academy of Pediatrics; 1993

30. Cushing AH, Samet JM. Indoor pollutants: how hazardous for children? *Contemp Pediatr.* 1991;8:109–127

31. Baum C, Shannon M. Environmental toxins: cutting the risks. *Contemp Pediatr.* 1995; 12:20–43

32. American Academy of Pediatrics, Committee on Injury and Poison Prevention. *Handbook of Common Poisonings in Children*. Elk Grove Village, IL: American Academy of Pediatrics; 1994

33. American Academy of Pediatrics, Committee on Environmental Hazards. Asbestos exposure in schools. *Pediatrics*. 1987;79:301–305

34. American Academy of Pediatrics, Committee on Environmental Hazards. Radon exposure: a hazard to children. *Pediatrics*. 1989;83:799–802

35. Centers for Disease Control and Prevention. CDC Surveillance Summaries. Youth risk behavior surveillance — United States, 1993. *MMWR Morb Mortal Wkly Rep*. 1995;44(SS-1):1–56

36. Preusser DF, Blomberg RD. Reducing child pedestrian accidents through public education. *J Safety Res*. 1984;15:47–56

37. Wilson MH, Baker SP, Teret SP, Shock S, Garbarino J. *Saving Children: A Guide to Injury Prevention*. New York, NY: Oxford University Press; 1991

38. American Academy of Pediatrics Committee on Injury and Poison Prevention. Firearm injuries affecting the pediatric population. *Pediatrics*. 1992;89:788–790

39. Robertson LS, Zador PL. Driver education and fatal crash involvement of teenaged drivers. *Am J Public Health*. 1978;68:959–965

40. Rosenberg ML, Mercy JA. Assaultive violence. In: Rosenberg ML, Fenley MA, eds. *Violence in America: A Public Health Approach*. New York, NY: Oxford University Press; 1991:14–50

41. Wilson-Brewer R, Spivak H. Violence prevention in schools and other community settings: the pediatrician as initiator, educator, collaborator, and advocate. *Pediatrics*. 1994;94:623–630

42. American Academy of Pediatrics, Committee on School Health. Medical guidelines for day camps and residential camps. *Pediatrics*. 1991;87:117–119

43. Maheady DC. Camp nursing practice in review. *Pediatr Nurs*. 1991;17:247–250

44. Lishner K, Busch K. Safe delivery of medications to children in summer camps. *Pediatr Nurs*. 1994;20:249–253

45. American Camping Association. *Standards for Day and Resident Camps: Accreditation Programs at the American Camping Association; Revised 1993*. Martinsville, IN: American Camping Association; 1990

46. Morrison ML, Fise ME. *Report and Model Law on Public Play Equipment and Areas*. Washington, DC: Consumer Federation of America; 1992

47. Tinsworth DK, Kramer JT. *Playground Equipment–Related Injuries and Deaths*. Washington, DC: US Consumer Product Safety Commission; 1990

48. Baker SP, Fowler C, Li G, Warner M, Dannenberg AL. Head injuries incurred by children and young adults during informal recreation. *Am J Public Health*. 1994; 84:649–652

49. US Consumer Product Safety Commission. *Handbook for Public Playground Safety*. Washington, DC: US Consumer Product Safety Commission; 1991

50. Sosin DM, Keller P, Sacks JJ, Kresnow M, van Dyck PC. Surface-specific fall injury rates on Utah school playgrounds. *Am J Public Health.* 1993;83:733–735

51. Jambor T, Palmer SD. *Playground Safety Manual.* Birmingham, AL: The Alabama Chapter of the American Academy of Pediatrics; 1991

52. American Academy of Pediatrics. *Playground Safety: Guidelines for Parents* (pamphlet). Elk Grove Village, IL: American Academy of Pediatrics; 1991

53. Gillis J, Fise MER. *The Childwise Catalog.* 3rd ed. New York, NY: HarperCollins; 1993

54. American Academy of Orthopedic Surgeons. *Play It Safe* (pamphlet). Rosemont, IL: American Academy of Orthopedic Surgeons; 1991

55. Transportation Research Board, National Research Council. *Improving School Bus Safety.* Special Report 222. Washington, DC: Transportation Research Board, National Research Council; 1989

56. National Highway Traffic Safety Administration. *Traffic Safety Facts 1993.* Washington, DC: US Department of Transportation; 1994

57. Widome MD. Pediatric injury prevention for the practitioner. *Curr Probl Pediatr.* 1991; 21:428–468

58. National Safety Council. *Accident Facts.* Itasca, IL: National Safety Council; 1994

59. American Academy of Pediatrics, Committee on School Health, Committee on Injury and Poison Prevention. School transportation safety. *Pediatrics.* 1996;97:754–757.

60. National Highway Traffic Safety Administration. *Traffic Safety Facts 1994: School Buses.* Washington, DC: US Department of Transportation; 1995;97:754–757

61. Federal Motor Vehicle Safety Standard 222 (School Bus Passenger Seating-Crash Protection-School Buses). *Code of Federal Regulations.* 49 Transportation, Part 571

62. National Transportation Safety Board. *Safety Study: Crashworthiness of Large Post-standard Schoolbuses.* Washington, DC: National Transportation Safety Board; 1987

63. Stewart DD. NTSB releases final report on Oklahoma school bus crash. *Safe Ride News.* 1995;14(3)

64. National Transportation Safety Board. *Highway Accident Report PB916204.* Washington, DC: National Transportation Safety Board; 1994

65. Stewart DD. Preschoolers on buses get NHTSA attention. *Safe Ride News.* 1994; 13(4):1

66. American Academy of Pediatrics, Committee on Injury and Poison Prevention. School bus transportation of children with special needs. *Pediatrics.* 1994;93:129–130

CHAPTER 6

Injuries in the Workplace

6.1 Scope of the Problem

Work is an important part of life for many adolescents. More than 5 million American children and adolescents are legally employed, and an additional 1 to 2 million are believed to be employed in violation of wage, hour, and safety regulations.[1] Efforts to improve school-to-work transitions are placing more teenagers into the workplace, while in some communities efforts to prevent gang activity and violence emphasize increasing work opportunities.

Despite protective laws, work continues to contribute to adolescent injury, mortality, and morbidity. The National Institute for Occupational Safety and Health has estimated that more than 70 American adolescents younger than 18 years die on the job every year.[2] A review of workers' compensation cases submitted to 24 states over 1 year included almost 24 000 occupational injuries to adolescents younger than 18 years.[3] Studies in relatively unpopulated states have documented hundreds of yearly occupational injuries to employed teenagers (S Pollack et al, unpublished data, 1997),[4–7] while larger and more populous states have observed injuries numbering in the thousands.[8–12]

These statistics underestimate the number of injuries for the following reasons:

1. Because people think of adolescents as students rather than employees, emergency medical service, emergency department, and trauma team personnel and coroners often assume injuries are not work related and may not ask before checking "not employed" on reporting forms, leaving surveillance efforts incomplete. For example, a 12-year-old girl who has been hit by a car while delivering newspapers on a bicycle route may not be asked if she was working at the time the injury occurred.

2. Reporting systems tend to record more severe injuries, whereas less severe but more frequent injuries may not be documented. For example, children who are burned while working at fast-food restaurants may receive no medical care or be treated in a physician's office if the burns are minor.

3. Some data about adolescent occupational injuries are derived from state workers' compensation reports, but pediatricians and teenage workers both tend to be unfamiliar with this system and how to gain access to it. Therefore some injuries to adolescents are not reported.

Table 6.1 gives representative numbers of injuries to teenage workers in various states.

Evidence accumulating across the United States supports the conclusion that occupational injuries are a serious problem among teenagers. Because injured youth do not usually receive treatment at pediatric offices or clinics, adolescent occupational injury has not been an obvious problem to most pediatricians. A study in Massachusetts of adolescent visits to emergency departments (EDs) for treatment of injuries, however, found that 24% of the injuries among 17-year-olds occurred at

TABLE 6.1.
Numbers of Working Teenagers Younger Than 18 Years Who Are Injured Annually

State	No. of Injuries
New York[8]	More than 1000 teens per year received workers' compensation benefits; more than 8 lost work days are needed to qualify
Texas[9]	More than 1000 injuries per year reported to the Workers' Compensation Commission
Connecticut[7]	Almost 800 injuries per year according to workers' compensation reports
Massachusetts[10]	About 400 injuries per year treated in emergency departments in the 5% of the state population under surveillance; potentially 8000 injuries per year
Minnesota[5]	Almost 750 injuries per year
Kentucky (S Pollack et al, unpublished data, 1997)	More than 400 injuries per year according to workers' compensation reports
Washington[11]	4450 injuries per year; data from accepted workers' compensation claims, children aged 11–17 years
California[12]	2104 injuries in 1991

work and that work was the most common location of injury in this age group.[10] An earlier nationwide estimate based on ED visits suggested that 75 000 annual occupational injuries occurred among American 16- to 17-year-olds,[13] while a survey of Saskatchewan (Canada) high school students also found that occupational injuries were the most common type of injury among 16- to 17-year-olds.[14] In the Massachusetts study, each year, one of every thirty 16- to 17-year-olds in the population received treatment in an ED for a work-related injury; in other words, each year, one student in every homeroom class in a high school will experience an occupational injury that requires medical care.

Opinions vary widely concerning the relative advantages and disadvantages of work as an influence on the moral development of youth.[15,16] More than 20 hours of employment per week is associated with declining school performance, and some studies suggest that effects are evident at 10 hours. Because adolescents continue to be injured and die on the job, it should be possible to unite people behind the injury prevention issues posed by youth employment. Pediatricians are a crucial link for advocacy on this issue. The original involvement of the American Academy of Pediatrics was prompted in part by two adolescents, employed in the same butcher shop in the early 1980s, who each had an arm amputated as a result of injuries that occurred several months apart. Despite considerable work by a small but growing number of people around the country, the largest fine levied for violation of child labor laws in 1994 was for the amputation of an adolescent's arm in a butcher shop. Assistance with occupational injury prevention is urgently needed from pediatricians and others who care for adolescents.

6.2 Background

The Fair Labor Standards Act (FLSA) of 1938 regulates conditions of youth employment. One part of the act limits the number of permissible work hours on school days and in a school week, derived from efforts to protect the education of working children. The other part of the act protects adolescent health and safety through "hazard" orders that prohibit work using dangerous machinery and exposure to hazardous chemicals.[17] Many states also have laws regulating child labor, which may be more current and in some cases more stringent than federal law (the most stringent law applies).

The practical result of these laws is that children younger than 12 years may legally deliver newspapers in many states, 14-year-olds may stock grocery shelves and ring up orders at the cash register (but are not permitted to work on deli slicers or paper balers and box crushers), and 16-year-olds may work in fast-food establishments. It is illegal, however, for anyone younger than 18 years to deliver pizza or newspapers by car. Using a motor vehicle for work is prohibited, as is work in mining and logging. Employment in industry other than agriculture is regulated to 18 years of age.[18] Agricultural employment is regulated only until 16 years of age,[19] and all work on family farms is exempt from regulations, as are baby-sitting, delivering newspapers, and some lawn care. On the basis of two assumptions, that the work is supervised in a training environment and that it occurs in a safe place, various types of vocational and technical education are also granted exemptions from the FLSA.

In many states, adolescents who want to look for a job must first secure a work permit, which is issued by the school. In some states the signature of a physician is also required, offering an opportunity to provide anticipatory guidance about work safety, injury prevention, and first aid.

Child labor laws are enforced by the federal and state departments of labor. Although some illegal child labor is performed by undocumented individuals who are in this country illegally, most illegal child labor involves youth who are US citizens and employed under conditions that violate the FLSA. With resources that were never abundant and have been cut under recent federal administrations, inspectors are responsible for enforcing wage, hour, and safety laws for all workers. Thus, most child labor is not investigated proactively, but only when a complaint is made, usually by a parent or occasionally by a legitimate business that is being undercut. The fines for child labor violations have historically been small compared with the savings made possible by the exploitation of children, although some states have recently increased fines, particularly for repeated violations. Two continuing widespread problems include keeping teenagers at work too late on school nights (hours violation) and having youth clock out at an appropriate time but stay without pay to finish work.

Perhaps the most critical aspect about violation of child labor laws relates to safety. Parents must understand why it matters when their child's work situation violates certain FLSA standards. If an employer does not abide by wage and hour laws, it is unreasonable to assume that the employer follows laws that are intended to protect the health and safety of the working teenagers; safe, legitimate work should be sought instead.

6.3 Patterns of Injury

National and state studies show that fatal injuries frequently occur when youth are engaged in work prohibited by law for safety reasons. In Suruda and Halperin's[20] study of 1984 to 1987 investigations by the Occupational Safety and Health Administration (OSHA) into adolescent fatalities, 41% of the deaths occurred while adolescents were engaged in work that was prohibited by the FLSA. In 70% of those investigations, OSHA issued citations to employers for safety violations. In a study based on medical examiner reports of North Carolina adolescent occupational fatalities, Dunn and Runyan[21] found that 86% of workers younger than 18 years who incurred fatal injury were engaged in work that seemed to violate the FLSA.

Even when boys and girls are employed in almost equal numbers, boys are injured more often than girls; most studies find a ratio of about 3:1. It is unclear whether this is because boys are employed in more hazardous occupations or whether boys engage in more high-risk behavior, resulting in higher numbers of injuries.

More older teenagers are injured when compared with younger teenagers. Although more older teenagers are employed, their rates of injury also rise for reasons that are unclear.[8,10]

While injuries among young adolescent workers are uncommon, some of the more serious injuries are incurred by younger workers, based on initial days lost from work and on the level of eventual disability (S Pollack et al, unpublished data, 1997).[8] In Suruda and Halperin's[20] analysis of adolescent OSHA fatality data, 13% of those injured were 15 years old or younger. More injuries occur during the summer months than at any other time.

Sprains or strains and lacerations are among the most common injuries in the workplace. Amputations and eye injuries also occur and may be associated with permanent disability. Although some burns are minor, others result in extensive surgery, disability, scarring, and permanent morbidity. Fractures are sometimes viewed as unimportant injuries that heal, but fractures through the growth plates in young adolescents may result in permanent discrepancies in limb length.

Head injuries are infrequent, but have major roles in mortality and may also be associated with severe morbidity, both directly and through secondary learning problems. (In New York State, approximately 10% of compensated adolescent occupational injuries involved the head. Head injuries alone, however, accounted for about 25% of fatalities and almost 50% of the fatalities when multiple trauma was considered.[8])

Restaurant employment is responsible for a large number of injuries, in part because the industry employs such a large number of youth. Many of these injuries occur in fast-food establishments.

Although few youth are employed on farms, rates of injury in the agricultural sector are among the highest. (In New York State, agriculture remains the most hazardous industry for 17-year-olds, as it is for adults.)

In several states, occupational fatalities in youth younger than 14 years are related to newspaper delivery. (This is one of the limited employment options open to young teenagers.)

Homicide has become the major occupational killer of teenage girls, as it is for women.[2]

6.4 Risk Factors

One of the most central occupational risk factors for adolescents is related to their desire to be good employees. Adolescents want to be considered competent, reliable, and responsible by adults. For this reason, some adolescents will do almost anything in the workplace that they are asked to do. It is therefore important that pediatricians are advocates for children to work in safe situations.

The combination of machinery use and inexperience creates risk for adolescents, resulting in occupational fatalities on farms, in supermarkets, and while driving vehicles to make deliveries.

Supervision seems to be an important issue. Other important issues, instruction and training, have not been fully explored.

Employment in isolated, high cash-flow businesses (eg, convenience stores and gas stations) is a risk factor for being a target of robbery or assault.

6.5 Injury Prevention by Occupation or Industry

Table 6.2, pp 126–127, outlines representative risks of injury associated with specific occupational activities in which adolescents commonly engage. Office-based counseling should emphasize industry-specific risks as adolescents enter the workforce. Adolescents also tend to have multiple tasks at a job; hence this table is meant to assist but is not all-inclusive. For example, many fast-food cooking jobs also involve clean up with attendant chemical exposures.

6.6 Intervention Strategies

The three major avenues for pediatrician involvement in occupational health and safety for adolescents include:

- Direct office-based counseling of adolescent patients — an additional reason pediatricians should see adolescents for annual health supervision visits
- Empowering parents and caregivers to make wise decisions about work for their teenagers
- Public advocacy and support for enactment and enforcement of child labor laws based on known injury risks and for occupational health and safety training

6.7 Recommendations for Pediatricians

For many pediatricians, occupational health and safety is new and unfamiliar. Although a practitioner's knowledge may be limited at first, the needs for knowledge and intervention are great. Practitioners are urged to choose from the following practical steps and incorporate them into their practice and community pediatrics efforts.

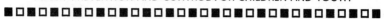
TABLE 6.2.
Issues and Risks in Representative Occupations and Activities

Job	Risk Issues and Preventive Measures
All	Transportation safety going to and from work, particularly at night; assure the vehicle is in safe operating condition, avoid driver fatigue, use safety belts or a bicycle helmet as appropriate
Newspaper delivery	Bicycle safety and helmet use as condition of employment (in some states, the newspaper industry has run bicycle safety courses and affixed registration cards to bicycles of teenagers who have completed the course); headphones should not be worn (so approaching vehicles can be heard); hats should be worn in cold weather instead of hoods that can obstruct vision; and appropriate behavior around dogs and what to do if bitten should be learned (Delivery of newspapers by car is illegal for adolescents younger than 18 years.)
Farm work and work in tree or yard service (see chapter 7)	Adequate training and continued supervision; tractors must have rollover protection, safety belts, working brakes, and properly inflated tires; devices to protect hearing are necessary when working on noisy farm machinery; use of hazardous machinery in bad weather and on uneven terrain should be avoided; caution must be exercised around large animals and animals with young; tetanus immunizations need to be current; be aware of hazards that can catch or trap hair, clothing, head, arms, legs, or fingers; use caution with long hair, scarves, loose sleeves, and shoe laces; do not take sibling riders on farm machinery; practice safety on highways; minimize the risk of nicotine poisoning during the tobacco harvest and the risk of falling in tobacco barns; most pesticide and chemical use is prohibited; use eye protection
Grocery store: stocking shelves	Avoid lacerations from box cutters[7]; proper body mechanics are necessary when lifting heavy or bulky objects and when reaching for objects on high shelves (Back supports do not protect against injury when too heavy a load is lifted or if improper body mechanics are used.); work on deli slicers is prohibited
Restaurants, including fast food	Prevent burns, especially from grease[22]; wear nonskid shoes and assure that floors are properly cleaned (falls lead to burns and other injuries); use sharp knives; avoid cuts during food preparation; do not use deli slicers; use proper body mechanics when lifting and carrying to avoid back strain, especially among wait staff and assistants
Pizza places	Prevent burns from hot ovens; know how to administer proper first aid if a burn occurs (Delivery by car is illegal for anyone younger than 18 years.)
Nursing homes and hospitals	Avoid back injuries by using proper body mechanics; use universal and other precautions to avoid or minimize exposure to bloodborne pathogens
Bakeries, donut or bagel stores	Avoid involvement in cleaning or operating industrial mixers

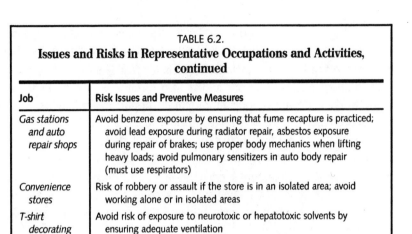

TABLE 6.2.
Issues and Risks in Representative Occupations and Activities, continued

Job	Risk Issues and Preventive Measures
Gas stations and auto repair shops	Avoid benzene exposure by ensuring that fume recapture is practiced; avoid lead exposure during radiator repair, asbestos exposure during repair of brakes; use proper body mechanics when lifting heavy loads; avoid pulmonary sensitizers in auto body repair (must use respirators)
Convenience stores	Risk of robbery or assault if the store is in an isolated area; avoid working alone or in isolated areas
T-shirt decorating	Avoid risk of exposure to neurotoxic or hepatotoxic solvents by ensuring adequate ventilation
Car wash	Do not permit adolescents to run or repair machinery

6.7.1 Patient-Directed Office-Based Strategies

- As in other emerging areas of pediatric practice (eg, learning disabilities and school health), physicians must first educate themselves about work and occupational injuries and illness as adolescent health issues and then educate patients and parents who come to the office.
- Know the state child labor laws. The state department of labor provides a one-page poster summarizing work hours, wages, and occupations permitted for adolescents of different ages. (This poster must be posted prominently in every workplace.) In some states, the state office of the US Department of Labor can also provide information.
- Know which patients work, where they are working, and exactly what they do on the job. The best source of this information is your patient. Obtain an occupational history: be alert to common hazards for teenagers employed in your area. Ask teenagers about their employers, what kind of training they have had, what they know about first aid, and who supervises them. Do they eat between school and work? Do they get an adequate amount of sleep and get their homework done? Do they wear a safety belt while driving to and from work?
- Inquire about possible chemical exposures in the adolescent's workplace. Occupational exposures are issues for employed youth, although far less is known about their extent than for other injuries. Youth employed in lawn care or on farms, including migrant farm

workers, may be exposed to pesticides. Nicotine poisoning, or green tobacco sickness, is an occupational hazard of harvesting tobacco.

- In the office literature, include booklets for teenagers and their parents about adolescent work and related hazards as well as benefits of work, choosing among employment opportunities, rights, and responsibilities. Some examples include booklets developed in New York State for schools and a booklet developed for teenagers in Kentucky (see Resources section).

- Consider the adolescent's occupation in the diagnosis of conditions. For example, a teenager who screens t-shirts and sleeps in the same enclosed room may be seen with fatigue caused by solvent intoxication.

- Consider the adolescent's occupation in the medical management of patients. If an adolescent with diabetes is going to school and working and has difficulty maintaining an appropriate blood glucose level, determine whether he or she has regular, adequate meal breaks, or perhaps is not eating until late at night after work.

- Consider possible occupations for adolescent patients with chronic disease, who, like many teenagers, want to work. It may be possible to have some influence on where they work and what types of work they do. For example, should a teenager with aplastic anemia work at a fast-food restaurant that requires long periods of standing or at a job that can be done sitting down? Exposure to air pollution at work could affect adolescents with cystic fibrosis. Secondhand smoke in restaurants may be a hazard for teenagers with asthma. At gas stations, is the potential exposure to benzene acceptable for a teenager who survived leukemia in the primary grades?

- Know about workers' compensation. Rules about such factors as who is covered and how many days of work must be missed before benefits begin differ from state to state. In many cases medical care for an injury incurred on the job should be paid by workers' compensation, and frequently a form must be filled out by the physician. Many agricultural injuries are not covered.

- For those who work in an ED or see injured teenagers:

Help improve surveillance by improving the quality of the history taken about the injury. Ask whether the injury is work related, and include as much detail as possible about the injury and job site.

Consider the occupational injury of a teenager a sentinel health event for other teenagers at risk in the same workplace and intervene rapidly by contacting appropriate state or federal agencies.

Maintain contact with state and federal agencies (eg, OSHA, the health department, and the department of labor) to enable rapid reporting of injuries so other at-risk youth in the same workplace are protected by a timely, thorough investigation. Some states (eg, Massachusetts) require reporting of occupational injuries.

Advocate for quality, age-appropriate rehabilitation for those injured on the job to ensure that optimal recovery is achieved. Be prepared for strong opposition. In many cases, workers' compensation should pay for the rehabilitation.

6.7.2 Empowering Parents to Make Informed Decisions About Their Adolescent's Safety

- Talk with parents about the risks and benefits of having their adolescent work. Many parents are unaware of the risks. Guide them in choices that help lessen those risks.

- Share information with parents about normal adolescent development and where their child fits into the spectrum. Wide ranges in individual size, strength, and emotional development and maturity among teenagers exist at any given age. Only half of boys have had their growth spurt by age 14 years. Youths who are small for their age may not be able to sit back far enough in the seat of a tractor to wear the safety belt and reach the pedals. Youths who are large for their age may be emotionally immature; an adolescent who is physically able to perform selected tasks cannot be expected to perform like an adult.

- Inform parents that they should ask potential employers what tasks their child will be doing. Parents should be concerned about issues such as supervision, job training, and safety instruction. It is important for parents to visit the workplace.

- Support parents in their decisions about safety, while realizing that responsibilities for teenagers should grow within safe limits. Parents faced with pressure from their children may doubt the wisdom of their own decisions. Support for safety is important as families weigh the appropriate limits of teenage independence with risk factors in the workplace.

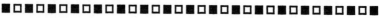
6.7.3 Public Advocacy

Laws and policy decisions made on local, state, and federal levels have profound implications for adolescent health and safety, yet most decision makers are unfamiliar with pediatric growth, development, and risk factors for and epidemiology of injury and do not receive input from pediatricians and others with expertise in these areas. Although pediatricians can continue to help patients during office visits, they need to be involved in law and policy decisions as advocates for pediatric and adolescent patients. They should:

- Become informed about and involved in the recurring debate about modification and revision of child labor laws. Through written and oral testimony, pediatricians can help balance economic arguments with a perspective of adolescent developmental needs and injury prevention.

- Support and become involved in local occupational safety training programs and organizations (eg, tractor training programs).

- Work to eliminate the "contract worker" status, to make someone clearly responsible for the safety of the adolescents who are hired.

- Work with the newspaper industry on programs for pedestrian safety, bicycle safety, and mandatory bicycle helmet use.

- Become a resource for local employers about first aid for burns, when to send for medical care, and other injury control issues.

- Become involved in school-to-work cooperative education programs. Advocate for occupational health and safety as a part of curriculum and practice.

- Advocate for engineering and environmental changes that would make a safer workplace. Such changes provide "automatic" protection so safety is not as dependent on daily behavioral changes by the employee or supervisor. This is a difficult issue because of its economic impact and need for specialized expertise. Roll-over protection on farm machinery is an example (see chapter 7, Agricultural Injuries).

Occupational health and safety is an important aspect of pediatric injury control that has been underappreciated by parents, the public, and health providers. While there are multiple avenues for effective involvement of pediatricians, the first step is to become knowledgeable about local employment patterns and conditions. Although productive employment should not be discouraged, the employment of youth entails special responsibilities that employers must understand. Physicians are encouraged to incorporate their developing expertise in this area into their routine health supervision and community pediatric activities.[1]

6.8 Resources

Resources for occupational safety and health are diverse. The following is a list of some of the resources available.

1. Department of labor for your state. Contact for information on child labor laws, wages, hours of work, safety regulations, and problems with any of those areas. In some states you will be told to call the local office of the US Department of Labor. Telephone numbers should be in all local telephone directories.

2. Occupational Safety and Health Administration (OSHA), the federal agency that deals with regulatory and enforcement issues. If a teenager comes to you and asks about a specific hazard, the patient (or you with permission) can call OSHA for assistance. This can be done anonymously, but sometimes an employee might still be identifiable. Consider this especially when you are concerned about imminent danger. For example, a patient who works in a fast-food restaurant tells you that a wire near her feet for the drive-through speaker has a short circuit and has been sparking whenever water is on the floor. This situation caused another employee to be shocked last week, but has still not been fixed. Telephone numbers for OSHA are in telephone directories.

3. National Institute for Occupational Safety and Health (NIOSH), the federal agency that deals with scientific, research, and educational aspects (800-356-4674). The Division of Safety Research in the Morgantown, WVa, NIOSH office has expertise in this area (304-285-5894); work is also currently being done through the Cincinnati, Ohio, NIOSH office. In May 1995, NIOSH published *Alert-Request for Assistance in Preventing Deaths and Injuries of Adolescent Workers.* This booklet (DHHS Publication No. 95–125, available from NIOSH at the above telephone numbers) has background information for you and a tear-out page to post in your office, copy for adolescent patients and their parents, or use for community injury prevention work. NIOSH can also direct you to your closest

ERC, the Educational Resource Center, that trains occupational medicine physicians and provides continuing education. Most such institutions are also a good source for finding or being referred to industrial hygienists.

4. The Child Labor Coalition, c/o the National Consumers League, Washington, DC, is a coalition of organizations and individuals (including consumer groups, medical professionals, universities, unions, religious organizations) interested in all aspects of international and US child labor. They have organized conferences, meet monthly, and maintain one of the most up-to-date watches on state child labor law changes as they evolve. For information, call 202-835-3323.

5. National Child Labor Committee, New York, NY, has existed since the 1800s and has much historical and legal information of help.

6. The Education Development Center is part of the Children's Safety Network, a group of organizations that provide technical assistance in child and adolescent injury control to states and others. Ask about availability of their 1995 resource guide, *Protecting Working Teens*[20]; it summarizes adolescent occupational injury and includes an extensive annotated resource list. The booklet or additional information can be obtained by calling 800-793-5076.

7. Several states have materials for adolescents dealing with employment/health and safety. In New York State, contact the Buffalo office of the state Department of Labor (716-847-7144) for booklets. The Kentucky Safety and Health Network has published a booklet that is available through the Kentucky Labor Cabinet (502-564-3070).

References

1. American Academy of Pediatrics, Committee on Environmental Health. The hazards of child labor. *Pediatrics*. 1995;95:311–313

2. Centers for Disease Control. Work-related injuries and illnesses associated with child labor — United States, 1993. *MMWR Morb Mortal Wkly Rep*. 1996;45:464–468

3. Schober SE, Handke JL, Halperin WE, Moll MB, Thun MJ. Work-related injuries in minors. *Am J Ind Med*. 1988;14:585–595

4. Parker DL, Carl WR, French LR, Martin FB. Characteristics of adolescent work injuries reported to the Minnesota Department of Labor and Industry. *Am J Public Health*. 1994;84:606–611

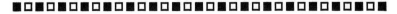
5. Parker DL, Carl WR, French LR, Martin FB. Nature and incidence of self-reported adolescent work injury in Minnesota. *Am J Ind Med.* 1994;26:529–541

6. Pollack SH, Landrigan PJ, Mallino DL. Child labor in 1990: prevalence and health hazards. *Annu Rev Public Health.* 1990;11:359–375

7. Banco L, Lapidus G, Braddock M. Work-related injury among Connecticut minors. *Pediatrics.* 1992;89:957–960

8. Belville R, Pollack SH, Godbold JH, Landrigan PJ. Occupational injuries among working adolescents in New York State. *JAMA.* 1993;269:2754–2759

9. Cooper SP, Rothstein MA. Health hazards among working children in Texas. *South Med J.* 1995;88:550–554

10. Brooks DR, Davis LK, Gallagher SS. Work-related injuries among Massachusetts children: a study based on emergency department data. *Am J Ind Med.* 1993; 24:313–324

11. Miller M. *Occupational Injuries Among Adolescents in Washington State, 1988–91: A Review of Workers' Compensation Data.* Olympia, WA: Washington State Department of Labor and Industries; 1995. Technical Report Number 35-1-1995: Safety and Health Assessment and Research for Prevention

12. Bush D, Baker R. *Young Workers at Risk: Health and Safety Education and the Schools.* Labor Occupational Health Program, Center for Occupational and Environmental Health, University of California at Berkeley; November 1994

13. Coleman PJ, Sanderson LM. Surveillance of occupational injuries treated in hospital emergency rooms — United States, 1982. *MMWR Morb Mortal Wkly Rep.* 1983; 32:31SS–37SS

14. Glor ED. Survey of comprehensive accident and injury experience of high school students in Saskatchewan. *Can J Public Health.* 1989;80:435–440

15. Bachman JG, Schulenberg J. How part-time work intensity relates to drug use, problem behavior, time use and satisfaction among high school seniors: are these the consequences or merely correlates? *Dev Psychol.* 1993;29:220–235

16. Steinberg L, Dornbusch SM. Negative correlates of part-time employment during adolescence: replication and elaboration. *Dev Psychol.* 1991;27:304–313

17. Fair Labor Standards Act of 1938, as Amended. Title 29, US Code, Section 201 et seq; 29 CFR § 570–580

18. US Department of Labor. *Child Labor Requirements in Nonagricultural Occupations Under the Fair Labor Standards Act.* Washington, DC: Employment Standards Administration, Wage and Hour Division; 1985. Child Labor Bulletin 101

19. US Department of Labor. *Child Labor Requirements in Agriculture Under the Fair Labor Standards Act.* Washington, DC: Employment Standards Administration, Wage and Hour Division; 1984. Child Labor Bulletin 102

20. Suruda A, Halperin W. Work-related deaths in children. *Am J Ind Med.* 1991; 19:739–745

21. Dunn KA, Runyan CW. Deaths at work among children and adolescents. *Am J Dis Child.* 1993;147:1044–1047

22. Hayes-Lundy C, Ward RS, Saffle JR, Reddy R, Warden GD, Schnebly WA. Grease burns at fast-food restaurants: adolescents at risk. *J Burn Care Rehabil.* 1991; 12:203–208

CHAPTER 7

Agricultural Injuries

Few settings in our nation are comparable to production agriculture when considering the horrific fatal and nonfatal injuries sustained by children. The impact of injury and death associated with farming in the United States is substantial. Although a variety of injury control methods have been suggested and implemented in the past, injuries continue to occur at an alarming rate as the most effective injury control interventions are sought. While significant strides have been achieved for childhood safety in the areas of motor vehicle restraints, helmet use or bicycling, and playground safety, the same cannot be said for agricultural safety. The 1992 Census of Agriculture reported a total of 1.93 million farms in the United States.[1] Although the total number of farms and farm workers has declined steadily since 1950, trauma and adverse exposures associated with production agriculture continue to persist. Production agriculture is one of the few industries in which children are victims of a relatively large proportion of traumatic injuries.

What is an agricultural injury? Confusion sometimes arises when the terms *agriculture* and *farming* are used synonymously and then cross-referenced with terms such as *industry, occupation,* and *lifestyle.* A farm is defined by the US Department of Agriculture as any place from which $1000 or more of agricultural products are produced and sold, or normally would have been sold during the census year.[1] Agriculture involves the production of crops and livestock (farming) including agricultural services, forestry (excluding logging), and fishing. *Production agriculture* is a preferred term that has replaced "farming" because it has broader application to the wide range of complex machinery, sophisticated crop and livestock management practices, and relationships with associated agricultural businesses.[2] A childhood agricultural injury is broadly defined as harm to an individual (younger than 18 years) that occurs on the agricultural work site (outside the home) or off agricultural property while conducting agricultural work. A person can be actively participating in work, observing work, or merely present in the production agriculture environment. The broad definition also encompasses harm caused by exposures to pesticides, dust, noise, and repetitive motion.

Who is affected? Children younger than 18 years are frequently the victims of unintentional agricultural injuries. Injuries occur across all age groups and mainly involve males. Studies have shown that from one third to half of nonfatal childhood agricultural injuries occur to children who do not live on farms.[3,4] Children of migrant and seasonal farm laborers, year-round employees, and visitors to farms can be exposed to agricultural hazards. Children can be injured as active participants in work, observers to work, or bystanders adjacent to work areas. Issues related to adult supervision, adequate training, family traditions, normative practices, peer pressure, and other factors are associated with injuries to children and can influence the success of prevention strategies. This chapter focuses on unintentional agricultural injuries to children younger than 18 years who are workers or bystanders to work, regardless of their relationship to the farm ownership.

7.1 Scope of the Problem

In 1991, 923 000 children younger than 15 years and another 346 000 children 15 to 19 years of age resided on US farms and ranches.[5] Given that up to half of the childhood agricultural injuries occurred to nonresidents, it is estimated that 2.5 million children are at risk of agricultural injury each year in the United States. Geographically, more than half of all farm residents live in the midwestern United States. This contrasts with the fact that only one quarter of the US population resides in this area. Published reports indicate that childhood agricultural injuries are most likely to occur on family owned farms compared with corporate multi-employee operated farms. However, the picture of the national experience seems inaccurate because there are few reports regarding the injuries experienced by children of migrant and seasonal farm workers (who make up nearly half of the agricultural labor force).

No annual US statistics of fatal and nonfatal childhood agricultural injuries exist because there is no national surveillance system. For different types of national data, sources include the Department of Labor's Bureau of Labor Statistics, the Consumer Product Safety Commission, and the Department of Health and Human Services' National Traumatic Occupational Fatality Systems. Other agricultural data sources include the National Safety Council's annual report, the Department of Commerce Bureau of Agricultural Census (which included two injury questions in 1992), state workers' compensation systems, and state and local surveillance or epidemiological studies. Limitations of the data are associated with difficulty in differentiating bystanders from workers; variations in age categories used in different databases; inconsistency n definitions of work, farm, farm-related, and child; and lack of a universal classification scheme of agricultural injuries.

7.1.1 Fatal Injury Estimates

In the absence of annual fatality rates of childhood agricultural injuries, the most frequently cited figure was reported in 1985, which estimated fatality rates for males 15 to 19 years old at 30.9 per 100 000 rural residents and a total of 300 children killed on farms annually.[6] Data on state fatalities have been collected from Wisconsin, with six deaths per year, to California, with an average of four deaths per year. These statistics, when joined with adult statistics, disclose that alarmingly, children account for approximately 10% of all agricultural fatalities. One can only imagine the reaction of our society if this occurred in any other industry.

7.1.2 Nonfatal Injury Estimates

Research suggests that an estimated 27 000 children younger than 20 years who live on farms and ranches are injured each year.[7] This number does not account for the injured children who do not reside on farms. A more recent report estimated that nearly 100 000 children sustain agricultural injuries annually.[3] When injuries specifically to youth (≥ 10 years old) involved as paid or nonpaid agricultural workers were studied, a 1993 report from the National Institute for Occupational Safety and Health (NIOSH) estimated nearly 13 000 injuries resulting in lost work time.[8] Of these injuries, nearly two thirds occurred during the months of June, July, and August, when children are typically out of school.

7.1.3 Societal Costs

The annual societal costs of childhood deaths and injuries on farms and ranches is around $3 billion, which involves an estimated $150 million in medical spending. The remaining costs are the value of lost future earnings and quality of life. More than one third of the earnings in quality of life lost result from fatal injuries.[3]

7.2 Risk Factors

7.2.1 Host

Data from the Traumatic Injury Surveillance Farmers' Survey (conducted by NIOSH) revealed that of the 12 873 occupational injuries among farm workers 10 to 19 years old, 89.2% were male. Analysis by race revealed 92.2% were white, 6.3% were Hispanic, and 1.5% were American Indian.[8] In both the United States and Canada, it has been shown that peak ages for agricultural trauma include early childhood years through 4 years of age and the period during middle adolescence. After the toddler age, males consistently experienced a greater rate of injuries than females.[9] A review of multiple studies[9] disclosed that minimal gender variation exists in agricultural trauma prior to the age of 5 years. After this age, the rate of injuries among males is greater overall in both fatal and nonfatal injuries. Females are mainly involved in certain types of nonfatal injuries, such as those associated with dairy cows and horses.

7.2.2 Agent of Injury

Tractors are the primary agents of fatal agricultural injury to children. A study of 460 Wisconsin and Indiana childhood farm fatalities during a 10-year period found that 50% were associated with tractors.[10] Among all working 16- and 17-year-olds in the United States during the years 1980 to 1989, 44% of the machine-related deaths were associated with tractors. Other motorized vehicles such as all-terrain vehicles (ATVs) and pickup trucks also account for many fatalities. Animals, machinery, tools, falls, and structures (ie, silos) account for both fatal and nonfatal injuries. In the midwest, nonfatal childhood agricultural injuries are most frequently associated with livestock, typically with injuries occurring during feeding, grooming, and standing in the vicinity of the animals.

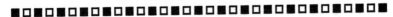
7.2.3 Environment

Both the physical and social/psychological environment create conditions associated with childhood agricultural injuries. The environment in which production agriculture occurs is comparable to any large industry with respect to the number of inherent hazards. Issues related to the physical environment include the condition of building structures and machinery; weather conditions; the personal health, energy level, and concentration of the child as well as the adult responsible for the child's care; the supervision of children; and the involvement of children in developmentally appropriate and age-appropriate tasks.

A myriad of factors are related to the psychological environment, such as the stress related to farm economics, work overload, cognitive and emotional coping skills of adults, and the unpredictable nature of farming. Adults and adolescents working in these conditions may compromise standards, especially regarding safe practices. Children under the care of adults in these conditions may suffer the consequences that such stressors place on adults. Additionally, children are unable to recognize when their working conditions do not meet ideal physical or psychological environmental standards. To date, studies have not depicted a strong relationship between socioeconomic status or education with the incidence of agricultural injuries. Also, among adult farmers, safety education has not been shown to be a protective factor.

7.3 Intervention Strategies

7.3.1 Education

To make a significant impact on the reduction of childhood agricultural injuries, an interdisciplinary, multifaceted approach is necessary. Education and training efforts, combined with engineering, public policy, and community-based interventions designed to change social norms, are required. For many years, education and training have focused primarily on teaching farm owner/operators the basic principles of safety in production agriculture. More recently, education programs targeted toward youth have been implemented. The efficacy of these educational programs, however, is unknown. As with other public health problems, educational interventions have their limitations. Studies have shown that farmers are knowledgeable of major safety risks to adults and children; yet, attitudes about farm safety do not equate with safe behaviors or a reduction in injuries.[11,12] Therefore, the problem of childhood agricultural injuries is analogous to other public health problems such as injuries caused by motor vehicles or firearms and transmission of communicable diseases; educational interventions alone do not have a significant impact.

7.3.2 Engineering

A number of engineering modifications have been implemented by major manufacturers to make equipment safer. Safety improvements in agricultural vehicles, machinery, and structures have been developed to provide both active and passive safety designs. Newer, safer equipment and structures have not been purchased by all farmers, however, often because of cost. At times, new equipment may actually encourage adults to involve children in farm work (to accompany parents during farm work) beyond the scope of the child's capabilities. Farm safety specialists and tractor manufacturers do not agree on the method to handle requests by farmers to introduce specific technology that ensures the safety of children present during farm work. For example, a passenger seat in the cab of tractors (a common practice in Europe) has been developed that could be used to place and restrain a child in the tractor cab while accompanying an adult during field work. Ideally, a child should never be placed on a tractor or in a tractor cab because of the risks associated with tractor runover or rollover or risks associated with noise, vibration, and exposure to airborne irritants. Yet, for reasons such as limited child care options, adults sometimes allow a child in the tractor cab.

7.3.3 Policy

The Occupational Safety and Health Act (OSHA) of 1970 mandated safety standards on workplaces throughout the United States including farms, regardless of size or type of enterprise. Shortly thereafter, farm owner/operators argued (through lobbying efforts of major farm organizations) that safety was a personal, economic issue, and therefore managerial freedom from government jurisdiction was warranted. In 1976, and every year since then, Congress has approved the exemption of farms with 10 or fewer workers from OSHA safety standards. Thus, the majority of farms on which children are exposed to hazards are not required to comply with OSHA safety regulations. In another public policy measure, the Fair Labor Standards Act of 1938 established minimum ages for engagement in hazardous agricultural activities unless a specific exemption applies. Again, children working on farms owned or operated by their parents or surrogates are not protected by these standards because of an exemption. Most parents are probably unaware of the specific safety standards or labor restrictions that apply to children and adolescents working on a farm.

The position of major farm organizations and most farm operators regarding involvement of children in hazardous farm work has hampered the likelihood of using federal public policy measures to protect children from dangers on the agricultural work site. The "agrarian myth" that has empowered farmers and farm organizations to be independent of government regulations is credited with the persistence of work environments and practices that put adults and youth at a high level of risk on farms.[13]

7.4 Recommendations for Pediatricians

A number of specific, targeted actions can be adopted by pediatricians to minimize the risk of agricultural injuries to children. Pediatricians and other primary care providers have unique opportunities to influence parental behavior.

Given the strong influence of community and social norms combined with traditional farm attitudes and practices, pediatricians are encouraged to model safe behaviors if personally involved in agricultural work. Another relatively simple action for practitioners is a media advocacy approach in dealing with injury events and safety messages. For example, pediatricians should respond to inappropriate depictions of children in high-risk situations (eg, a 9-year-old driving a tractor) on the local news, in agricultural journals, and in other media. The editor or station manager should be provided facts about risk and injuries from pediatricians. These approaches should be used routinely to counteract the depiction of unsafe behaviors. Specific steps for utilizing a media advocacy approach have been outlined for health promotion activities.[14]

Physicians and other health care providers should keep the following principles in mind regarding the prevention of childhood agricultural injuries:

- There is no such thing as a "farm accident"…each event is predictable and preventable.

- The farm should be viewed as a dangerous, adult occupational work site. The presence of children in any adult work site must be avoided or carefully monitored by adults.

- Federal child labor laws place specific restrictions on children's work prior to the age of 12 for low-risk jobs (eg, paper route, golf caddie) and age 16 for most other jobs. Parents should try to equate specific farm tasks to their child's developmental level to reduce risk of injury.

- Parents tend to think their own child is smarter and better skilled than other children, and parents who are farmers typically believe their children have much more common sense than city children. Studies show that parents underestimate the real risk of injury to their own children and judge the decisions of other parents more critically.

- Parents who are farmers are under tremendous stress to maintain an economically viable operation and sometimes feel they need to have children involved in the work. Yet, parents who have had a child killed in a farm-related injury will tell you they would readily give away their farm to have the life of their child back.

- Parents who are farmers should remember that to their child the farm is like a giant playground. Parents need to be creative in developing options to safeguard their young children, such as day care centers, neighborhood babysitting cooperatives, and fenced-in play yards where an adult can supervise.

Individual patient counseling and presentations to parent groups should incorporate the following specific safety messages promoted by agricultural safety specialists and child safety advocates.

- Appreciate the contributions that children bring to a fulfilling family life and preserve the legacy of farming by protecting children from known hazards.

- Parents, caregivers, and employers should serve as role models of safe behaviors and be active in community efforts to promote agricultural safety.

- Establish meaningful roles for children working in an agricultural setting that are age- and developmentally appropriate. Recognize that sometimes children do not have a role.

- Because children almost always want to engage in high-risk, challenging activities, parents should *not* decide what type of work their child should be involved in based on the child's desires.

- Provide safe play areas and protective barriers from hazards (eg, large animals, heavy items in storage, sources of electricity, areas of production, and machinery).

- Ensure that children avoid exposure to chemicals and fuels during their application, use, and in storage.

- Establish parental expectations that are clearly communicated, continually reinforced, and monitored by adults.

- Know the agricultural safety standards and child labor laws that affect children.

- Protect the heads of children (with helmets, ear plugs, eye shields, masks) and extremities (with long sleeves/long pants, gloves, proper shoes) during the operation of recreational and work machinery such as ATVs, lawn tractors, or power tools. Children should not operate powered equipment or vehicles.

- Maintain an adequate, accessible supply of personal protective equipment for children to use, including sunscreen and sunglasses.

- Emphasize that children should not be present during tractor operation.

- Provide guidelines and orientation to young children whose parents work on a farm or who are visiting a farm.

- Celebrate the uniqueness, richness, and variety afforded in an agriculturally based lifestyle.

7.5 Resources

For information on planning childhood agricultural injury prevention programs or to obtain patient education resources (eg, fact sheets, brochures, videotapes), contact:

1. Your local county extension office — public health nurse, 4-H agent, agricultural agent

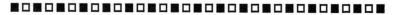
2. Farm Safety for Just Kids
   110 S Chestnut Ave
   PO Box 458
   Earlham, IA 50072-0458
   515-758-2827
   515-758-2517 (fax)

3. Your state agricultural safety specialist, located at the land grant university

4. National Safety Council
   National Headquarters/Central Region
   1121 Spring Lake Dr
   Itasca, IL 60143-3201
   800-621-7615
   630-285-0797 (fax)

5. Children's Safety Network
   National Farm Medicine Center
   1000 North Oak Ave
   Marshfield, WI 54449
   715-389-4999
   715-389-4999 (fax)
   nikolaic@mfldclin.edu (e-mail)

6. Children's Safety Network
   Education Development Center
   55 Chapel St
   Newton, MA 02158-1060
   617-969-7100
   617-244-3436 (fax)
   csn@edc.org (e-mail)

References

1. US Department of Commerce. *Census of Agriculture.* Washington, DC: US Department of Commerce, 1994. Report No. AC92-A-51, 1994:1

2. Murphy DJ. *Safety and Health in Production Agriculture.* St Joseph, MI: American Society of Agricultural Engineers; 1992

3. Miller T. Unpublished tabulation and analysis of 1987–1992 National Health Interview Survey data. Landover MD: National Public Services Research Institute, Children's Safety Network Economics and Insurance Resource Center, 1995.

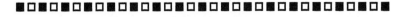

4. Stueland D, Aldrich R. All-terrain vehicle injuries in central Wisconsin: a continuing problem. *Wis Med J.* 1991;90:275–278

5. Dahmann DC, Dacquel LT. *Residents of Farms and Rural Areas: 1991.* Washington, DC: US Bureau of Census; 1993

6. Rivara FP. Fatal and nonfatal farm injuries to children and adolescents in the United States. *Pediatrics.* 1985;76:567–573

7. Gerberich SG, Gibson RW, Gunderson PD, et al. The Olmsted agricultural trauma study (OATS): a population-based effort. 1991. A report to the Centers for Disease Control, Mar 1991. The estimate was developed using data from pages 38–40 by staff at the National Farm Medicine Center and uses denominators constructed from baseline data compiled from Rural and Rural Farm Population: 1988, 1989

8. Myers JR. *Traumatic Injury Surveillance of Farmers: 1993 Statistical Abstract.* Washington, DC: National Institute for Occupational Safety and Health; 1995. US Dept of Health and Human Services publication NIOSH 95–116

9. Purschwitz MA. *Fatal Farm Injuries to Children.* Marshfield, WI: Wisconsin Rural Health Research Center; 1990

10. Sheldon EJ, Field WE. Fatal farm work-related injuries involving children and adolescents in Wisconsin and Indiana. In: McDuffie HH, Dosman JA, Semchuk KM, Olenchock SA, Senthilselvan A, eds. *Agricultural Health and Safety: Workplace, Environment, Sustainability.* Boca Raton, FL: Lewis Publishers; 1995:355–362

11. Hawk C, Donham KJ, Gay J. Pediatric exposure to agricultural machinery: implications for primary prevention. *J Agromedicine.* 1994;1:57–74

12. Murphy DJ. Farm safety attitudes and accident involvement. *Accid Anal Prev.* 1981; 13:331–337

13. Kelsey TW. The agrarian myth and policy responses to farm safety. *Am J Public Health.* 1994;84:1171–1177

14. Wallack L, Dorfman L, Jernigan D, Themba M. *Media Advocacy and Public Health: Power for Prevention.* Newbury Park, CA: Sage; 1993

CHAPTER 8

Violence

Traditionally, injury has been classified as either "intentional" or "unintentional." Such a simple classification has been criticized on several counts. First, intent is often uncertain, ambiguous, or unknowable. What was the intent of an angry parent who "inadvertently" let discipline get out of hand? What was the "intent" of the depressed and drinking teenager who was killed when his car veered off the road and into a tree? What was the "intent" of the 6-year-old who shot his younger brother with his parent's handgun? The second argument claims that such a classification ignores the commonality of injury mechanism and preventive countermeasures to both sets of injuries. In each case, there is the issue of energy transfer and the various strategies to prevent, reduce, or modify that transfer of energy (see chapter 1.2).

Nevertheless, there are certain injuries (and far too many fatalities) that can be grouped as being the result of violence. Violence is the purposeful excessive use of force to a destructive (often self-destructive) end. In this chapter, the topic is divided into the areas of child abuse, suicide (and suicide attempts or self-inflicted injury), peer violence, and violence as portrayed in the popular media. Sexual abuse, war, and other forms of observed violence are not discussed. Pediatricians need to address certain psychosocial symptoms present in various forms of violence. Because these injuries tend to cluster in malfunctioning individuals and families, they require a broad-based multidisciplinary approach to prevention. Homicides and suicides are becoming more common among youths, and child abuse is more frequently being recognized. In 1992, nearly 7000 children from birth to 19 years of age died violent deaths. This represented more than a third of all deaths from injury in this age group and more than a fifth of all deaths to pediatric patients after their first birthday.

In the preface to the book *Violence in America*,[1] Dr William Foege points out that throughout history, the two leading causes of early death have been infection and violence. While much of the scourge of infection has come under control in the last century, the control of violence has been resistant to our better standard of living, scientific sophistication, and improved health care. Dr Foege states: "…violence has defied the best minds in health, politics, religion, and law enforcement, and therefore has often appeared inevitable. This and other forms of fatalism must be actively opposed. That we live in a cause-and-effect world is as true with violence as with infectious diseases, an important observation for both public health people and educators."[1]

Pediatricians are in a key position to recognize persons at risk of violent injury and intervene in a preventive capacity. The following sections reflect the growing understanding that many of these injuries are, in fact, preventable through screening, early identification of risk, and intervention. Pediatricians have the opportunity to intervene at the office level, at the public and community health levels as educators, and as advocates.

8.1 Abuse

This section addresses the prevention of intentional physically abusive injuries that affect infants and young children. The most promising interventions are also likely to prevent many unintentional injuries.

The preventive methods for reducing interpersonal violence between peers who are children but who emulate adult violent behaviors are likely to be somewhat different than the prevention of child abuse and are addressed in section 8.3. Promising methods for the prevention of sexual abuse are also somewhat different.

8.1.1 Definition

Separate streams of research and practice

Describing how to prevent intentional and abusive injuries is easier in practice than in theory because the theories of injury prevention and child abuse prevention have been developed in different ways using different terminology. In practice, however, certain factors correlate strikingly in both types of injuries, and certain interventions hold great promise of being capable of preventing both types of injuries.

Child abuse research has been inhibited by lack of funding and a lack of trained researchers.[2] It has also been slowed by a lack of standardized research definitions[3] and by the inherent difficulties of recognizing the incidence of injuries that happen privately.

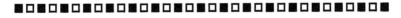

The problem with the term "intentional"

Shortly after the original description of the battered child syndrome,[4] some of the early researchers met to develop a definition that could be used in reporting. The term "intentional" was considered but rejected because the diagnosis did not involve "intent" but rather "mechanism of injury." Eventually the term "other than accidental" was adopted, which is still used in most child abuse reporting laws. In medical practice the term was changed to "nonaccidental trauma," or "NAT," which is now widely used in hospital pediatric services. Meanwhile, researchers divided all injuries into the two classes, intentional and unintentional, ignoring the earlier misgivings about defining and ascertaining intent.

Researchers from both fields need to resolve this problem in nomenclature; fortunately, it is possible to accomplish a great deal in the prevention of injuries without resolving the theoretical issues.

Age-related definitions

The intentional (or nonaccidental or inflicted) injuries that affect infants and young children often differ markedly from those that affect older children and adolescents. Injuries in older children are often inflicted abusively by adults, whereas many of the intentional injuries inflicted by peers occur in violent interactions similar to those between adults of roughly equal strength. Weapons are commonly used. In contrast, injuries to infants and young children are inflicted with the use of hands, feet, or implements that are found in almost any home and not normally used as weapons.

The violent interactions of older children, adolescents, and young adults combined produce far more serious injuries and deaths than injuries inflicted by caregivers on young children. This does not mean, however, that they should receive disproportionately greater resources for prevention. Protection of very young children from avoidable harm is important because research suggests that physical abuse early in life contributes substantially to a later propensity for violence toward others.[5]

Similarities and differences

Sociodemographic factors

Unintentional and abusive injuries of children are highly associated with low income and with living in low-income areas,[6,7] which suggests that prevention efforts should target specific neighborhoods. A history of abuse in childhood appears to be a distinct (but not absolute) predictor of abusive behavior toward children, suggesting that individually oriented healing efforts provided to children growing up with abuse may help stop the cycle of abuse.[8]

Event-related factors

Events related to abusive and unintentional injuries differ markedly. Isolation of the abuser and the child is common during severe physical abusive events, whereas unintentional injuries often occur on the street, outside of buildings, and in other public settings. Intentional injuries affecting infants and young children are often preceded by irritating (albeit normal) behaviors, while unintentional injuries are more likely to be preceded by circumstances that suggest lack of supervision.

Avoidability, responsibility, culpability, and condoning

Abusive injuries are considered to be clearly avoidable. The avoidability of unintentional injuries varies with circumstances and perception. Caregivers are held responsible and considered culpable when they cause the injury. Caregivers may or may not be regarded as negligent when unintended injuries occur. The acts of inflicting injuries on infants and young children are regarded almost universally as inexcusable, while the infliction of injuries by older children on their peers is often condoned and even encouraged at least by peer groups.

8.1.2 Scope of the Problem

The incidence of physical abuse

Before intervention measures for undesirable events are put in place, the incidence of these events must be established. In the case of intentional injuries affecting young children, the actual events are usually not witnessed and are difficult to document. Injuries to children are counted when they are reported to the appropriate agencies. In the United States, these agencies include state and county departments of social services and law enforcement agencies, which collect the reports, investigate them to determine their accuracy, and provide necessary interventions to assure the safety of the child.

States report their data on child abuse to the National Child Abuse and Neglect Data System, which produces consolidated reports for the

United States.[9] The national reporting rate of all forms of child abuse in 1993 was 43 reports per 1000 children. About half of these reports are "substantiated." Physical abuse accounts for about 25% of these cases.

The survey method of Straus and Kantor[6] yielded an incidence of abusive events about four times higher than the incidence of reported physical abuse obtained by counting reports, although both methods reveal astonishingly high incidences. Neither method produces data that classify the types and severity of injury, and, unfortunately, neither the US Public Health Service, state, or local health departments have established data systems that provide this type of information.

Incidence of serious injuries resulting from physical abuse

The precise incidence of serious intentional injuries affecting young children is not known. Some information from organized local trauma services is available that may be utilized to evaluate local programs. Such a trauma system exists in San Diego (Calif) County, a jurisdiction with a total population of about 2.6 million persons and about 0.5 million children. All children with serious injuries who are alive are brought to the Children's Hospital and either admitted or treated and released from the emergency department. While there are precise definitions of injury mechanism, injury severity, and injury type, a number of children who have less serious injuries may not be recognized by the system, although virtually all life-threatening injuries are recorded.

The San Diego Children's Trauma Center sees about 1000 seriously injured children each year. Of these injuries, 4% or about 40 are recognized as nonaccidental trauma or intentional, yielding an incidence for serious abusive injury of about 15 per million total population, or 75 per million children per year. When this incidence is compared with the Straus and Kantor survey data indicating that 14% of children are hit, kicked, or struck with objects each year, the ratio of assaultive events to serious injuries is almost 2000:1.

For jurisdictions of more than 1 million total population, the incidence of serious injuries attributed to child abuse could be a useful marker for the evaluation of prevention programs and is likely to be much less confounded than either the reports of physical abuse to the public social agency or self-reporting in response to telephone surveys. It is a clear marker for the cases that require immediate use of health care resources, but is not an indicator of the overall individual psychological harm and predisposition for later violence that may be induced by early physical abuse. The incidence of injuries caused by child abuse probably relates directly to the overall incidence of violent events occurring in family settings.

Incidence of death from physical abuse

Until recently, the incidence of death of infants and young children from intentional injuries was uncertain because of differences in the definition of intentional injury and because in many jurisdictions autopsies were infrequently performed. The expansion of child death review teams into 40% of US jurisdictions[10] has produced increasingly reliable data in recent years. It now seems that the annual national incidence of deaths from child abuse is about 2000, or about 8 deaths per million total population per year. Because most of these deaths affect very young children, they can be considered a component of infant mortality, in which case they would contribute about 0.5 deaths per 1000 live births per year. These estimates are considerably higher than the 831 deaths for children from birth to 4 years of age recorded as either homicides or of unknown intent by the National Center for Health Statistics for the year 1992 (see Appendix A).

8.1.3 Risk Factors

A number of general risk factors for physical abuse and other adverse events have been identified. The approach to prevention involves altering these risk factors to reduce the future risks for injury.

Income

While the association of poverty with child abuse and all forms of injury is strong, it is far from absolute. Straus and Kantor[6] found that for families with incomes greater than $22 000 a year (1985), there was a 14% incidence of abusive events compared with about 25% for families with incomes less than $9000 a year, although most experienced clinicians have encountered very serious cases in high-income families as well. Furthermore, the move to eliminate poverty as a national policy priority was abandoned in the late 1970s and has never seemed more remote than at present. Such a goal is certainly beyond the resources of the health system. The elimination of poverty is therefore not a realistic short-term preventive strategy.

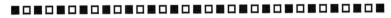
Neighborhood

A federal initiative currently affecting states and localities encourages combining funds from health, justice, and social services to increase prevention services in neighborhoods where possible. Whether this approach reduces injuries is uncertain. It seems more likely to be effective in reducing the public violence than the private violence that occurs in homes; however, it may be helpful for both. It seems reasonable to base preventive services close to the families who may benefit from them and to apply such services under the direction of persons who know the neighborhoods. However, some important lessons were learned during the "war on poverty" when major resources were placed in the hands of persons who had not been trained to use them well.

Alcohol and other drug abuse

Substance abuse, especially alcohol abuse, appears to be a component of many cases of child abuse and other forms of violence in families. Prevention programs that provide support to families must attempt to provide treatment for persons who abuse alcohol and other drugs.

Absence of protective factors: attachment

In the late 1970s, Gray and colleagues[11] demonstrated that serious abusive physical injuries in early infancy could be predicted by relatively inexpensive screening measures and prevented by health care measures that were easily available (at that time). A number of predictive methods were useful, but the most powerful one was the observation of the attachment of parents during the minutes and hours following birth. A simple questionnaire was also effective, although less so. The effective preventive intervention was continuous and attentive health care by a pediatrician supplemented by weekly home visits by a nurse.

This study supported a theory that affectionate attachment of an adult to an infant is highly protective. Theoretically, parents who are attached to their children do not injure them or allow anyone else to do so. Conversely, the absence of attachment puts infants at risk.

Personal history of abuse of a parent or caregiver

The intergenerational transmission of many forms of abusive behaviors toward infants and children is well-established.[12] However, many previously abused parents are competent and nonabusive. Thus, although a history of abuse does not disqualify a person from being a good parent, it suggests the need for some special attention. From a public health standpoint, these observations suggest that children who are recognized as being abused or neglected should receive special attention aimed at blocking the cycle of abuse.

Isolation

Isolation may be the most important single factor predisposing to intentional physical injury. Isolation is mentioned in the early work of Steele and Pollock,[13] in the survey data of Straus and Kantor,[6] and in many other sources. Short-term, event-related isolation of the caregiver as well as long-term social isolation of the family unit are problematic. Thus serious physical injuries by isolated family day care providers are frequently seen, whereas serious physical injuries (intentional or otherwise) are rare in day care centers with multiple caregivers.[14] The reduction of isolation is a complex intervention and a part of every program that has reported benefit.

Victim age

Victim age is a factor related more to severity than to incidence of intentional injury. Infants and young children can easily be killed by adults, but with increasing size the danger of being killed declines. For this reason, many departments of social services sharply focus their interventions on families in which young infants have been abused. This makes sense from the standpoint of the prevention of death and serious injury; however, the long-term societal effects of ongoing physical abuse of older children may be equally deleterious. The psychological vulnerability of *infants* to ongoing physical abuse is another consideration, but little has been written in this area.

Event-related factors

Behaviors that provoke abuse

Event-related factors that lead to inflicted injuries affecting young children are difficult to study. Because abusive events occur in isolation, most of the time the only person who knows what happened is the person who inflicted the injury. Accounts given by abusers of events related to injuries are notoriously unreliable even after legal risks have passed. Information from confessions indicates that many cases involve some behavior on the part of the infant or child that provokes the attack. Generally the behavior is one that is fairly common, if not typical for the age of the victim, such as crying or enuresis. Therefore, the pathway to prevention must include informing parents and caregivers that these behaviors are normal for their infant and suggesting responses that are not abusive. Such anticipatory guidance is suggested in Schmitt's victim-blaming title, "The Seven Deadly Sins of Childhood."[15] Anticipatory guidance as a method for preventing inflicted injuries seems to be good in theory, although it has not been systematically studied.

Immediate stressors

A fairly common event preceding abuse is some type of abandonment by a partner or caregiver, such as a mother who is left alone with a crying infant after an argument with her husband. Here again, anticipatory guidance seems to be one of the few avenues of prevention.

8.1.4 Intervention Strategies

Prevention of specific forms of abuse

Shaken infant syndrome (SIS)

This term, coined by Caffey, describes a specific form of physical abuse.[16] Caffey himself and other writers considered a theory that many instances of SIS occurred because parents and caregivers did not know that shaking an infant was dangerous. This theory of ignorance is almost entirely untested, but has nevertheless given rise to many programs that attempt to educate the public about the dangers of shaking infants.[17] To date, no evidence exists that these programs are effective.

Burns

Children are sometimes intentionally burned with hot water, curling irons, pressing irons, cigarette lighters, and cigarettes. Feldman et al[18] found that 28% of children hospitalized for tap water scald burns were the victims of intentional scalding. It has been pointed out by the American Academy of Pediatrics that scalds (whether intentional or not) can be greatly reduced, in severity if not number, if the maximum temperature of hot water at the tap is adjusted to 120°F (see chapter 11).

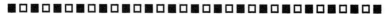

Abuse by various implements

Implements used for child abuse are common objects found in most homes or available to most persons. For this reason, in contrast to vectors of unintentional injury, the modification of implements offers little opportunity for reducing the incidence or severity of injury.

Sadistic abuse

The diagnosis of sadistic physical abuse is considered when evidence exists that the person who inflicts the injuries derives positive reinforcement from the process, particularly when the abuse occurs repeatedly over time and the injuries are multiple. Perhaps one in 10 serious inflicted physical injury cases shows these features, and many involve fatalities. Opportunities for primary prevention are limited. Intervention can be provided in families with mentally ill or drug-abusing parents. Child care workers should be carefully screened for previous legal and/or mental problems. Nonfatally injured victims of sadistic abuse must be recognized by health care and social service personnel.

An approach to primary prevention: risk assessment plus family support

In recent years, empirical evidence has been accumulating to support the hypothesis that a combination of relatively simple risk assessment procedures and acceptable and affordable interventions may prevent a great deal of physical abuse. The feasibility of this approach was demonstrated on a small scale by Gray et al[11] soon after it was first described by Kempe.[19,20] Sia described the first statewide application of these principles in Hawaii.[21]

During the 1980s, small parent-aide programs appeared in many communities that provided home visiting services to families at risk for a variety of problems. Many were inspired by the writings of Kempe, but others eschewed the "medical model" and were not connected to health systems of any kind. Because these programs were not systematically evaluated, their effectiveness was never demonstrated.

In 1986, Olds and Henderson described a randomized trial of home visitations that demonstrated a reduction in verified child abuse and unintentional injuries and improved health care utilization.[22] In 1992, following additional study, Olds published a review paper discussing the technical and policy issues related to home visitation and the prevention of abuse.[23] He pointed out that well-designed home visiting programs prevented *many* adverse events. Such programs tended to reduce smoking and drinking during pregnancy, to increase the intervals between pregnancies, and to reduce *all* forms of childhood injuries including intentional injuries. Olds demonstrated cost-benefits only for programs that utilized nurses for home visitors and for programs that targeted families with significant risk factors such as poverty and young maternal age.

The rigorous approach by Olds, which proved that home visiting could be cost-beneficial and prevent many problems, gave great impetus to the development of policies to apply these methods more widely. Simultaneously, the state of Hawaii moved to establish the first statewide program for home visitation, called Hawaii Healthy Start. The Hawaii program has been in place about 7 years (as of 1996) and is being rigorously evaluated by several investigators. The Hawaii program, like many of the small parent-aide programs that began during the 1970s and 1980s, utilizes paraprofessional home visitors instead of nurses, but includes the medical home component advocated by Sia.[21] The high level of interest in home visiting and related family support programs led to the publication of *The Future of Children*,[24] in which 12 papers explore various aspects of current policy and home visitation practice.

Although a number of methodological questions about the content of family support programs remain unresolved, the general principles of program design are well established, and research is in progress to address these unresolved issues.

Primary prevention program guidelines

The following guidelines are suggested for programs to prevent child abuse, neglect, and intentional and unintentional injuries and to improve many other health outcomes.

Target services

Although the idea of universal service available to all families with young children has great appeal, currently it may not be economically feasible to implement such programs. For this reason, programs should target high-risk groups, families, and individuals.

Criteria for services

All programs need protocols that list risk factors and indicate which families qualify for services. About 10% of families having babies is a reasonable estimate for planning purposes.

Streamlined risk assessment

Risk assessment should be a relatively simple, economical process and should be applied as early as possible during a pregnancy (although late prenatal care is a risk factor that should be included). Income, neighborhood, maternal age, parity, alcohol or other drug use, smoking, and social network can be assessed quickly. After delivery, birth weight and gestational age become factors. Maternal attachment behavior can be observed by delivery room and postpartum care nurses after patient education and seems to be an important determining factor of risk.

Standards

All programs should attempt to meet standards that ensure effectiveness. The task of disseminating standards and accrediting training programs has been assumed by the National Committee for the Prevention of Child Abuse (NCPCA), 332 Michigan Ave, Suite 1600, Chicago, IL 60604.

Provision of preventive services

Engagement

Generally, family support service programs are voluntary, and families must choose to participate in them. When the choice is voluntary and when the home visitor is well-trained and experienced, well over 90% of families are accepting of services.

Types of services

Three basic classes of service are present in all promising programs: home visitations, parents' groups, and parent education. The home visitor facilitates all other services, including the vital service of assuring that the client family is connected to a continuous source of health care. The home visitor must be able to deal with many issues of caring for infants and children. Many programs have required that home visitors be parents. The content of home visits addresses the different needs of each family, but almost always involves issues of family life and parenting.

In addition to the three basic services, many families benefit by connection to additional services, the most generally useful of which may be developmental enhancement services (infant stimulation and early intervention services) that involve the parent in the process. Many families also need transportation, especially for purposes of health care, but sometimes also for general household needs. Child care services may also be an important consideration in the prevention of abuse.

The financing of prevention programs

State and federal funds

The Hawaii program has been primarily funded from state appropriations administered through the Department of Health. In many states small programs have been funded through state "Children's Trust Funds," which often utilize birth certificate fees. Few, if any, states will be able to establish full statewide programs on the Hawaii model from that source. However, in some cases federal funds designated to states as "Family Preservation" funds can be used for prevention services. A limiting factor in funding programs has been their past conceptualization as child abuse prevention programs; however, recent studies indicating that a large number of adverse health events are also prevented by these services may remove this barrier.

Health funding streams

There are two major reasons why family support programs as described here should be linked to health funding streams or appropriated monies earmarked for health services. The first is that most of the benefits achieved (including reduced numbers of injuries) are health benefits. The second is that the health components of the programs contribute significantly to the success of the programs. Many programs successfully operate from hospitals, and all programs should be closely linked to both primary health care for the clients and to public health departments for quality control and assessment of effects.

Managed care

As more and more health care becomes prepaid, prevention programs that utilize multiple services should be brought into the managed care funding streams and should be administered by managed care organizations. Based on 1995 information, it seems likely that managed care organizations that have contracted to provide care to Medicaid clients will save money by establishing a home visitation program based on one of the models described in this chapter that meets NCPCA standards.

8.1.5 Recommendations for Pediatricians

1. Pediatricians should be aware of the risk factors for child abuse (prematurity, disability, isolation, substance abuse, spousal abuse, a parent who was a victim of child abuse) in order to identify, monitor, and appropriately counsel such families.
2. Pediatricians should remain knowledgeable about, and responsive to, the signs and symptoms of child maltreatment.
3. Pediatricians should inquire about disciplinary strategies used by parents and should promote nonassaultive methods of discipline.
4. Pediatricians should become aware of, and take advantage of, social service agencies, child protection teams, and child protective agencies in their communities in order to protect children who have been subject to abuse or who are at high risk of abuse.
5. Pediatricians should be aware of, and comply with, state reporting requirements for suspected child abuse and neglect.
6. Pediatricians should support and serve as a resource to primary prevention programs such as home visitation programs and advocate that they are carefully designed and properly evaluated.

8.2 Suicide

8.2.1 Scope of the Problem and Risk Factors

Suicide is one of the three leading causes of death among adolescents and young adults, the other two being unintentional injury and homicide. At least some — perhaps most — deaths from suicide are preventable. In 1992, more than 2100 children and teenagers took their own lives in the United States, and an estimated half-million teenagers attempt suicide and survive annually. Of particular concern is the increase in teenage suicide rates in recent decades. Furthermore, suicide is emerging as a preteen problem as well. In 1992, there were 304 reported suicides among 10- to 14-year-olds. This section on suicide highlights the major issues and provides relevant sources[25,26] for further information.

Attempting suicide vs committing suicide

When all ages are considered, including adults and older persons, there are 10 suicide attempts for every committed suicide, but for 15- to 25-year-olds, the ratio is 100 to 1. Thus, there is much interest among adolescent health providers in the study and treatment of adolescents who attempt suicide. It is particularly important not to dismiss attempted suicides as merely gestures by individuals seeking attention. Suicide attempts not taken seriously may result in the adolescent trying a more lethal method the next time an attempt is made. Therefore, clinicians should avoid using the term "gesture" when discussing the prevention of suicide with families.

It is a bad prognostic indicator if the family fails to take an attempt seriously. Any suicide attempt is an indicator of serious psychological difficulty, either within the family or for the adolescent in some aspect of his or her life. Suicide attempts place a strain on families as well as others who are close to or know the adolescent. Parents, siblings, grandparents, and close friends are most affected by suicides, but students in an entire school can experience the consequences of such events. These reactions to suicide attempts must be channeled productively to assure that the individual and family receive help, and interventions should at least be considered at the school and community level. A first suicide attempt identifies the young person as statistically at risk for subsequent attempts and for later death by suicide.[27] A suicide attempt in adolescence indicates the need for psychosocial intervention for the adolescent and parents. Prompt psychiatric evaluation is usually important, often followed by psychotherapy, family counseling, and possibly a trial of antidepressant medication for the adolescent.

Gender

In adolescence, three times as many females attempt suicide as males. This ratio is reversed, however, for successful suicides, with three times as many males committing suicide. The higher death rate among males results from more lethal methods being used, such as shooting or hanging themselves; females tend to choose less lethal methods, such as taking an overdose of drugs or cutting their wrists. It is unclear to what degree the choice of methods by males represents "style" as opposed to a deeper wish to succeed in killing themselves.

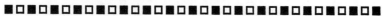
Frequency/incidence

The incidence rate of suicide increases with age and is highest in older persons (Fig 8.1, p 163). Death by suicide is thus less common in adolescence and young adulthood than later in life. However, the incidence rate of suicide attempts, unlike the steadily rising curve of successful suicides, peaks between 15 and 25 years of age and then falls off. Because suicide attempts in adolescents and young adults have such a great impact on public consciousness, it is often a surprise to learn that the rate of successful suicides is lower in this age group than in later life. Nevertheless, the high numbers of attempted suicides in young people emphasize how many teenagers are crying for help.

8.2.2 Intervention Strategies

Efforts to prevent suicide among adolescents have focused in at least five general areas[28]: (1) basic education about suicide directed to the general public through such avenues as high school classes and television programming, (2) screening programs to identify individuals at high risk for suicide, (3) training of health care and community providers who serve as gatekeepers for intervention services, (4) treatment programs for those who have attempted suicide, and (5) efforts to address firearm availability as a risk factor for suicide.

Basic education about suicide

Educational programs about suicide generally teach about the extent of the problem, the warning signs, and how to obtain help for yourself or for someone known to be at risk. Such programs aimed at general populations are of questionable value. When measured in terms of attitudes, these types of programs have had disappointing results.[29] Efforts to measure change in suicide rates following such interventions are burdened by many statistical and methodologic difficulties resulting from low incidence rates and insufficient sample size. Efforts to measure effects on rates of attempted suicides are hampered because of the high number of attempts that are concealed. Some studies suggest that well-intended suicide prevention telecasts may be followed by a temporary increase in adolescent suicide rates.[30,31]

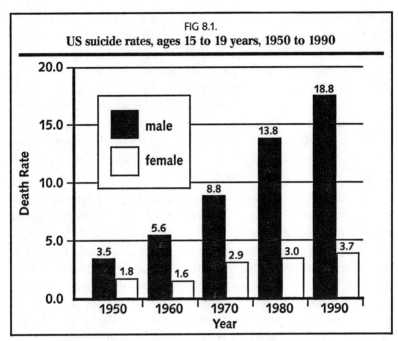

FIG 8.1.
US suicide rates, ages 15 to 19 years, 1950 to 1990

Data from the National Center for Health Statistics.[28] Rates are per 100 000 persons.

Screening programs

Screening tools, such as questionnaires and structured interviews, to select adolescents at high risk for suicide are currently being developed.[29] Identification of a population of troubled adolescents (who are impulsive, abuse substances, and have conduct disorders), which statistically contains adolescents at higher risk for suicide attempts, may be a useful effort. However, the population of adolescents with conduct disorders is very large, and therapeutic work with that group has, in general, been discouraging.[31] There are reliable screening tools available to the clinician to identify depression, although these have been greatly underutilized, particularly because depression is common among adolescents.[32(p177)]

Use of gatekeepers

Adolescents who have attempted suicide frequently report that they had seen a physician during the weeks and months just prior to the attempt.[33] Often such visits are precipitated by somatic complaints, such as headaches or abdominal pain, where underlying depression, distress, or suicidal thoughts were not overt and needed to be discovered through skillful clinical assessment. Similarly, among the behaviors associated with risk for suicide are truancy, failure in school, drug abuse, social isolation, and delinquency. Adolescents involved in such behaviors often come to the attention of health professionals in the community as well as to school guidance personnel, human services providers, and individuals working within the juvenile justice system. Prevention of suicide requires that professionals identify and appropriately refer young people at risk.

For health care providers, the interview with an adolescent should include screening for such at-risk behaviors and include questioning regarding mood and thoughts about suicidal behavior. Such questioning is neither complex nor time consuming. Inquiries should be made as to whether teenagers sometimes find themselves feeling especially sad and what circumstances are precipitating those feelings. Have there ever been thoughts that maybe "life sometimes seems more trouble than it's worth?" Health care providers may then ask the following questions of the adolescent if they are receiving affirmative answers. "Have you ever *thought* of maybe doing something about that? Have you ever actually done anything? How about right now, as we speak, or earlier today, or earlier this week? *Might* you actually *do* something to hurt yourself. Today? Tomorrow? This week?" If the answers are yes, immediate action must be taken, which may include hospitalization or obtaining an urgent mental health consultation with someone experienced in evaluating suicide-prone adolescents, or both. Confidentiality restrictions against informing parents do not apply for suicide ideation. Sometimes an experienced outpatient psychotherapist is willing to accept responsibility for the patient, but the potential severity of such situations requires great caution.

In such directed interviews, the full range of responses should be anticipated — from young people who have never thought of hurting themselves to adolescents who have attempted suicide and require immediate psychiatric attention and hospitalization. Between these extremes are adolescents who admit to thinking about suicide but who do not appear to be at serious risk. Once identified, those adolescents should be referred for mental health services, often with their families. Direct inquiries regarding thoughts of self-injury do not increase the risk of self-injury, but failure to ask direct questions may result in missed opportunities for intervention and prevention for at-risk adolescents.

Prevention of repeated attempts at suicide

One of the most important opportunities for preventive efforts against suicide occurs immediately after a survived attempt. This is a critical time for two reasons. First, the risk for future attempts is clear. The rate of successful suicide for those who attempt suicide again is 2% to 5%, compared with .01% for the general population. Furthermore, a history of previous attempts has been noted to be as high as 40% in those who commit suicide.[34] Second, this is a time of vulnerability, when the patient may be particularly open or responsive to intervention efforts. Hospitalizing individuals who have attempted suicide makes them a "captive audience" for further assessment, mental health consultation, and development of a therapeutic plan. It also places the individual in a safe environment, greatly reducing the immediate risk for further suicide attempts.

Hospitalization may be either in a general pediatric unit or in a psychiatric service, depending on local resources. The main requisites of hospitalization are the ability to maintain the safety of the patient (preventing elopement and/or further attempts in the hospital), the ability to treat the medical condition after the attempt (overdose, injury), and the availability of mental health specialists (social workers and/or psychiatrists) to conduct a psychosocial evaluation of the adolescent and the family to develop a therapeutic plan. Hospitalization after a suicide attempt can also be a prime opportunity to provide brief psychotherapy and/or initiate longer term therapy.[35,36]

Hospitalization should focus on several key issues. Those adolescents at continuing risk for suicide need to be identified and transferred to a psychiatric hospital. For those patients who regret the attempt and/or claim no further risk, it is important to address the seriousness of their behavior and assure that a follow-up plan is in place — who to call for help — should the impulse to commit suicide recur. The plan should also include appropriate mental health follow-up. It should not be assumed that the risk is resolved.

In-hospital assessment and intervention must also focus on the family. Family stresses and recurrent strains in parent-adolescent relationships are typically critical proximal factors leading to suicide attempts.

Adolescents often feel disconnected, misunderstood, or unappreciated by their parents, whether justified by parental behavior and attitudes or not. Interventions need to address these feelings and identify and respond to conflict areas where they exist.

All therapeutic interventions initiated in the hospital *must* be linked to a clear plan for follow-up, whether on an inpatient or outpatient basis. Follow-through of this plan must be monitored and reinforced.

Firearms and adolescent suicide

To date, restriction of access to firearms has unfortunately not been a major focus of suicide prevention efforts despite empirical evidence of its effectiveness.[28] Guns are twice as likely to be found in homes of adolescents who commit suicide as in homes of those who attempt suicide.[37] Two thirds of the suicides in 15- through 19-year-olds are accomplished with firearms (Table 8.1). Use of firearms accounted for 81% of the increase in successful suicides in this age group that occurred between 1980 and 1992.[38] The presence of a firearm can make the difference between a successful or unsuccessful attempt. If no firearm is available, the adolescent may choose a less lethal method or may go through an episode of anger and depression without attempting suicide. This is particularly important given the transient nature of anger and distress frequently seen in adolescence. Adults, however, more typically attempt suicide in the context of a more enduring state of depression.

TABLE 8.1.
Means of Suicide in Pediatrics, United States, 1992*

Means	10- to 14-Year-Olds No. (%)	15- to 19-Year-Olds No. (%)
Firearms	172 (56.6)	1251 (67.7)
Suffocation and hanging	96 (31.6)	333 (18.0)
Poisoning: solid and liquid	26 (8.6)	121 (6.6)
Poisoning: gas and vapor	4 (1.3)	71 (3.8)
Falls	1 (0.3)	28 (1.5)
Other	5 (1.6)	43 (2.3)
Total	**304 (100)**	**1847 (99.9)**

*Data from the National Center for Health Statistics, courtesy of Lois Fingerhut.

When working with adolescents identified as at risk for suicide, clinicians should take the initiative and parents should be *strongly* directed to remove all guns from the home. (Likewise, toxic medications should be secured.) Data have shown that firearms thought to be locked up and secured were involved in adolescent suicides as frequently as firearms identified as not locked up. It may not be possible to transform the mindset or mental attitude of high-risk adolescents, but it is certainly possible to remove firearms in the home.

8.2.3 Recommendations for Pediatricians

1. Utilize health supervision visits to screen for depression and suicidal ideation in adolescent patients. Such screening should be done privately.
2. Be alert for adolescents at risk for self-harm during their visits for illness. Recognize that depressed patients often present with somatic rather than affective complaints. Large percentages of adolescents who attempt suicide have had recent contact with a health professional.
3. Refer patients at risk for suicide to the appropriate mental health professional for further diagnosis and treatment. Timeliness and monitoring of these referrals are crucial.
4. If firearms are kept in the home, encourage parents to keep them locked up or to remove them, particularly in situations involving impulsive, depression-prone persons, or families with histories of depression, substance abuse, alcohol abuse, or other mental health and behavioral difficulties.
5. Following a suicide attempt, exercise your authority and influence to ensure that the patient and family take the situation seriously, and define a plan for follow-up intervention that is monitored.
6. Prescribe medications judiciously, considering the potential for intentional overdose for at-risk patients and siblings.
7. Serve as an educational resource to community groups and schools about adolescent suicide and its prevention.

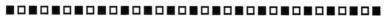
8.3 Peer Violence

8.3.1 Scope of the Problem

Perhaps no segment in our society is touched as extensively and repeatedly by violence as our youth. Homicide is the principal cause of injury death in the first year of life and the second leading cause of death for all young people in America. It is the principal cause of death for poor Americans younger than 19 years. It is also the leading cause of death in young African-American men and women. Between 1985 and 1991 the homicide rate for 15- to 19-year-old boys increased 154%, surpassing for the first time the rates for 25- to 29-year-olds and 30- to 34-year-olds.[39] Of 12- to 19-year-olds, 9.7% of boys and 3.1% of girls report having been the victim of a violent crime (crimes involving use of physical force) in the last year (the highest rate for any age group). A 1993 survey of high school seniors found that 16.4% reported having been purposefully injured by another person in the last year, and 31% reported having been threatened with injury. Nationally, 22% of adolescents report a fear of being attacked at school, and 14% fear going to and from school. Six percent avoid places at school because of fear of violence.[40]

Adolescents are also perpetrators of violence. One in five adolescents reports having engaged in a serious fight in school or at work in the last year, and 13% report having hurt someone badly enough that bandages or a physician's attention was required. Between 1984 and 1993 the number of violent crimes committed by those younger than 18 years increased by 67.6% (in 1993 there were 119 678 arrests of adolescents for violent crimes). The rate of arrests for murder in boys younger than 18 years increased between 1992 and 1993 by 13.5% (2966 in 1993), and in girls the rate increased by 17.9% (184 in 1993).[40]

Although a high proportion of youth participate as perpetrators or victims of violence, many more witness violence. This exposure may be important for the mental health of children and adolescents and as an independent risk factor for future perpetration. A recent study of 225 African-Americans 11 to 19 years of age living in urban public housing in Augusta, Ga, found that self-reported use of violence was strongly associated with exposure to violence and personal victimization.[41]

Witnessing of violence is widespread and begins early in life. The impact of violence in the media is reviewed later in this chapter. Other, more immediate exposures are also frequent. Of a selection of fifth-graders in New Orleans, La, 98% reported hearing about violence and 91% had witnessed violence. Parents of first- and second-graders in Washington, DC, reported that 84% of their children had witnessed violence and 21% had been victims of violence. In Baltimore, Md, 42% of adolescents had seen someone shot, and 23% had witnessed a murder. In a Maryland resort community, 75% of adolescents reported either having witnessed or fallen victim to violence, or knew someone who was a victim of violence. In suburban Philadelphia, 43% of sixth-graders reported having seen someone beaten up, and 3% had witnessed a murder. One in 50 American children has a parent who is in prison.

8.3.2 Risk Factors

Most of the work that has been done to identify risk factors for violence has focused on perpetration of violent acts. This is in part because the field of "violence research" was, until recently, principally the province of criminal justice professionals who were more concerned with crime and "delinquency," than with injury or victimization. Recent work from the field of public health has also provided a focus on "fighting behaviors," where violent injury results from mutual conflict rather than predatory behavior. While fighting behaviors likely result in many serious injuries, it is not yet clear what factors have the most impact on fighting. International reports suggest that fighting is common in adolescence. What is unusual in the United States is that adolescent fighting results in death. This is clearly related to the use of weapons, particularly firearms, by youth in this country. The issue of firearm use is addressed in chapter 12.

Unlike the literature on fighting behaviors, which is in its early development, literature on delinquency has matured over the past 3 decades. Researchers who have studied delinquency have identified a long list of factors that predispose children and adolescents to the perpetration of violent acts and law-breaking.[42] These factors are shown in Table 8.2, p 170. While this list may be useful for the pediatrician, only a few of the factors are likely to be particularly relevant in the office setting. Others may be influenced by advocacy efforts.[43]

TABLE 8.2.
Factors Predisposing Children and Adolescents to the Perpetration of Violent Acts and Law-Breaking

Biology	Genetics, fetal environment, birth events, brain injury, hormonal effects
Social/economic factors	Poverty, racism, economic opportunity, cultural values of fighting
Parenting	Discipline, corporal punishment, abuse, effectiveness of patrolling/monitoring
Home environment	Witnessing violence, television, crowding
Behavioral factors	Peer group, substance use, failure in school, conflict resolution skills, life skills
Environmental factors	Lighting, architecture, policing, hot weather
Alternatives	Employment, recreation, school hours, prison
Weapons	Availability, ability to conceal, lethality
Deterrents	Legal penalties, law enforcement
Other factors	

The area of the biology of violence has received growing interest in the past two decades. As brain chemistry is better elucidated and pharmacologic manipulation becomes possible in coming years, it will be increasingly important for the pediatrician to understand the precise physiologic etiology of violence. Currently, scientists have a concept of how dopaminergic and serotonergic neurons affect animal behavior related to aggression, but human models are still crude. Studies of the genetics of aggression have as yet proven to be unrevealing.[42] It has been suggested that "antisocial tendencies" may be more common in certain, rare genetic syndromes, but few chromosomal patterns have been identified. Rather, recent work suggests that there may be some inheritability of aggressiveness or predisposition toward delinquency, but the genetics of this phenomenon is not understood. Given the lack of current knowledge, one ought to be extremely cautious in reaching conclusions about the genetics of behavior.

Brain injury, particularly that affecting the limbic areas, may have an impact on aggressive behavior, although the few human studies of brain injury and violence have not been conclusive. The long-held belief that seizure disorder is associated with violent or aggressive behavior has been investigated, but results are mixed. The elimination of other factors associated with epilepsy has been particularly difficult. Factors such

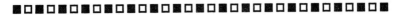
as lead exposure, birth trauma, and head injury also may have an impact on aggressiveness.[43] Evidence from both longer term follow-up of exposed children and those who have suffered severe injury suggests that this association is valid, although no methods exist to predict which children will be at highest risk for violent behavior after a brain insult. Also, this and other biological risk factors may contribute a relatively minor portion of the total risk for violent behavior.

Social and economic factors have long been associated with violent behaviors. The many stresses associated with poverty and the often coincident impacts of racism, joblessness, and poor economic life prospects have been linked to violence. These factors are often used to explain the higher rates of violence in urban areas. Many well-done empirical analyses have shown that the correlation often described in the popular press between race itself and violence disappears when economic factors are accounted for.

Perhaps the areas with the greatest interest to pediatricians include parenting and the home environment. Many studies link delinquency with parental styles of discipline that are either coercive and harsh or lacking in positive reinforcements.[44]

Similarly, parents who do not monitor their children's behavior and those whose adolescents spend a great deal of unsupervised time out of the home have been shown to have children who are more likely to engage in delinquent acts.[45] In long-term cohort studies, both the regular use of corporal punishment and the witnessing of parental violence (separate from child abuse) have been found independently to predispose to later violent behaviors.[44]

The impact of associating with a peer group that engages in antisocial activities is a key factor in adolescence. A series of cohort studies following up children from age 7 to 17 years in three US cities in the 1980s found participation in a delinquent peer group to be the strongest time-linked predictor of later delinquent behaviors.[46] These same studies confirmed often-reported associations between substance abuse and failure in school and later delinquency. Similarly, early delinquency predicts substance abuse and failure in school. Lack of skills, which is often cited as a reason why youths engage in peer violence, has not been empirically shown to have an impact on levels of violent activity or delinquency. This cause is included in the list because it is frequently mentioned and a locus for intervention with high-risk youths.

Studies of crime involving adults have shown that a range of situational factors in the environment correlate with violent crime, including poor outdoor lighting, building construction that creates places to hide or shadows, the absence of a visible police presence, and temperature (violent events are more common in the summer months in temperate climates). The way in which a number of these factors affect crime and violent events seems obvious.

While unemployment has been shown to increase the rate of delinquency, youth in cohort studies who are employed have been found to have higher rates of delinquent offenses. In fact, as the number of hours worked increases, the amount of criminal activity increases.[46] While these two findings about employment appear contradictory, it has been hypothesized that unemployment rates are markers for poverty and disadvantage at a community level, whereas adolescent employment likely reflects being a school dropout, which strongly correlates with delinquency.

A few studies have looked systematically at the role of recreation in preventing delinquency; historically recreational activities were considered an empirical method to prevent youth criminal activity. More work is needed to link the promotion of recreational activities and crime prevention. Likewise, other activities that youths engage in have been thought to reduce the rate of delinquency. Again, little carefully researched evidence has been generated to substantiate this assertion.

As discussed elsewhere in this manual, firearms have been found to correlate with increasing levels of the most serious violent injuries. In general, youth involvement with firearms increases with age, with knives becoming popular slightly earlier than firearms. Studies on delinquency have shown that possession of a legal firearm (ie, one obtained from a parent for sporting purposes or protection) does not correlate with violent crime. However, possession of an illegal firearm correlates strongly with violent criminal activities.[46]

8.3.3 Intervention Strategies

Many interventions have been tried to reduce the toll of peer violence on children and youth. These strategies have generally focused on one or more of the previously described risk factors. Perhaps the most pop-

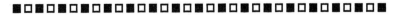
ular interventions among health professionals have involved school curricula to teach conflict resolution, peer mediation, or life skills. These curricula have been developed for all grade levels, though those focusing on high school or middle school have been more common than curricula for elementary school.[47,48] Data that evaluate these curricula are sparse. While a few curricula have been found to reduce reported fighting or school suspension for a short time after their implementation, rarely have they been found to have an impact on violent injuries occurring either within or outside the school building.[49]

Juvenile justice approaches have focused on incarceration and probation. The few controlled evaluation trials have shown high rates of repeated offending, and there have not been good data to suggest that common policies that stress deterrence make a difference for youth violence.

Some success has been found with parent-based interventions for chronic young juvenile offenders (7 to 11 years of age). These approaches have stressed teaching parents how to monitor their children's behavior and how to set limits effectively using both positive and negative reinforcement. Since the mid-1970s data have shown that these approaches can reduce rates of repeat offending in the short term. The longer term impact of parent training has not been as positive.

Weapons-related policy interventions (eg, gun control) generally have not been evaluated by looking specifically at their impact on youth violence. School-based metal detectors have been widely implemented to reduce weapon carrying in schools. While these strategies have not been implemented in a controlled way, quasi-experimental data from New York suggest that the use of metal detectors may not have an impact on either weapon carrying or on violence and fighting. However, students report feeling safer in schools with metal detectors than in schools without.

Community-based efforts have been established during the past decade in a number of urban and suburban areas. These interventions have combined a number of modalities, including conflict resolution and other curricula, town watches, community policing, interagency conferencing, and juvenile justice policies. Only anecdotal data, however, have suggested the positive impacts from these interventions.

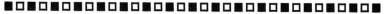
8.3.4 Recommendations for Pediatricians

The scarcity of sound outcome-related data may be discouraging to the pediatrician who wishes to make an impact on peer violence. However, office-based intervention trials or experiments where pediatricians combine efforts with others to have an impact on youth violence are not included in the previously described programs. It is important to recognize that a number of the factors that may increase the risk of violent or delinquent behaviors are frequently discovered during pediatric visits and may be influenced through office-based intervention.[50]

Parenting factors

Poor parenting practices, particularly those related to supervision and discipline in early childhood, are important in promoting delinquency. Pediatricians often encounter parents who do not have knowledge of appropriate disciplinary practices or those who use only harsh punishment (physical, verbal, or both), rather than a balance of punishment and reward. Either office-based or community-based interventions to teach parenting skills related to effective supervision and balanced disciplinary practices may hold promise as a means of preventing future delinquent behaviors.

Similarly, identifying families in which children witness violence, particularly domestic violence, and strongly urging counseling for the parents and supportive intervention and counseling for the child appear to be effective interventions.[51,52]

Biologic factors

Given the lack of strong evidence of a link between specific biologic factors and long-term violent activities, recommendations for intervention must be made with great caution. However, sufficient evidence exists for pediatricians to at least anticipate and monitor for aggressive behaviors in children who have experienced brain insults, including children with fetal or birth trauma, those exposed to toxins including lead, and those with brain injury. Pediatricians need to be vigilant for early evidence of aggressive behavior in these children and can work with parents to assist them in managing these children with patience and understanding. At the same time, unnecessary labeling of aggressive behavior must be avoided for fear that parental expectation may lead to undue punishment or a sense of futility.

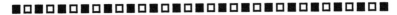
Behavioral factors

The link between delinquent activity and antisocial peer groups, substance abuse, and failure in school has been well established. They are key predictors of adolescent mental health, and the American Academy of Pediatrics (AAP) has gone far in advocating better training for pediatricians in managing failure in school and substance abuse. Techniques for identifying these problems and working through interdisciplinary approaches to assist families in combating them may result in a reduction in violent activities as well. The special factor of antisocial peers, which is independently linked to failure in school and substance abuse, needs to be particularly highlighted, and exploration of peer groups should be part of the routine history taking of school-age and adolescent patients.

Alternatives to violence

The value of recreation for children has been a key belief of child health professionals for many years. Both the value of exercise and the mental health impacts of play have been clear in the pediatric literature. As public sector expenditures are reduced, it will be important for pediatric professionals, particularly those serving disadvantaged communities, to advocate for adequate recreational opportunities for children and youth.

Social and economic factors

Pediatricians have historically been advocates for the welfare of children and families. The strong links between disadvantage and violence reinforce the need to strengthen advocacy efforts. It has been suggested that delinquency and youth homicide are largely diseases of poverty.

A century ago, the principal killer of adolescents and young adults was tuberculosis. It was known to be a problem that was strongly linked to poverty and disadvantage, more common in crowded communities and urban areas. Washington, DC, had some of the highest rates of tuberculosis up to the late 1970s. It was not until the 1950s that we had effective antimicrobial treatment for tuberculosis, yet through public health and office-based identification and education the rates of tuberculosis fell dramatically through the early decades of this century.

By the year 2000, violence may well be the principal killer of young people in this nation. It is anticipated that more young people will soon be dying from firearm injuries than from motor vehicle crashes. Violence is concentrated among the disadvantaged and is particularly prevalent in crowded, urban communities. Washington, DC, has the highest rates of youth homicide of any city in the nation. Although medications that alter brain chemistry to prevent violent behaviors are not available, pediatricians, in partnership with nurses, social workers, mental health professionals, police, attorneys, educators, and parents, will have an impact on this problem. The many dimensions of violent behavior need to be understood to' achieve long-term success in its reduction over the next several decades.

8.3.5 Resources

Children's Defense Fund
25 E Street, NW
Washington, DC
202-628-8787
Good source for statistics, information on local programs, up-to-date reports on congressional action regarding juvenile justice.

The Center for the Study and Prevention of Violence
University of Colorado, Boulder Campus
Box 442
Boulder, CO 80309-0442
303-492-1032
303-433-3297 (fax)
Information on programs and curricula that have been tried and are available around the nation for violence prevention. Articles are available on various topics related to youth violence and its prevention.

National Crime Prevention Council
1700 K Street, NW, Second Floor
Washington, DC 20006-3817
202-466-6272
202-296-1356 (fax)
Resources, materials, and information about youth crime prevention nationwide are available. Good source of brochures and information for parents and community groups, including posters, leaflets, and newsletters.

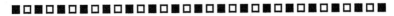

8.4 Media Violence

8.4.1 Scope of the Problem

Children and adolescents in America are victims of violence, not only at home, at school, and in the streets, but also in front of the television set or video arcade screen. By watching television alone, young people will witness 12 000 violent acts each year, or more than 200 000 violent acts before they reach age 18 years.[53] As one critic observes: "Our entertainment, like our society, is the most violent in the world. Somehow the idea has taken hold that bodies shot to pieces, women stalked and sliced, murder, and terror are entertainment."[54]

Numerous well-designed studies from many disciplines confirm the association between heavy viewing of media violence in childhood and subsequent violent or antisocial behavior. Although there are many causes of violence — poverty, racism, firearm availability, and family dysfunction — media violence may be the most easily remediable.

Because of its ubiquitous nature, television is the most concerning and well-studied of the media. As Gerbner notes, television is our cultural storyteller, "that ritual myth builder," that teaches us right from wrong, defines our heroes, and is "totally involving, compelling, and institutionalizing as the mainstream of the socializing process."[55] Television violence teaches and models to children and adolescents that violence is the first solution to a conflict, violence is frequently rewarded, violence is entertaining, and violence is justified, since both the "good guys and bad guys" use it. Television violence is common and without consequence; there is no pain, suffering, or remorse. Although both men and women commit violent acts on the screen, men are far more likely to be powerful, aggressive, and successful with violence. Women and minority characters frequently are cast as victims of violence. American media glamorize weapons, especially firearms, offering dangerous scenes of deadly, desirable behaviors to children and adolescents.

Viewers of heavy amounts of television violence tend to develop these dysfunctional patterns of thought or behavior:

- Aggressive or violent behavior toward others
- A view of the world as hostile ("mean and scary world")

- A greater acceptance of violence (desensitization)
- An increased appetite for violence

Evidence exists that television may also offer scripts of violent behavior to a few particularly vulnerable viewers, for example, copy cat murders and suicides after programs with graphic violent content. More research is needed in this critical area.

Some children and adolescents are more susceptible than others to violence in the media, specifically, those who experience or witness violence in their homes or neighborhoods. Violence on television tends to reinforce the violence elsewhere in the lives of these vulnerable young people. Additionally, young children (<8 years old) have difficulty separating fantasy from reality; therefore scripted, repetitive violence in the media may more profoundly affect this group.

Prime-time dramatic shows contain 5 to 12 violent episodes per hour. Cartoons, a favorite viewing pastime of young children, have even more violence — 20 or more acts per hour.[56] Promotions for upcoming features on television are among the most violent offerings and are often aired during children's peak viewing hours. The frequency of violent acts on television is a powerful influence on viewers.

8.4.2 Research Support

Thousands of studies in several fields and reports from the US Surgeon General, the National Institute of Mental Health, and the American Psychological Association have reached the identical conclusion: violence on television is associated with subsequent violent behavior in children. As one researcher recently concluded: "There can no longer be any doubt that heavy exposure to televised violence is one of the causes of aggressive behavior, crime, and violence in society. The evidence comes from both laboratory and real-life studies. Television violence affects youngsters of all ages, of both genders, at all socioeconomic levels and all levels of intelligence. The effect is not limited to children who are already disposed to being aggressive and is not restricted to this country. The fact that we get this same finding of a relation between television violence and aggression in children in study after study, in one country after another, cannot be ignored."[57]

Early laboratory experiments by Bandura[58] concluded that young children learn aggressive behavior when it is modeled by attractive adult role models, such as those they see on television. Longitudinal studies are particularly powerful in determining that heavy viewers of television in childhood demonstrate more aggressive behavior 10 and 22 years later.[59] (The converse is not true, however; violent behavior does not seem to lead to an increased appetite for viewing violent television). Naturalistic studies, which examine communities before and after the introduction of television, also find a significant upswing in aggressive and antisocial behaviors.[60] Meta-analyses of large numbers of studies also establish the cause-and-effect relationship. Centerwall[61] examined homicide rates in the United States, Canada, and South Africa and found significant increases 15 years after the introduction of television into each country — precisely what theory would predict.[61] The research is conclusive.[62,63] Even if the research were not conclusive, "there would still be ample reason to oppose violent programming based on common sense, philosophical, humanistic, or aesthetic grounds."[64]

8.4.3 Implications for Media Other Than Television

Many researchers believe that findings associated with the well-studied effects of television violence can be readily extrapolated to video games, movies, music videos, and software. However, because television viewing predominates in the lives of young people, it is by far the most influential medium. Movies can be more graphic than television, but only several movies may be viewed weekly, compared with 23 to 28 hours of television. The impact of violent media likely varies according to the amount of time a child spends viewing violence in programs.

Youth spend a significant amount of time listening to rock music and watching rock music videos on television, up to 2 or more hours daily. More than 50% of music videos contain violent content. No study has established a relationship between this medium and aggressive behaviors in youth, although some impact on attitude toward violence has been noted. Research has shown that music videos are self-reinforcing (hearing a song recalls the visual imagery of the video).[65]

Researchers are becoming increasingly interested in the effects of violent video games and computer games. Preliminary research "suggests a possible relationship between playing violent video games and subsequent aggressive behavior, at least for young children in a laboratory setting."[66] Research is urgently needed in this area as the popularity of playing these games increases.

8.4.4 Response/Intervention Strategies

Violence in society — with media violence as one contributing cause — must be viewed as a public health problem. A public health approach involves broad educational programs with the goal to change the public's attitude and behavior regarding violence in general, and media violence specifically. Intervention must be implemented widely and involve parents, schools, the community, government, pediatricians, and the media industry. Parents, schools, and communities need to "(1) minimize the impact of the media on children and adolescents and (2) maximize their resistance to its influence."[62]

Parents should limit their children's television viewing to 2 hours or less per day and should actively watch and discuss programming to help their children interpret what they see. Parents should be aware of the violent content of television, movies, and other media, the association between viewing violence and aggressive behavior, and the important role they can play in intervention.

Schools and communities should promote media literacy campaigns and curricula, some of which have been proven beneficial. Community-based groups should hold local television affiliates to the letter of the Children's Television Act, which mandated positive programming for children as a requirement for re-licensure. Many communities have successfully sponsored "Turn Off the Violence" days or weeks, providing families with creative, alternative pastimes to television viewing. Schools and communities should also promote exercises in conflict resolution for young people to reduce the impact of the negative lessons learned from television, movie, or video screens.

Many experts decry legislative attempts to deal with media violence because it may infringe on First Amendment rights. Instead, they call upon the media industry to act voluntarily to address the problem. Adherence to the standards proposed by the networks in 1992 (Table 8.3, p 181), a rating system, warning labels, and agreeing to work constructively with child health experts (including the AAP) would be positive steps. Continued debate on the appropriateness of legislative or regulatory interventions should also continue as evidence grows about the relationship between violence in the media and violent behavior.

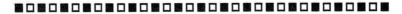

TABLE 8.3.
Joint Network Standards on Television Violence*

Voluntary Limits On:
- Gratuitous or excessive violence
- Glamorous depictions of violence
- Scenes showing excessive gore, pain, or physical suffering
- Scenes showing use of force that are "on the whole" inappropriate for a home viewing medium
- Replicable, unique, or "ingenious" depictions of inflicting pain or injury
- Portrayals of dangerous behavior or weapons that invite imitation by children
- Realistic portrayals of violence that are unduly frightening in children's programs
- Gratuitous depiction of animal abuse

Encourage:
- Portrayal of the consequences of violence
- Scheduling all programs with regard for the likely composition of the intended audience

Urge Caution:
- In stories and scenes using children as victims
- In themes, plots, or scenes that mix sex and violence (eg, rape)

---

*From Network Television Association, New York, 1992.

8.4.5 Recommendations for Pediatricians

Because of their developmental expertise, pediatricians can play a pivotal role in the area of media violence and its effect on the children and adolescents they serve.[67] Ideas for pediatric intervention include:

1. Working directly with the entertainment industry in a constructive manner to advocate for children and adolescents. This includes urging positive, educational programs for children on a local and national basis and encouraging the realistic depiction of the consequences of violence and firearm use.

2. Urging the network and cable television industries to adhere to their recently published guidelines regarding violent programming.

3. Working with musicians and music producers, software developers, screen writers, directors, and producers to voluntarily create nonviolent entertainment products.

4. Urging all media to sponsor and honor a 1-day moratorium on violence in their programming each October during Child Health Month.

5. Providing teaching and support for parents, schools, and communities regarding the effects of media violence on children and adolescents and working actively with these groups to devise strategies to address the problem.

6. Communicating with government agencies (eg, the FCC) to enforce strictly the Children's Television Act of 1990 and the local and national legislatures to continue strong support for public television and radio.

7. Continuing to educate colleagues and other professionals about the negative effects of media violence on children and adolescents and actively joining the debate on strategies to reduce the amount of violence shown. There is no substitute for reducing both the amount and the graphic nature of current media violence on television, in movies, and in video games.

Evidence is compelling that violence in the media plays a significant role in promoting aggressive attitudes and behavior in children and adolescents. Television is a powerful medium that "leads and mirrors society." The issue of media violence demands a unified, strong public health response from all sectors of society. The reader is referred to the recent AAP policy statement on this subject.[68]

References

1. Foege W. Preface. In: Rosenberg ML, Fenley MA, eds. *Violence in America: A Public Health Approach.* New York, NY: Oxford University Press; 1991:7–11

2. Sirotnak AP, Krugman RD. Physical abuse of children: an update. *Pediatr Rev.* 1994; 15:394–399

3. National Research Council, Panel on Research on Child Abuse and Neglect. *Understanding Child Abuse and Neglect.* Washington, DC: National Academy Press; 1993

4. Kempe CH, Silverman FN. The battered-child syndrome. *JAMA.* 1962;181:17–24

5. Widom CS. Child abuse, neglect, and adult behavior: research design and findings on criminality, violence, and child abuse. *Am J Orthopsychiatry.* 1989;59:355–367

6. Straus MA, Kantor GK. Stress and child abuse. In: Kempe RS, Helfer RE, eds. *The Battered Child.* 4th ed. Chicago, IL: University of Chicago Press; 1987:42–59

7. Durkin MS, Davidson LL, Kuhn L, O'Connor P, Barlow B. Low-income neighborhoods and the risk of severe pediatric injury: a small-area analysis in northern Manhattan. *Am J Public Health.* 1994;84:587–592

8. Kaufman J, Zigler E. Do abused children become abusive parents? *Am J Ortho-psychiatry.* 1987;57:186–192

9. US Department of Health and Human Services, National Center on Child Abuse and Neglect. *Child Maltreatment 1993: Reports From the States to the National Center on Child Abuse and Neglect.* Washington, DC: 1995

10. Durfee MJ, Gellert GA, Tilton-Durfee D. Origins and clinical relevance of child death review teams. *JAMA.* 1992;267:3172–3175

11. Gray JD, Cutler CA, Dean JG, Kempe CH. Prediction and prevention of child abuse and neglect. *J Soc Issues.* 1979;35:127–139

12. Oliver JE. The intergenerational transmission of child abuse: rates, research, and clinical implications. *Am J Psychiatry.* 1993;150:1315–1324

13. Steele B, Pollock CB. A psychiatric study of parents who abuse infants and young children. In: Helfer RE, Kempe CH, eds. *The Battered Child.* Chicago, IL: University of Chicago Press; 1968:103–147

14. Chadwick DL, Salerno C. Likelihood of the death of an infant or young child in a short fall of less than 6 vertical feet. *J Trauma.* 1993;35:968

15. Schmitt BD. The seven deadly sins of childhood: advising parents about difficult developmental phases. *Child Abuse Negl.* 1987;11:421–432

16. Caffey J. The whiplash shaken infant syndrome: manual shaking by the extremities with whiplash-induced intracranial and intraocular bleedings, linked with residual permanent brain damage and mental retardation. *Pediatrics.* 1974;54:396–403

17. Showers J. Shaken baby syndrome: the problem and a model for prevention. *Child Today.* 1992;21:34–37

18. Feldman KW, Schaller RT, Feldman JA, McMillon M. Tap water scald burns in children. *Pediatrics.* 1978;62:1–7

19. Kempe CH. Approaches to preventing child abuse: the health visitors concept. *Am J Dis Child.* 1976;130:941–947

20. Kempe CH. Child abuse: the pediatrician's role in child advocacy and preventive pediatrics. *Am J Dis Child.* 1978;132:255–260

21. Sia CC. Abraham Jacobi Award Address: April 14, 1992. The medical home: pediatric practice and child advocacy in the 1990s. *Pediatrics.* 1992;90:419–423

22. Olds DL, Henderson CR Jr, Chamberlin R, Tatelbaum R. Preventing child abuse and neglect: a randomized trial of nurse home visitation. *Pediatrics.* 1986;78:65–78

23. Olds DL. Home visitation for pregnant women and parents of young children. *Am J Dis Child.* 1992;146:704–708

24. Center for the Future of Children. *The Future of Children: Home Visiting.* Los Altos, CA: The David and Lucile Packard Foundation; 1993;3

25. Weiner IB. Suicidal behavior. In: *Psychological Disturbance in Adolescence.* 2nd ed. New York, NY: John Wiley and Sons; 1992:357–383

26. Busch KA, Clark DC, Fawcett J, Kravitz HM. Clinical features of inpatient suicide. *Psychiatr Ann.* 1993;23:256–262

27. O'Carroll PW, Rosenberg ML, Mercy JA. Suicide. In: Rosenberg ML, Fenley MA, eds. *Violence in America: A Public Health Approach.* New York, NY: Oxford University Press; 1991:184–196

28. Centers for Disease Control. Programs for the prevention of suicide among adolescents and young adults. *MMWR Morb Mortal Wkly Rep.* 1994;43(RR-6):1–7

29. Shaffer D, Garland A, Gould M, Fisher P, Trautman P. Preventing teenage suicide: a critical review. *J Am Acad Child Adolesc Psychiatry.* 1988;27:675–687

30. Hazell P. Adolescent suicide clusters: evidence, mechanisms and prevention. *Aust N Z J Psychiatry.* 1993;27:653–665

31. Kazdin AE. *Conduct Disorders in Childhood and Adolescence.* Newbury Park, CA: Sage Publications; 1987

32. Wilson MH, Baker SP, Teret SP, Shock S, Garbarino J. *Saving Children: A Guide to Injury Prevention.* New York, NY: Oxford University Press; 1991

33. Hawton K, O'Grady J, Osborn M, Cole D. Adolescents who take overdoses: their characteristics, problems and contacts with helping agencies. *Br J Psychiatry.* 1982; 140:118–123

34. Harris JC. Suicide. In: Oski FA, ed. *Principles and Practice of Pediatrics.* 2nd ed. Philadelphia, PA: JB Lippincott Co; 1994:725–727

35. Dulit E. Immediately after the suicide attempt: evaluation and brief therapy on a medical ward. In: Zimmerman JK, Asnis GM, eds. *Treatment Approaches With Suicidal Adolescents.* New York, NY: John Wiley and Sons; 1995:91–105

36. Marks A. Management of the suicidal adolescent on a nonpsychiatric adolescent unit. *J Pediatr.* 1979;95:305–308

37. Brent DA, Pepper JA, Allman CJ, Moritz GM, Wartella ME, Zelenak JP. The presence and accessibility of firearms in the homes of adolescent suicides: a case-control study. *JAMA.* 1991;266:2989–2995

38. Centers for Disease Control. Suicide among children, adolescents, and young adults — United States, 1980–1992. *MMWR Morb Mortal Wkly Rep.* 1995;44:289–291

39. Centers for Disease Control. Homicide among 15- to 19-year-old males — United States, 1963-1991. *MMWR Morb Mortal Wkly Rep.* 1994;43:725–727

40. Flanagan TJ, Maguire K, eds. *Sourcebook of Criminal Justice Statistics, 1992.* Washington, DC: US Department of Justice, Bureau of Justice Statistics, US Government Printing Office; 1993

41. Durant RH, Pendergrast RA, Cadenhead C. Exposure to violence and victimization and fighting behavior by urban black adolescents. *J Adolesc Health.* 1994;15: 311–318

42. Reiss AJ Jr, Miczek KA, Roth JA, eds. *Understanding and Preventing Violence, Vol. 2: Biobehavioral Influences.* Washington, DC: National Academy Press; 1994

43. Rivara FP, Farrington DP. Prevention of violence: role of the pediatrician. *Arch Pediatr Adolesc Med.* 1995;149:421–429

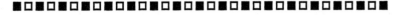
44. Strauss MA. Discipline and deviance: physical punishment of children and violence and other crime in adulthood. *Soc Probl.* 1991;38:133–154

45. Patterson GR. Orderly change in a stable world: the antisocial trait as a chimera. *J Consult Clin Psychol.* 1993;61:911–919

46. Huizinga D, Loeber R, Thornberry TP, eds. *Urban Delinquency and Substance Abuse.* Washington, DC: US Department of Justice, Office of Juvenile Justice and Delinquency Prevention; 1993

47. Earls FJ. Violence and today's youth. *Crit Health Issues Child Youth.* 1994;4:4–23

48. Webster DW. The unconvincing case for school-based conflict resolution programs for adolescents. *Health Affairs.* 1993;12:126–141

49. Tolan P, Guerra N. *What Works in Reducing Adolescent Violence: An Empirical Review of the Field.* Boulder, CO: Center for the Study and Prevention of Violence, University of Colorado; 1994

50. Slaby RG, Stringham P. Prevention of peer and community violence: the pediatrician's role. *Pediatrics.* 1994;94(suppl):608–616

51. Wolfe DA, Korsch B. Witnessing domestic violence during childhood and adolescence: implications for pediatric practice. *Pediatrics.* 1994;94(suppl):594–599

52. Zuckerman B, Augustyn M, Groves BM, Parker S. Silent victims revisited: the special case of domestic violence. *Pediatrics.* 1995;96:511–513

53. Huston AC, Donnerstein E, Fairchild H, et al. *Big World, Small Screen: The Role of Television in American Society.* Lincoln, NE: University of Nebraska Press; 1992

54. Berkson SJ. TV violence is abuse of network privileges. *Star Tribune.* Minneapolis, MN; July 6, 1993

55. Gerbner G. Society's storyteller: how television creates the myths by which we live. *Media and Values.* 1992;59:8–9

56. Gerbner G, Morgan M, Signorelli N. *Television Violence Profile No. 16: The Turning Point.* Philadelphia, PA: The Annenberg School of Communication; 1992

57. Eron LD. Violence and the media. Testimony of Leonard D. Eron, PhD, on behalf of the American Psychological Association before the US Senate Committee on Government Affairs. March 31, 1992. Washington, DC: US Government Printing Office; 1993

58. Bandura A. *Social Foundations of Thought and Action: A Social Cognitive Theory.* Englewood Cliffs, NJ: Prentice Hall; 1986

59. Eron LD. Media violence. *Pediatr Ann.* 1995;24:84–87

60. Williams TM, ed. *The Impact of Television: A Natural Experiment in Three Communities.* New York, NY: Academic Press; 1986

61. Centerwall BS. Television and violence: the scale of the problem and where to go from here. *JAMA.* 1992;267:3059–3063

62. Comstock G, Strasburger VC. Media violence: Q & A. *Adolesc Med.* 1993;4:495–509

63. American Psychological Association. *Summary Report of the American Psychological Association Commission on Violence and Youth.* Washington, DC: American Psychological Association; 1993

64. Gadow KD, Sprafkin J. Field experiments of television violence with children: evidence for an environmental hazard? *Pediatrics.* 1989;83:399–405

65. Hendren RL, Strasburger VC. Rock music and music videos. *Adolesc Med.* 1993; 4:577–587

66. Funk J. Video games. *Adolesc Med.* 1993;4:589–598

67. Sege R, Dietz W. Television viewing and violence in children: the pediatrician as agent for change. *Pediatrics.* 1994;94(suppl):600–607

68. American Academy of Pediatrics, Committee on Communications. Media violence. *Pediatrics.* 1995;95:949–951

Suggested Reading

Physician Guide to Media Violence. Chicago, IL: American Medical Association; 1996

CHAPTER 9

Motor Vehicles

After the first year of life, mechanical energy transmitted from motor vehicles is the leading cause of death and serious injury in children and adolescents. More than 8000 children and adolescents die each year in the United States because of motor vehicle injuries sustained in traffic, and more than 800 000 young people are injured.[1] Motor vehicle–related injuries are the most costly of all pediatric injuries, with direct medical costs approaching $3 billion annually and total lifetime direct and indirect costs exceeding that figure fourfold.[2]

While pedestrian fatalities caused by impact with the outside of the vehicle are relatively evenly distributed over the pediatric age range, the number of fatalities of motor vehicle occupants (generally caused by impact with the interior structures of the vehicle, but also by ejection from the vehicle) greatly increases through early and midadolescence. Control of injury is complex and involves each of the three Es: education, enforcement, and engineering. Pediatricians can have an impact in the office and the community only if they are well-informed about the epidemiologic factors of motor vehicle–related fatalities and the effectiveness of various interventions (Fig 9.1, p 188). (Bicycle injuries are covered in chapter 17.)

9.1 Motor Vehicles: Occupant Protection

Proper use of safety belts and child restraint devices (CRDs) and the implementation of laws in all 50 states that require children to be restrained while riding in motor vehicles have resulted in a substantial reduction in injuries and deaths on our nation's highways.[3–5] Use of CRDs by infants and children has been estimated to reduce fatal injuries by 69% and 47%, respectively.[5]

Despite the presence of legislation and the effectiveness of CRDs, many children continue to be needlessly killed or seriously injured each year while riding in motor vehicles. In 1995, 616 motor vehicle occupants younger than 5 years died.[5] For every child occupant killed, about 100

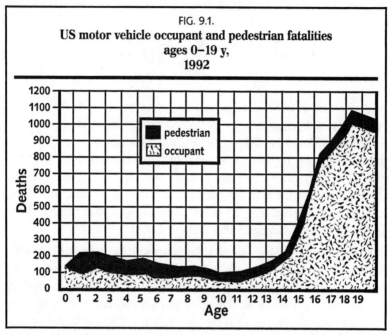

FIG. 9.1.
US motor vehicle occupant and pedestrian fatalities ages 0–19 y, 1992

Data from the National Center for Health Statistics. Occupants include passengers and drivers of motor vehicles excluding motorcyclists and their passengers. Pedestrians include those killed in traffic and nontraffic settings. Fatalities of motorcyclists and pedal cyclists are not included in the data.

additional children are injured in crashes.[6] More than half of the children killed were not restrained. Had all young children in 1994 been using CRDs, another 200 lives could have been saved. Pediatricians can help save hundreds of lives — and reduce or eliminate thousands of injuries each year — by counseling parents about the importance of using CRDs and safety belts correctly and by providing up-to-date, suitable information for parents about selecting a CRD.[7] They can also improve child safety by strengthening the existing occupant protection laws that vary from state to state.[8,9] Specific information about each state's law can be obtained from the state highway safety office (Table 9.1, p 189).

9.1.1 Protection From Injury in an Automobile Crash

To recognize the necessity for using a CRD or safety belt correctly, the basics of the crash must be understood. When a crash occurs, there are

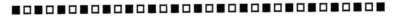

> **TABLE 9.1.**
> **Child Passenger Protection Laws: Gaps in Coverage**
>
> ---
>
> Only young children are covered by the law.
>
> A safety belt may be substituted for a car seat for toddlers.
>
> Primary enforcement of safety belt use is not part of the law applicable to older children; the driver may be cited only if stopped for another offense.
>
> Some laws apply only to parents, guardians, or drivers licensed in that state, rather than to all drivers.

two collisions. In the first collision, the vehicle strikes an object. The vehicle occupants, if unrestrained, continue to travel forward. In the second collision, the occupants strike the interior of the vehicle or another occupant or are ejected from the vehicle and strike the roadside or other object. Likewise, the second collision might occur when the occupant strikes an ill-fitting or loose safety belt or when an airbag strikes a rear-facing CRD. The *second* collision causes personal injury.

The primary function of a CRD is to secure the child to the vehicle so that the full impact of the second collision is lessened after a crash. The CRD limits the forward motion of the child's head in a frontal crash, prevents the child from striking the interior of the vehicle, and, most important, prevents the child's ejection from the vehicle. The CRD also broadly distributes the forces of the crash to the skeletal areas that are more capable of withstanding those forces and minimizes hyperextension or hyperflexion of the spinal column. In a frontal crash, the front end of the vehicle, which is designed to crush on impact, absorbs much of the energy for properly restrained occupants. For CRDs to be effective, children must be properly positioned in the device, which is firmly attached to the vehicle via the safety belt (or integrated restraint device, see section 9.1.2).

9.1.2 Restraint Devices and Seating Position

A variety of CRDs are available to accommodate passenger size and vehicle model. They are intended to biomechanically link the child to the automobile's seat belt in a biomechanically appropriate fashion. Child restraint devices are primarily designed to protect the brain and spinal cord in a severe frontal crash. Protection of the skeleton and viscera and protection in side and rear impacts are secondary design considerations.

Parents frequently ask, "Which car seat is best for my child?" The correct answer is that there is no one perfect CRD. Child restraint devices, vehicle seats, and automobile safety belts vary from vehicle to vehicle, so the best CRD is one that is easy for parents to use, fits the automobile's seats and safety belts, and is the right size for the child.[10] Child restraint devices must also meet or exceed federal motor vehicle safety standard 213 (FMVSS 213). All CRDs manufactured after January 1, 1981, meet those standards. Although the standard did not change between 1981 and 1996, many improvements have been made in the seats over those years, making the newer seats easier to use. The standard was substantially changed for seats manufactured on or after January 1, 1996. To encourage use of the rear-facing riding position up until the child's first birthday, the new standard provides for testing rear-facing CRDs with a 20-lb dummy the size of a 9-month-old and labeling of such CRDs for infants weighing up to 22 lb. The new standard also provides for testing of booster seats with a dummy the size of a 6-year-old in addition to the dummy the size of a 3-year-old that was previously required. Parents should refer to the manufacturer's instructions for recommended weights for the seat they intend to purchase and use.

A label on CRDs gives the date of manufacture and the model number. Such labeling allows parents to determine whether a CRD has been recalled by the manufacturer. When a new CRD is purchased, it comes with a registration card that should be completed and returned to the manufacturer. If the seat is recalled, the registered owner of the CRD is notified.

Air bags and children

Beginning in 1997, all new passenger vehicles are equipped with passenger-side air bags. Although air bags were designed to save lives, they pose a very serious risk to children. In 1995 alone, 500 drivers' lives were saved by air bags; eight children died from air bag–related injuries during this same period — all of whom were improperly restrained or not restrained at all. With increased exposure to air bags, more are at risk. As of December 1996, the total number of reported deaths of children is 31.

Children are at increased risk for air bag–related injuries because of their size. The vehicle seat belts, when worn, do not fit most children correctly. As a result, children often place the shoulder belt behind them and perch on the edge of the vehicle seat. This positioning, combined with the child's short stature, places the child's face and neck directly in the path and full velocity of the deploying air bag. This turns a minor 10-mph impact into a 140-mph head impact with the passenger-side air bag. The risk of death in a crash of a vehicle with a passenger-side air bag is extremely high for unrestrained children and for infants in rear-facing child seats.

In light of the above information, the American Academy of Pediatrics (AAP) recommends the following:

- The safest place for infants and children to ride is in the back seat of the vehicle. Children riding in the front seat are at risk if they are improperly restrained, out of position, or too small for the safety belt to fit correctly. In a crash, children can easily slide forward on the seat, and the inflating air bag can hit them in the head or neck. Whether the vehicle has an air bag or not, children are up to 29% safer riding in the back seat, as compared with the front seat. The National Highway Traffic Safety Administration currently recommends placing all children age 12 and younger in the rear seat. The AAP advises that the most important factor is the size (height and weight) of the child to ensure proper fit of the seat belt (see Fig 9.2, p 192).

- In an emergency, if a child *must* ride in the front seat, make sure he or she is correctly restrained and then move the vehicle seat back as far as possible, away from the air bag.

- *Never* put an infant in the front seat of a vehicle equipped with a passenger-side air bag. An infant weighing under 20 lb or younger than 1 year must *always* ride in a rear-facing child safety seat in the back seat of the vehicle.

- The child should be properly secured in the back seat of the vehicle in a child safety seat, a booster seat, or shoulder/lap belt correct for his or her size.

Infant-only CRDs

Infant-only devices are designed for infants who weigh up to 17 to 22 lb and are up to 26-in long and must be used rear-facing. (With 1996

FIG 9.2.

Selecting an appropriate type of infant and child restraint

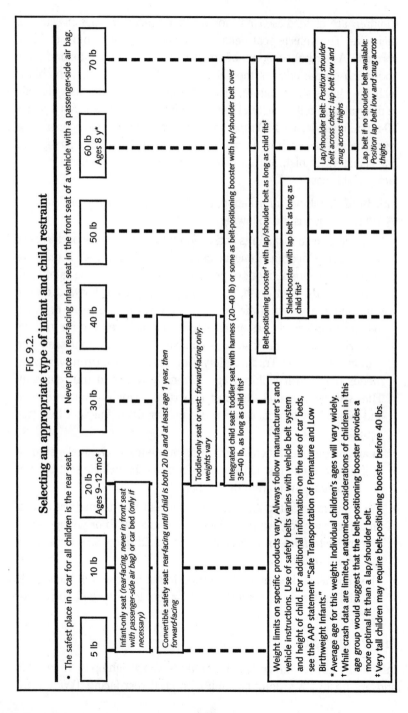

- The safest place in a car for all children is the rear seat.
- Never place a rear-facing infant seat in the front seat of a vehicle with a passenger-side air bag.

| 5 lb | 10 lb | 20 lb
Ages 9–12 mo* | 30 lb | 40 lb | 50 lb | 60 lb
Ages 8 y* | 70 lb |

Infant-only seat (rear-facing, never in front seat with passenger-side air bag) or car bed (only if necessary)

Convertible safety seat: rear-facing until child is both 20 lb and at least age 1 year, then forward-facing

Toddler-only seat or vest: forward-facing only; weights vary

Integrated child seat: toddler seat with harness (20–40 lb) or some as belt-positioning booster with lap/shoulder belt over 35–40 lb, as long as child fits‡

Belt-positioning booster† with lap/shoulder belt as long as child fits‡

Shield-booster with lap belt as long as child fits‡

Lap/shoulder Belt: Position shoulder belt across chest; lap belt low and snug across thighs

Lap belt if no shoulder belt available: Position lap belt low and snug across thighs

Weight limits on specific products vary. Always follow manufacturer's and vehicle instructions. Use of safety belts varies with vehicle belt system and height of child. For additional information on the use of car beds, see the AAP statement "Safe Transportation of Premature and Low Birthweight Infants."

* Average age for this weight: Individual children's ages will vary widely.
† While crash data are limited, anatomical considerations of children in this age group would suggest that the belt-positioning booster provides a more optimal fit than a lap/shoulder belt.
‡ Very tall children may require belt-positioning booster before 40 lbs.

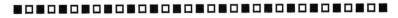

changes in FMVSS 213, parents should refer to instructions about the upper weight limit.) The rear-facing position provides distribution of forces in a frontal crash over the long axis of an infant's body. The restraining harness in an infant-only device is intended *only* to keep the infant in place, not to absorb crash forces. Therefore, an infant-only seat should never be used in the forward-facing position. *Additionally, an infant-only CRD must never be used in the front seat of a car that has a passenger-side frontal air bag.* Air bags inflate at speeds of 100 to 200 mph and can kill or seriously injure infants in rear-facing seats.

Infants are safer in the rear seat of a vehicle. Some parents are uncomfortable with not being able to see the infant easily. Such parents should be counseled that unattended normal infants properly restrained in the rear seat are safer than infants within their view in the front seat.

A rear-facing CRD should be used until the infant is about 1 year of age and weighs about 20 lb. Infants who outgrow their infant seats because of length should most appropriately graduate to convertible seats in the *rear-facing* position until they are at least 20 lb or outgrow the rear-facing position in that device. Infants who reach 20 lb well before their first birthdays, occasionally before 6 months of age, should be kept in a rear-facing CRD as long as they fit comfortably. These infants still have relatively heavy heads and weak necks, making them more prone to cervical spinal cord injury if they are facing forward in a frontal crash. (New amendments to FMVSS 213, effective in January 1996, increase the 20-lb limit labeling to 22 lb.)

Convertible CRDs

Convertible restraints are designed for children who weigh up to 40 lb and are 40 in tall. They are used rear-facing for infants up to 20 to 22 lb and forward-facing for children who weigh more than 20 lb. Although these restraints are usable for newborns, they do not fit smaller infants well, and given a choice, an infant-only CRD may work better for the first few months of life. Convertible restraints are designed with three basic styles of internal restraint: five-point harnesses, "T" shields, and tray shields. The latter two styles are convenient but are not recommended for newborns or small infants because the child's face or neck could contact the shield during a crash, and the harness straps do not fit snugly.

In the forward-facing position, the restraining straps are designed to absorb and distribute crash forces. Therefore, the straps must be used correctly and according to the manufacturer's instructions. Five-point harnesses and harness-shield combinations are equally effective. Parents should make sure that the shoulder straps are threaded through the *top* set of slots on the seat back when the seat is used in the forward-facing position; the lower set (or sets) of slots intended for a rear-facing position may not be strong enough to restrain the child in a forward-facing position. Many models include a retaining clip to keep the shoulder straps in place. This clip should be positioned on the child's chest at the level of the armpit so it does not contact the child's throat during a crash.

Toddler CRD–belt-positioning booster seats

Several manufacturers offer new designs in CRDs that combine a forward-facing toddler seat (with a harness system) and a booster seat (with belt-positioning guides for the vehicle's lap-shoulder belt). In general, the toddler configuration can be used after the infant's first birthday and until the child weighs about 45 lb, whereas the belt-positioning configuration is appropriate for children who weigh between 30 and 60 lb. These hybrid CRDs are rapidly evolving to meet consumer interest and demand. Manufacturers' instructions, which vary from model to model, should be consulted to ensure proper use.

Integrated safety seats

Integrated safety seats are offered by some automobile manufacturers in vans and mid- to full-sized cars. These devices have much to recommend them, compared with separate CRDs. During a crash, the integrated seats limit movement of the child's head better than a separate CRD. Also, compatibility between the vehicle and the device is not an issue with integrated safety seats. Currently, integrated seats are designed only for children older than 1 year (and over 20 pounds) who can ride facing forward in the vehicle. Some seats can be used with a harness system until the child weighs 40 lb, and some may be used for older children as belt-positioning booster seats until the child weighs 60 lb. The vehicle owner's manual should always be checked for exact weight requirements.

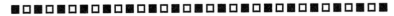

Booster seats

Booster seats are designed for children who weigh more than 40 lb who have outgrown convertible car seats. Booster seats provide added height for children and allow correct positioning of safety belts until they are large enough to be adequately restrained by the lap-shoulder belts alone. The two types of booster seats include belt-positioning booster seats, used with combination lap-shoulder belts only, and shield booster seats, used if only a lap belt is available.

Of the two styles of booster seats, the belt-positioning seat is preferable because it provides upper-torso restraint that limits forward motion of the child's head. A seating position with a three-point harness (a lap-shoulder belt) is required. The shield booster seats are preferable to a lap belt alone for the 40- to 60-lb children who have outgrown their convertible CRDs, because the lap belt may ride up on the abdomen and cause abdominal and spinal injury during a crash.

Parents should use only booster seats designed for use in motor vehicles (labeled as meeting or exceeding federal safety standards); they should not use aftermarket devices or objects such as pillows, books, or household booster seats.

Used CRDs

Many families choose to buy a used CRD, which is risky. The buyer has no knowledge of whether the safety seat has been involved in a crash and whether parts are missing. Used CRDs may be safe only if the following criteria are met:

- A certification label states that the device meets or exceeds the requirements of FMVSS 213.
- A label indicates the model number and date of manufacture.
- The device was manufactured after January 1, 1981 (CRDs made before that date did not meet stringent current standards and may not be crashworthy).
- No parts are missing according to the instructions. (If the instructions are missing, contact the manufacturer to obtain a copy.)
- The device has no visible cracks in the plastic shell or other noticeable damage.

- The harness straps are not frayed or damaged. (Although straps can often be replaced, only replacements intended for the particular seat and that meet federal safety standards should be used.)
- The device has not been involved in a crash.
- The device is not under recall, or the recall problem has been remedied. (To determine whether the seat has been recalled, call the Auto Safety Hotline at 800-424-9393.)

Safety belts

Safety belts are used when a child outgrows a booster seat, usually when the child weighs about 60 lb or when the child's ears show above the seat back of the vehicle. Although safety belts do not provide optimal protection for small children, they are preferable to using no restraints.

Upper-torso restraint is very important to prevent forward motion of the child's head and chest and to prevent head impact and flexion injury to the lumbar spine in a crash. Therefore, one should make every effort to make a lap-shoulder belt fit the child — with or without a belt-positioning booster seat before resorting to restraining a child with a lap belt alone.

Safety belts must be worn low and flat across the hips, across the chest, and fastened snugly. Children should sit up straight, firmly against the vehicle back seat. Shoulder harnesses may touch the side of the neck, but should not cross the front of the throat. The shoulder belt should *never* be placed under the child's arm. When no belt-positioning booster seat is available and the shoulder belt is too high, the shoulder belt, as a last resort, should be tucked behind the child's back. However, children should *never* be placed in the front seat in this configuration (lap belt only) if there is a passenger-side air bag.

Transition from one system to the next

The recommended weights and ages for changing the style of restraint system used are somewhat arbitrary. The transition involves trade-offs and compromises in the degree of protection provided. Biomechanically, rear-facing devices are safer than forward-facing devices, and five-point harnesses are more protective than two- and three-point harnesses. Therefore, generally it is best to delay use of the next larger restraint system for as long as is practical. A 1-year-old who weighs less than 22 lb and still fits in a rear-facing convertible seat should continue riding in

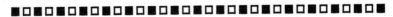

that CRD — folding an infant's legs is not harmful. Although parents often want to begin using a booster seat with their first child when a second child is born (some booster seats are labeled for use beginning at 30 lb), continued use of the forward-facing convertible car seat is best until the child is closer to 40 lb and has physically outgrown it. The factors that usually indicate that a change is needed in the restraint system are shown in Table 9.2.

Restraints for children with special needs

Children with temporary or permanent special needs resulting from prematurity, respiratory problems, developmental disabilities, a cast, or other conditions may not be safely transported in conventional CRDs. Special restraints exist but may not be widely available for children who need them.[11] Restraints for children with special needs who have outgrown regular CRDs also are available but parents often do not know where or how to obtain them.

The AAP has specific recommendations for the transportation of high-risk infants, including infants born at less than 37 weeks' gestation or infants with medical conditions that place them at high risk for apnea, bradycardia, or oxygen desaturation.[12]

Current information suggests that high-risk infants be observed in a CRD before discharge from the hospital to monitor for possible apnea, bradycardia, or oxygen desaturation. Infants with documented oxygen

---

TABLE 9.2.
Factors Usually Precipitating Transition to Next Larger Restraint System

From rear-facing to forward-facing CRD*	Child's head reaches top of seat shell; leg length
From forward-facing to booster seat	Length of the shoulder straps The CRD is too narrow for the child Child's shoulders are above the insertion slots of the shoulder straps
From booster-seat to seat belt	Child's ears extend above the seat back (preferable option is to use a high-backed belt-positioning booster) In the case of small shields, make the transition as soon as an available lap-shoulder belt fits reasonably across the child's hips and shoulder

*CRD indicates child restraint device.

desaturation, apnea, or bradycardia in an upright position should travel lying down in an alternative CRD such as a car bed that meets the requirements of FMVSS 213.[13,14]

The positioning of premature or small infants in CRDs presents special problems. For a very small infant, rolled towels or blankets may be used in the crotch area and along the sides of the infant's torso to reduce slouching. A device in which the harness straps fit properly across the shoulders should be selected. The retainer clip, which rests on the infant's chest, keeps the harness on the infant's shoulders and should not touch the infant's neck. The clip may be removed until the infant is larger if a proper fit cannot be obtained. Likewise, devices with shields or arm rests that may contact the infant's head or neck during a crash should not be used. An appropriate safety seat should have 5½ in or less between the crotch strap and the seat back and 10 in or less between the shoulder strap slots and the seat bottom. If the infant's head droops forward because the position of the seat is too vertical, a rolled towel or blanket should be wedged under the base of the car safety seat (beneath the infant's feet) to tilt the seat back slightly at a 45° angle.

Additional information about transportation of children with special needs may be obtained from the Automotive Safety for Children Program at James Whitcomb Riley Hospital for Children. (See Resources section.)

9.1.3 Patterns of Use, Misuse, and Special Precautions

Use of child-restraint devices decreases as children get older. A recent observational study by the US Department of Transportation revealed the following percentages of occupants using restraints by age group[15]: infants (younger than 1 year), 88%; toddlers (1 through 4 years), 61%; youths (5 through 15 years), 58%; young adults (16 to 24 years), 53%; and adults (older than 24 years), 59%.

In addition to the lack of restraint system use, incorrect use is a major problem. Estimates have been made that two thirds or more of CRDs are misused. The five major misuses of car seats are listed as follows:

• Placing an infant in a forward-facing position

- Failure to secure the car safety seat to the automobile correctly with the automobile's seat belt according to the manufacturer's instructions, or inability to secure the safety seat firmly because of hardware incompatibility
- Failure to position the child snugly in the car safety seat with the harness system according to the manufacturer's instructions
- Failure to use a safety seat that is appropriate for the child's age and weight
- Placing a child in a safety seat in the front seat of a car with a passenger-side air bag

Serious incompatibility problems that occur between the design of the vehicle seat, seat belt, and child safety seat may increase the risk of injury or death. A properly secured child safety seat should not move more than a fraction of an inch in any direction. If the safety seat is loose after installation, parents should carefully consult the warning labels on the seat belts, the vehicle owner's manual, and the manufacturer's instructions for the safety seat. (Older vehicles do not always provide warnings or instructions about CRD incompatibility.)

Seat belts that emerge forward of the junction of the seat back and cushion or those that are on a stiff plastic stalk may not work well with rear-facing infant seats. A combination lap-shoulder belt with a freely sliding latch plate does not hold a CRD tightly unless a standard 2½-in locking clip is used to keep the latch plate from sliding. Some lap belts have emergency locking retractors that lock tight only in a crash, not during normal driving. Safety seats used in that situation require a special 3-in heavy-duty locking clip to shorten the belt. *Automatic lap-shoulder belts — those that attach to the door frame and automatically slide into place as the car door is closed — are incompatible with CRDs.* Restraint devices can be used safely in vehicles with automatic safety belts only when a separate manual lap belt is used. Some manufacturers provide special belts and buckles to secure CRDs in front seats with automatic belts. In all cases, the vehicle manual and the CRD manual should be consulted.

Given the complexity of incompatibility of CRDs with automobile seats, impetus is growing to inform and educate parents more fully. New programs and educational efforts are emerging to address the issue, but more important, CRD and vehicle manufacturers are beginning to collaborate to make child safety devices and vehicles more compatible.

During extreme weather conditions, child safety seats may become too hot or too cold, posing potential risk to the child. Parents should protect the seat from direct exposure to the sun or extreme cold and check the seat and harness buckles before placing the child in the seat. Children should never be left unattended in a CRD.

9.1.4 Distribution Programs

The cost of a CRD, even a used CRD, may be too high for some families. Community distribution (loan or low-cost purchase) programs may be available to assist those families. The functions of such programs vary, and different programs use different criteria to evaluate a family's eligibility for services. Some programs require a deposit for the seats, and others provide the seats free of charge. Information about local programs may be obtained from the state's highway safety office.

9.1.5 Pickup Trucks

Almost one third of registered passenger vehicles in 1993 were minivans, utility vehicles, and light trucks.[16] Children are at great risk riding unrestrained in nonstandard seating areas in motor vehicles, such as in enclosed or open cargo areas.[17-19] During a crash, children are tossed against and injured on the interior surfaces of the vehicle and may risk death or severe injury because they are ejected from the vehicle, the vehicle rolls over, or part of the vehicle, such as the shell of a pick-up truck, comes off and crushes them. Children riding under a canopy in the rear of a pickup truck are also at risk of carbon monoxide poisoning.[20] Each year, about 200 persons in the United States are killed while riding in the backs of pickup trucks; most of these fatalities are children and teenagers. As of 1995, 28 states and the District of Columbia permitted passengers to ride in the bed of a pickup truck without restrictions. Most state laws restrict passengers only from riding in open cargo beds. Such an unsafe practice is common in rural areas, particularly in the south and west, where two-seat trucks are used as business and family vehicles. Regrettably, the practice is also common among families who have other, larger vehicles. Pediatricians should support state legislation prohibiting children from riding in the cargo areas of pickup trucks.[19]

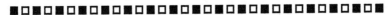
9.1.6 Motorcycles

Data from the National Highway Traffic Safety Administration indicate that in 1993 about 13 000 people younger than 21 years were injured riding motorcycles; 3000 were 15 years old or younger. About 350 motorcycle-related pediatric deaths occurred in the same period.[1] One out of five motorcyclists killed is a teenager. A motorcyclist is five times as likely to be injured and 20 times as likely to be killed as an automobile passenger when a comparison is made on a per-mile basis. For this reason, motorcycle use by young people should be discouraged. Helmets are estimated to be 29% effective in preventing fatalities. About half of those fatally injured are riding without helmets. State helmet laws that apply to riders of all ages should be supported because in states with such laws, helmet use is almost 100%. In states with helmet laws that apply only to young riders, only about 50% of all riders comply with the laws. In such states, fewer than 40% of fatally injured minors are not wearing helmets when they are killed, even though the law requires them to do so.[21]

9.1.7 Air Travel

Although all child restraints manufactured since 1985 are labeled "certified for use in motor vehicles and aircraft," recent tests by the Civil Aeromedical Institute of the Federal Aviation Administration suggest that most child safety seats are not effective in airplane crashes, although they may prevent injury during turbulence. The rear-facing infant seat is the only type of restraint that performs satisfactorily in a crash. Forward-facing, convertible, and toddler restraints allow too much forward motion of the head. The designs of airplane seats and seat belts do not allow proper installation of child safety seats, especially in the economy section of the aircraft. Shield booster seats should not be used because the aircraft seat back tends to flex forward from the movement of the passenger behind the seat. These problems are currently under evaluation, and new requirements and recommendations may be developed.[22]

9.1.8 Adolescent Drivers

Young drivers 16 to 20 years old have the highest crash and fatality rates of any age group, and males are twice as likely to die in automobile crashes as are females.[5] Inexperience and risk-taking behaviors, including low rates of safety belt use, along with the use of alcohol and other drugs, are major factors contributing to the high rate of injury and death in this population.[23]

Parental and community interventions can effectively lower crash rates for teenage drivers. Proposals under consideration in some states include graduated licensing systems, nighttime driving curfews, and more stringent laws for use of safety belts. Students Against Driving Drunk (SADD) provides peer-to-peer education and programs that promote alternatives to high-risk driving.

Physicians can provide anticipatory guidance for parents and teens by addressing risk factors including driving while impaired or nighttime driving. Two brochures for parents include "The Teen Driver," available from the AAP, and "Beginning Drivers: Helping Them Make It Home," available from the Insurance Institute for Highway Safety (see Resources section).

Physicians can also support community initiatives including alcohol-free social events, chauffeuring of adolescents to high-risk events (ie, parties, particularly at night where fatigue, possible alcohol use, a recreational atmosphere, and the likelihood of multiple teen passengers with a teen driver combine to increase risk), and parent-teen contracts. High school driver education does not seem to be an effective intervention. Students who take driver education have crash experience no different than those who learn to drive from parents or other sources. To the extent that driver education programs facilitate and encourage licensure at age 16 (as opposed to 1 or 2 years later), they may actually be increasing teen fatality rates.[24]

Local, state, and federal legislative advocacy is important for reducing motor vehicle crashes. Primary safety belt use laws, nighttime driving curfews (about half of all teenage motor vehicle deaths occur between 9 pm and 3 am), limiting the number of nonadult vehicle occupants, zero alcohol tolerance laws (a blood alcohol concentration of 0.02% or less), and the documentation of a safe driving record before granting full licensure are among measures proved effective.[25] An outline of strategies to reduce teenage highway injury is shown in Table 9.3, p 203. Counseling guidelines are outlined in Table 9.4, p 204.

TABLE 9.3.
Selected Strategies for Reducing Teenage Highway Injuries and Deaths*

Strategy	Rationale
Limit the numbers of teenage passengers in automobiles driven by teenagers	Multiple teenage passengers distract the driver and promote high-risk recreational driving. Sixty-five percent of deaths of teenage passengers occur in crashes in which another teenager is driving.
Curfews on nighttime driving	Late-night driving is demanding for inexperienced drivers; the driver is fatigued, and the driving tends to be "recreational." About half of teenage highway fatalities occur between 9 pm and 3 am.
Limit the legal blood alcohol concentration to near zero tolerance (under 0.02%) for teenage drivers.	Tolerance for alcohol is less in teenagers than in adults, so lower blood alcohol concentrations increase risk.
Graduated licensing system that requires that licensed teens drive only under adult supervision for a specified period and/or have restrictions on nighttime driving before being granted unrestricted licenses.	This would provide inexperienced drivers with an increased amount of learning time.

*For further details see Insurance Institute for Highway Safety.[77]

9.2 Pediatric Pedestrian Injuries

Pedestrian injuries are the leading cause of traumatic death for children 5 to 9 years of age, with the number of 1- to 4-year-olds killed each year nearly the same. Pedestrian injury rates for nonwhite children are 1.5 times the rates for white children.[26] Police reports give a national estimate of approximately 51 000 nonfatal injuries annually.[26] Studies suggest that this may be an underestimate, primarily because of underreporting, especially of events that occur in nontraffic locations, such as driveways or parking lots.[27,28] Pedestrian injuries are more severe and have a higher case-fatality rate than other types of motor vehicle–related injuries.[26]

TABLE 9.4.
Counseling Suggestions to Promote Safety
of Teenagers in Automobiles

Caution 13- to 15-year-olds and their parents about the risks of riding in automobiles with recently licensed older teens, riding at night, or with teenage drivers who may be impaired.

Promote consistent seat belt use for the entire family.

Encourage parents to ride with, monitor, supervise, and continue to coach their newly licensed teenagers.

Parents should institute "driving curfews" for new drivers. For example, after dark, new drivers should drive only when a parent is in the car.

Teenagers should be cautioned about driving under the influence of alcohol or other drugs and the hazards of accepting a ride from an impaired driver.

Parents should set limits on driving or riding with multiple teenage passengers.

Consider the safety of the vehicle for teenage drivers; a car with air bags is ideal. Large cars — even old "clunkers" — are preferable to small cars.

Teenagers should accept some financial responsibility for driving, such as insurance, gasoline, and maintenance costs.

Parents should deny driving privileges when teenagers ignore safety rules.

Adapted from Widome.[78]

9.2.1 Developmental, Gender, and Age-Related Risks of Pedestrian Injuries

Gender and age influence the risk for and types of pedestrian injuries to children.[26,29,30] Pedestrian injury and fatality rates are consistently higher among boys. Limited research has been conducted related to exposure,[31,32] but studies by Routledge et al[33,34] and Howarth et al[35] did not support the hypothesis that boys have increased exposure. A study in Canada indicated that when exposure is considered, the highest level of risk for pedestrian injury is for 3- to 12-year-olds and the elderly.[36]

Infants (younger than 1 year)

Infants are considered "pedestrians" when they are carried or transported, for example, in a stroller, by a caregiver. The risk of injury is related to the risk of injury to the child's caregiver. For example, a caregiver who jaywalks puts the infant at the same risk of injury. Fortunately, pedestrian injuries to infants are rare.

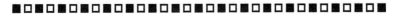
Toddlers (1 to 2 years)

Toddlers are more likely to be injured in nontraffic locations, although this is not always reflected in the data because of errors in coding, or recording the injuries (Fig 9.3, p 206). Pedestrian injuries in toddlers most frequently occur when they are hit by a vehicle, such as when a family member backs a car out of a driveway without seeing the child.[37] These serious and fatal injuries are unique to young children. Residential driveways are also hazardous because of pedestrian injuries related to the use of automatic garage doors. Children may also cause an unattended vehicle to move (by releasing a brake, for example), which may run over a pedestrian. Toddlers are not safe near motor vehicles because they are not easily seen by motorists and they do not have the developmental skills to protect themselves from being injured. Toddlers should therefore be kept away from motor vehicles, eg, with a fence and gate, and must be actively supervised when they are near traffic.

Preschool-age children (3 to 4 years)

Most pedestrian injuries among 3- and 4-year-olds result from children darting into traffic at midblock from between parked cars on residential streets.[26,38,39] Most of these children are playing near their homes, alone or with other children, and are unsupervised by adults. Children 3 and 4 years old are too young to play responsibly, alone or with other children, in or near traffic. They are unlikely to remember to stay out of the street when they are engrossed in play. They focus on only one task at a time and have little ability to inhibit impulses. Their ability to perform the tasks necessary to deal with traffic is inconsistent and unreliable. Preschool children are unlikely to have effective protective reactions to moving vehicles. They cannot be taught to cross the street safely; they lack the cognitive awareness to be responsible pedestrians.

School-age children (5 to 9 years)

Most pedestrian injuries among 5- to 9-year-olds result from children darting out into traffic at midblock from between parked cars on residential streets, as with 3- and 4-year-olds. After-school hours and early evening are periods of high exposure to traffic. School-age children are increasingly mobile, play with others, use bicycles and other recreational vehicles, and travel further from home. When they are playing they are not focused on crossing streets safely. Perceptual skills relevant for

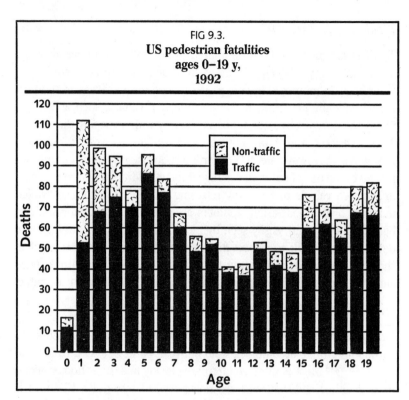

FIG 9.3.
**US pedestrian fatalities
ages 0–19 y,
1992**

Data from the National Center for Health Statistics, courtesy Lois Fingerhut.

Editor s note: It is likely that substantial incorrect coding occurs of nontraffic pedestrian fatalities of young children as traffic fatalities. See Brison et al.[37] Therefore, a larger percentage of pedestrian fatalities may be occurring in nontraffic situations, for example, as a result of driveway incidents. The above data for nontraffic fatalities include pedestrian-train fatalities, although the number of such fatalities is small.

pedestrian behavior, such as peripheral vision, depth perception, and assessment of hazards, are still developing. Knowledge of traffic patterns, street signs, and rules of the road is often insufficient. School-age children should not be relied on to cross streets safely, yet parents and drivers often unrealistically expect such an ability.

Preadolescents and young adolescents (10 to 14 years)

Of all pediatric age groups, 10- to 14-year-old children are at least risk for pedestrian injury. Their judgment and skills in dealing with traffic when involved in pedestrian activity and at play are markedly improved compared with younger children. They are more experienced in an environment with traffic. However, more children in this age group are injured on busier streets further from home. Lapses in judgment, distractions, and substance use place the young adolescent at risk for pedestrian injury. The decrease in pedestrian injuries in this age group may be partly related to a decrease in pedestrian activity. Compared with younger children, preadolescents and young adolescents more frequently ride bicycles and may more often travel in motor vehicles.

9.2.2 Pedestrian Skills

The ability of a pedestrian to deal with traffic safely is complex and requires as many as 26 tasks.[40] Numerous studies have confirmed that young children are not physically, behaviorally, or cognitively able to be safe pedestrians.[41-43] Young children are difficult for drivers to see in time to stop the vehicle, especially when they dart out suddenly from between parked vehicles. The peripheral vision of children younger than 8 years is more restricted than that of adults, making it difficult for them to see oncoming vehicles. Depth perception, which is needed to judge the distance and speed of an oncoming vehicle, is not as well developed in young children. Likewise, localization of the vehicle sound (interpreting distance and location of a vehicle) is less well developed. Cognitive abilities of young children are more limited than those of adults for recognizing hazards; children are more impulsive and less cautious and cannot concentrate on multiple tasks at once, for example, playing and paying attention to the roadway. Children on skates, bicycles, skateboards, or other moving toys are at further risk for pedestrian injury (see chapter 17).

Skills learned in programs designed to teach crossing streets safely will not necessarily be applied by children playing in or near the street.

9.2.3 Parents' Perceptions and Expectations

Parents frequently are unaware of the potentially serious nature of pedestrian injuries.[44] Rivara et al[45] and Dunne et al[46] have demonstrated that the perceptions and expectations of parents about their children's pedestrian capabilities and skills are often inappropriate and unrealistic; thus parents allow children to be involved in pedestrian situations that require skills beyond their capabilities. Adults often place children at risk by allowing them to walk to school or allowing play in and near streets without adequate supervision.[32,47] Additionally, parents do always not set examples of safe pedestrian behavior for children.[48] Behavior modeling by parents must be addressed in this context.

9.2.4 Socioeconomic and Environmental Factors

Socioeconomic and environmental factors are associated with increased risk for pedestrian injury. Studies have found that low-income, densely populated areas with high traffic volume have a higher incidence of pedestrian injuries. Other factors associated with pediatric pedestrian injuries include the following[30,49–53]:

- Number of parked vehicles on the street
- Neighborhoods with a greater proportion of children
- Neighborhoods with a greater proportion of nonwhite residents
- Household crowding
- Female heads of household

Preliminary studies of road size, traffic density, and traffic patterns suggest that "traffic calming" measures offer the potential for decreasing risk of pedestrian injury. These measures include lowering speed limits in residential areas, redirecting through traffic away from residential areas, installation of sidewalks, use of warning signs, prohibiting parking in areas where visibility of pedestrians, especially children, would be obstructed, regulating vendors (eg, ice cream trucks) and strengthening enforcement of pedestrian safety laws.

9.2.5 Driver Factors

Driver inattention, speeding, substance use, and failure to follow the rules of the road are related to risk of pedestrian injury. Some studies have found a high proportion of young male drivers involved in these events.[30,54] The degree to which drivers have been found responsible ranges from 21% to 46% in different studies.[55] Other studies have found that drivers take minimal evasive action to avoid striking child pedestrians.[47,56]

9.2.6 Interventions

Education

Most interventions aimed at preventing pediatric pedestrian injuries have been educational, focusing on teaching knowledge, behavior, and skills to school-age children with an emphasis on crossing streets safely.[57-59] The results of these efforts have been variable; knowledge is increased, but behavioral changes have been more difficult to achieve.[26,53,55,58,60-63] While these programs may help increase skills for safe intentional street crossing, the skills needed by children during play to prevent them from darting into the street have not been proved to be affected. A limited number of programs have been designed to address pedestrian injuries in preschool children,[64] with emphasis on street avoidance (ie, not playing in or near the street or wandering into the street during play) and safe crossing skills.[65,66] Evaluation of these programs has found them to be minimally effective; these results indicate that the message or the target is inappropriate or that the evaluation methods are not sensitive enough to detect changes.[57,64,65] Many programs for preschool and school-age children have emphasized the importance of parent involvement to reinforce and enhance the education.[58,65-66] Educational programs directed toward Hispanics have not been developed with the exception of a public service announcement in Spanish aired in Los Angeles. Time-series analysis showed an 18% reduction in pedestrian injuries involving individuals with Hispanic surnames after the message was aired, suggesting that positive outcomes can be achieved.[67-69]

Parents or caregivers of young children must be made aware of the hazards of the driveway for young children. The issue of adequate supervision must be emphasized, because in many cases children are in the company of adults at the time they are injured. Ideally, the driveway should be separated from the house, and play in the driveway or in adjacent unfenced front yards should be prohibited.[70]

The role of parents in preventing pedestrian injury

Parents must be role models for safe pedestrian practices. However, they must neither expect the preschool-age child or early elementary school child to behave as a responsible pedestrian nor give the child such responsibility. Supervision of children in these age groups must be active and continuous near roadways and traffic.

Increasing a child's visibility to the motorist is no substitute for careful parental supervision. However, use of retroreflective clothing (using retroreflective tape or fabric) and bright neon colors can add an additional level of protection for children in or near traffic, particularly in low-light conditions.

Driver-related injuries

Little attention has been given to programs aimed at educating drivers at special risk for involvement in pedestrian injuries. Drivers must learn to expect the unexpected and drive more slowly and cautiously in residential communities. They must anticipate that children will dart into the street and be prepared to stop suddenly and within a short distance.

Vehicle modification

Interventions aimed at modification of vehicle design (such as lower, cushioned bumpers) to reduce the severity of pediatric pedestrian injuries have not been particularly fruitful.[55,71]

Legislative and environmental modifications

As with other injury control measures, legislative and environmental modifications that would eventually separate children from traffic would seem to have the greatest effect.[26] The concept of traffic calming has recently been introduced into injury control interventions for pedestrians and bicycle riders. Measures that require major changes in street configuration (eg, cul-de-sacs, specific play streets, and restricted access areas) are best built into communities at the time they are planned. The effectiveness of many of these measures remains to be proved.[38,72–75] Some of these measures are considered in the development of new communities; however, changes are unlikely to occur in the near future for the communities in the United States at high risk for pedestrian injuries (high density, low income, residential urban areas with high traffic volume).[38,76] Therefore, community-based programs, advocacy, and traffic calming measures must be the focus in existing communities.

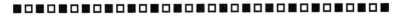
9.2.7 Role of the Pediatrician

Pediatricians, family physicians, and other health care providers can assume leadership in the prevention of pedestrian injuries at several levels. First, pediatricians who work with all family members can increase an awareness of the hazards related to traffic that children face at each stage of development. Counseling should emphasize key messages (Table 9.5, p 212). These messages also apply to the prevention of other causes of injury. Second, health care providers can become advocates for child pedestrian safety by participating in community coalitions, educating public policy makers such as city planners and members of legislative bodies, and becoming recognized as advocates for pediatric injury prevention.

9.3 Resources

1. American Academy of Pediatrics
   141 Northwest Point Blvd
   PO Box 927
   Elk Grove Village, IL 60009-0927
   800-433-9016

   Ask for the current year's Family Shopping Guide to Car Seats. This provides guidance for correct use and lists the available seats and their important features. Educational materials are also available about topics such as "One-Minute Safety Check Up" and "Teens Who Drink and Drive."

2. Automotive Safety for Children Program
   James Whitcomb Riley Hospital for Children
   702 Barnhill Dr, S-139
   Indianapolis, IN 46223
   317-274-2977

   A variety of up-to-date information and educational materials are available regarding vehicle occupant protection for children with special needs and low-birth-weight infants.

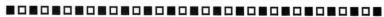
TABLE 9.5.
Key Pedestrian Messages for Parents and Communities

Reduce Exposure to Traffic
Create vehicle-free environments where children can play.
Separate children from traffic by use of fencing and physical distance of play areas from the roadway.
Discourage through traffic in residential areas.

Encourage Traffic Calming Measures
Enforce reasonable speed limits in residential areas.
Consider speed bumps or other engineering measures to control traffic speeds near areas where children play.
Create neighborhood and community awareness of pedestrian safety issues.

Increase Child's Visibility to the Motorist
Modify hazards (eg, eliminate shrubbery that obstructs view of child).
Alter parking patterns to increase visibility of children darting into street.
Use bright or retroreflective clothing at dusk.

Provide Adequate Supervision
Supervision of young children must be active.
Designated supervisor is essential.
Older children may not be appropriate supervisors.

Increase Parental Awareness of the Ability of Children to Deal With Traffic
Preschoolers and young elementary school children should not cross the street alone.
Individualize the age when independent crossing is allowed, but not before age 7 years.
All children should be taught to *stop at the curb.*
Skills must be repeatedly *demonstrated* before unsupervised crossing is allowed.
Initially limit unsupervised crossing to familiar, calm, two-lane streets.

Recognize the Hazards of the Driveway
Do not allow toddlers and preschoolers to use the driveway for a play area.
Do not allow children to play in parked cars.
Do not allow young children access to the electric garage door opener.
Check behind vehicles before backing up.
Be aware that children playing in the yard may inadvertently end up playing in a driveway or street.

Assume a Proactive Role in Community Groups
Promote education of motorists to understand the limited abilities and unpredictability of children near traffic.

Selected references for review include Brison et al,[37] Winn et al,[39] Vinje,[43] Dunne et al,[46] and National Highway Traffic Safety Administration.[64]

■□■□■□■□■□■□■□■□■□■□■□■□■□■□■□■

3. Insurance Institute for Highway Safety
1005 North Glebe Rd, Suite 200
Arlington, VA 22201
703-247-1500

This insurance industry–supported institute publishes *Status Report*, a newsletter that serves as a good general source of highway safety information. Also ask for *Fatality Facts*, a data packet reviewing the epidemiologic factors associated with highway deaths.

4. Midas Project Safe Baby
225 N Michigan Ave
Chicago, IL 60601
800-868-0088

Wholesale-priced convertible child safety seats are available through Midas retail outlets. Consumers may obtain a free child safety seat educational brochure in English or Spanish. The same information is available on video tape for the cost of shipping and handling.

5. National Highway Traffic Safety Administration
Office of Occupant Protection
400 Seventh St, NW
Washington, DC 20590
Auto Safety Hotline: 800-424-9393
DC Metro Area: 202-366-0123
Hearing Impaired: 800-424-9153

Handles consumer inquiries about CRD safety problems and recalls. (See section 9.1.2.)

6. Pediatric Injury Prevention Research Program
Health Policy Research
University of California, Irvine
714-824-7410

Based on pedestrian research in the Hispanic-Latino population, has developed a Spanish-language *fotonovela* aimed at prevention of pedestrian injuries in young children.

7. *Safe Ride News*
   5223 NE 18th St
   Lake Forest Park, WA 98135
   206-364-5696

   Published by the American Academy of Pediatrics from 1982 until 1995, it is an excellent ongoing source of child traffic safety information for the interested practitioner. The quarterly publication is now published by its editor, Deborah Stewart, and is available by subscription at the above address for $25 per year.

8. SafetyBeltSafe USA
   PO Box 553
   Altadena, CA 91003
   800-745-SAFE
   800-747-SANO (Spanish)

   Responds to consumer questions about child safety seats. Brochures (including tip sheets on incompatibility of car seats and automobiles) are available in English, Spanish, and many other languages.

References

1. National Highway Traffic Safety Administration. *Traffic Safety Facts 1993: A Compilation of Motor Vehicle Crash Data from the Fatal Accident Reporting System and the General Estimates System.* Washington, DC: US Department of Transportation; 1994

2. Rice DP, Mackenzie EJ, and Associates. *Cost of Injury in the United States: A Report to Congress.* San Francisco, CA: Institute for Health and Aging, University of California and Injury Prevention Center, and The Johns Hopkins University; 1989

3. Agran PF, Dunkle DE, Winn DG. Effects of legislation on motor vehicle injuries to children. *Am J Dis Child.* 1987;141:959–964

4. Margolis LH, Wagenaar AC, Liu W. The effects of a mandatory child restraint law on injuries requiring hospitalization. *Am J Dis Child.* 1988;142:1099–1103

5. National Highway Traffic Safety Administration. *Traffic Safety Facts 1995: Occupant Protection.* Washington, DC: US Department of Transportation; 1996

6. National Highway Traffic Safety Administration. *General Estimates System 1990: A Review of Information on Police-Reported Traffic Crashes in the United States.* Washington, DC: National Highway Traffic Safety Administration; 1991

7. American Academy of Pediatrics. 1995 Family Shopping Guide to Car Seats (pamphlet). Elk Grove Village, IL: American Academy of Pediatrics; 1995

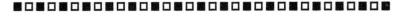

8. National Highway Traffic Safety Administration. State traffic data. In: *Traffic Safety Facts 1993: A Compilation of Motor Vehicle Crash Data from the Fatal Accident Reporting System and the General Estimates System.* Washington, DC: US Department of Transportation; 1994

9. Teret SP, Jones AS, Williams AF, Wells JK. Child restraint laws: an analysis of gaps in coverage. *Am J Public Health.* 1986;76:31–34

10. American Academy of Pediatrics, Committee on Injury and Poison Prevention. Selecting and using the most appropriate car safety seats for growing children: guidelines for counseling parents. *Pediatrics.* 1996;97:761–763

11. American Academy of Pediatrics, Committee on Injury and Poison Prevention. Transporting children with special needs. *Safe Ride News.* 1993;Winter

12. American Academy of Pediatrics, Committee on Injury and Poison Prevention and Committee on Fetus and Newborn. Safe transportation of premature and low birth weight infants. *Pediatrics.* 1996;97:758–760

13. Willett LD, Leuschen MP, Nelson LS, Nelson RM Jr. Ventilatory changes in convalescent infants positioned in car seats. *J Pediatr.* 1989;115:451–455

14. Bass JL, Mehta, KA, Camara J. Monitoring premature infants in car seats: implementing the American Academy of Pediatrics policy in a community hospital. *Pediatrics.* 1993;91:1137–1141

15. National Highway Traffic Safety Administration. Research Note: *National Occupant Protection Use Survey, Controlled Intersection Study.* Washington, DC: US Department of Transportation; 1995

16. Shelton TST. *Revised Vehicle Miles of Travel for Passenger Cars and Light Trucks, 1975 to 1993. Research Note.* Washington, DC: National Highway Traffic Safety Administration; September 21, 1995

17. Agran PF, Winn DG, Castillo DN. Pediatric injuries in the back of pickup trucks. *JAMA.* 1990;264:712–716

18. Woodward GA, Bolte RG. Children riding in the back of pickup trucks: a neglected safety issue. *Pediatrics.* 1990;86:785–787

19. American Academy of Pediatrics, Committee on Injury and Poison Prevention. Children in pickup trucks. *Pediatrics.* 1991;88:393–394

20. Hampson NB, Norkool DM. Carbon monoxide poisoning in children riding in the back of pickup trucks. *JAMA.* 1992;267:538–540

21. National Highway Traffic Safety Administration. *Traffic Safety Facts 1995: Motorcycles.* Washington, DC: US Department of Transportation; 1996

22. Federal Aviation Administration. *The Performance of Child Restraint Devices in Transport Airplane Passenger Seats, Final Report.* Washington, DC: US Department of Transportation; 1994

23. Brown RC, Sanders JM, Schonberg SK. Driving safety and adolescent behavior. *Pediatrics.* 1986;77:603–607

24. Robertson LS, Zador PL. Driver education and fatal crash involvement of teenaged drivers. *Am J Public Health*. 1978;68:959–965

25. American Academy of Pediatrics, Committee on Injury Prevention and Committee on Adolescence. The teenage driver. *Pediatrics*. 1996;98:987–990

26. Rivara FP. Child pedestrian injuries in the United States: current status of the problem, potential interventions and future research needs. *Am J Dis Child*. 1990;144: 692–696

27. Teanby D. Underreporting of pedestrian road accidents. *BMJ*. 1992;304:422

28. Agran PF, Castillo DN, Winn DG. Limitations of data compiled from police reports on pediatric pedestrian and bicycle motor vehicle events. *Accid Anal Prev*. 1990; 22:361–370

29. Children's Safety Network. *A Data Book of Child and Adolescent Injury*. Washington, DC: National Center for Education in Maternal and Child Health; 1991

30. Lapidus G, Braddock M, Banco L, Montenegro L, Hight D, Eanniello V. Child pedestrian injury: a population-based collision and injury severity profile. *J Trauma*. 1991; 31:1110–1115

31. Stevenson MR. Analytical approach to the investigation of childhood pedestrian injuries: a review of the literature. *J Safety Res*. 1991;22:123–132

32. Van Der Molen HH. Child pedestrian exposure, accidents and behavior. *Accid Anal Prev*. 1981;13:193–224

33. Routledge DA, Repetto Wright R, Howarth CI. A comparison of interviews and observation to obtain measures of children's exposure to risk as pedestrians. *Ergonomics*. 1974;17:623–638

34. Routledge DA, Repetto Wright R, Howarth CI. The exposure of young children to accident risk as pedestrians. *Ergonomics*. 1974;17:457–480

35. Howarth CI, Routledge DA, Repetto Wright R. An analysis of road accidents involving child pedestrians. *Ergonomics*. 1974;17:319–330

36. Jonah BA, Engel GR. Measuring the relative risk of pedestrian accidents. *Accid Anal Prev*. 1983;15:193–206

37. Brison RJ, Wicklund K, Mueller, MB. Fatal pedestrian injuries to young children: a different pattern of injury. *Am J Public Health*. 1988;78:793–795

38. Wade FM, Foot HC, Chapman AJ. Accidents and the physical environment. In: Chapman AJ, Wade FM, Foot HC, eds. *Pedestrian Accidents*. New York, NY: John Wiley and Sons; 1982:237–264

39. Winn DG, Agran PF, Castillo DN. Pedestrian injuries to children younger than 5 years of age. *Pediatrics*. 1991;88:776–782

40. Van Der Molen HH, Rothengatter JA, Vinje MP. Blueprint of an analysis of the pedestrian's task: I. *Accid Anal Prev*. 1981;13:175–191

41. Sandels S. Young children in traffic. *Br J Educ Psychol*. 1970;40:111–116

42. David SS, Foot HC, Chapman AJ, Sheehy NP. Peripheral vision and the etiology of child pedestrian accidents. *Br J Psychol*. 1995;1:112–115

43. Vinje MP. Children as pedestrians: abilities and limitations. *Accid Anal Prev.* 1981; 13:225–240

44. Eichelberger MR, Gotschall CS, Feely HB, Harstad P, Bowman LM. Parental attitudes and knowledge of child safety: national survey. *Am J Dis Child.* 1990;144:714–720

45. Rivara FP, Bergman AB, Drake C. Parental attitudes and practices toward children as pedestrians. *Pediatrics.* 1989;84:1017–1021

46. Dunne RG, Asher KN, Rivara FP. Behavior and parental expectations of child pedestrians. *Pediatrics.* 1992;89:486–490

47. Thackray RM, Dueker RL. *Child Pedestrian Supervision Guidance.* Washington DC: US Department of Transportation, National Highway Traffic Safety Administration; 1983

48. Van der Molen HH. Behavior of children and accompanying adults at a pedestrian crosswalk. *J Safety Res.* 1982;13:113–119

49. Mueller BA, Rivara FP, Lii SM, Weiss NS. Environmental factors and the risk for childhood pedestrian-motor vehicle collision occurrence. *Am J Epidemiol.* 1990; 192:550–560

50. Joly MF, Foggin PM, Pless IB. Geographical and socio-ecological variations of traffic accidents among children. *Soc Sci Med.* 1991;33:765–769

51. Braddock M, Lapidus G, Gregorio D, Kapp M, Banco L. Population, income, and ecological correlates of child pedestrian injury. *Pediatrics.* 1991;88:1242–1247

52. Pless IB, Verreault R, Tenina S. A case-control study of pedestrian and bicyclist injuries in childhood. *Am J Public Health.* 1989;79:995–998

53. Rivara FP, Barber M. Demographic analysis of child pedestrian injuries. *Pediatrics.* 1985;76:375–381

54. Stevenson MR, Lo SK, Laing BA, Jamrozik KD. Child pedestrian injuries in the Perth metropolitan area. *Med J Aust.* 1992;156:234–238

55. Malek M, Guyer B, Lescohier I. The epidemiology and prevention of child pedestrian injury. *Accid Anal Prev.* 1990;22:301–313

56. Howarth CI. Interactions between drivers and pedestrians: some new approaches to pedestrian safety. In: Evans L, Schwing RC, eds. *Human Behavior and Traffic Safety.* New York, NY: Plenum Press; 1985:171–188

57. Race KE. Evaluating pedestrian safety education materials for children ages five to nine. *J School Health.* 1988;58:277–281

58. Rivara FP, Booth CL, Bergman AB, Rogers LW, Weiss J. Prevention of pedestrian injuries to children: effectiveness of a school training program. *Pediatrics.* 1991; 88:770–775

59. Grayson GB. The identification of training objectives: what shall we tell the children. *Accid Anal Prev.* 1981;13:169–173

60. Fortenberry JC, Brown DB. Problem identification, implementation and evaluation of a pedestrian safety program. *Accid Anal Prev.* 1982;14:315–322

61. Rothengatter JA. The influence of instructional variables on the effectiveness of traffic education. *Accid Anal Prev.* 1981;13:241–253

62. Singh A. Pedestrian education. In: Chapman AJ, Wade FM, Foot HC, eds, *Pedestrian Accidents*. New York, NY: John Wiley and Sons; 1982:71–108

63. Rothengatter T. A behavioral approach to improving traffic behavior of young children. *Ergonomics*. 1984;27:147–160

64. National Highway Traffic Safety Administration. *Literature Review on the Preschool Pedestrian*. Washington, DC: US Department of Transportation; 1985

65. Embry DD, Malfetti JL. *Reducing the Risk of Pedestrian Accidents to Preschoolers by Parent Training and Symbolic Modeling for Children: An Experimental Analysis in the Natural Environment*. Research Report Number 2. Lawrence, KS: Safe-Playing Project; 1980

66. Limbourg M, Gerber D. A parent training program for the road safety education of preschool children. *Accid Anal Prev*. 1981;13:255–267

67. Los Angeles County Department of Health Services. *Pedestrian Injuries in Los Angeles County*. Los Angeles, CA: Los Angeles County Department of Health Services, Data Collection and Analysis Unit, Injury Prevention and Control Project; 1992

68. Michon JA. Traffic education for young pedestrians: an introduction. *Accid Anal Prev*. 1981;13:163–167

69. Pruesser DF, Blomberg RD. *Development and Validation of a Road Safety Public Education Process*. Walfeboro, NH: Van Gorcum; 1987

70. Roberts I, Norton R, Jackson R. Driveway-related child pedestrian injuries: a case-control study. *Pediatrics*. 1995;95:405–408

71. Robertson LS. Car design and risk of pedestrian deaths. *Am J Public Health*. 1990; 80:609–610

72. Rivara FP, Reay DT, Bergman AB. Analysis of fatal pedestrian injuries in King County, WA, and prospects for prevention. *Public Health Rep*. 1989;104:293–297

73. Zegeer CV, Zegeer SF. *Pedestrian and Traffic-control Measures*. Washington, DC: Transportation Research Board, National Research Council; 1988

74. Pitt R, Guyer B, Hsieh CC, Malek M. The severity of pedestrian injuries in children: an analysis of the pedestrian injury causation study. *Accid Anal Prev*. 1990;22:549–559

75. Reiss ML, Shinder AE. *School Trip Safety and Urban Play Areas: Volume VII-Guideline for the Creation and Operation of Urban Play Streets*. Washington, DC: US Department of Transportation, Federal Highway Administration; 1975

76. Christoffel KK, Schafer JL, Jovanis PP, Brandt B, White B, Tanz R. Childhood pedestrian injury: a pilot study concerning etiology. *Accid Anal Prev*. 1986;18:25–35

77. Insurance Institute for Highway Safety. *Fatality Facts, 1994 Edition*. Arlington VA: Insurance Institute for Highway Safety; 1994

78. Widome MD. Pediatric injury prevention for the practitioner. *Curr Probl Pediatr*. 1991; 21:428–468

CHAPTER 10

Water Safety

10.1 Scope of the Problem

Drowning is defined as death resulting from immersion injury within 24 hours of the event. *Near-drowning* is an immersion injury in which the person survives for at least 24 hours.[1] More than 1400 children and adolescents (from birth to 19 years of age) drown in the United States each year. More than 600 of those are infants and preschoolers and another 500 are teenagers[2] (Fig 10.1, p 220). After motor vehicle–related injuries, drowning ties with fires as the second leading cause of unintentional injury-related death to pediatric patients. In Alaska, Arizona, California, Florida, Hawaii, Montana, Nevada, Oregon, Utah, and Washington, drowning has been the leading cause of injury-related death for children from birth to 14 years of age.[3] For every drowning death, approximately four substantial but nonfatal submersion injuries occur.[4] The economic costs to families and to society are large. Direct annual medical costs to care for children from birth to 14 years of age who are injured by drowning and near-drowning have been calculated at $34 million. Including indirect costs to society (lost present and future productivity), the figure approaches $400 million per year.[5] The emotional costs to families and communities cannot be calculated.

10.2 Age-Related Issues and Interventions

Efforts to prevent drowning are most easily understood by studying the underlying epidemiologic factors for each age group. The places and ways in which children drown are related to the developmental stage and the opportunities offered by the environment. However, the causes of and factors related to drowning vary greatly by gender, geography, season, race, and economic status.[6] Anticipatory guidance in the office must be based on the age of the patient and on local patterns of exposure and injury.[6]

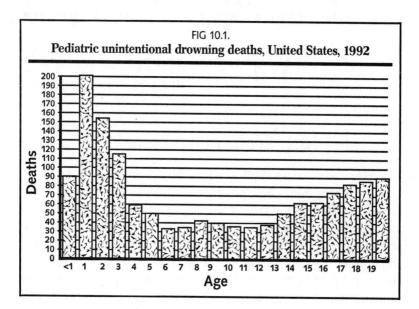

FIG 10.1.
Pediatric unintentional drowning deaths, United States, 1992

10.2.1 Infants, Tubs, and Buckets

Infants most commonly drown in bathtubs or other fluid-filled containers such as 5-gallon scrub buckets found in the home. Bathtubs are the site of 8% of all childhood drownings.[7] In a recent study in Utah, all but one bathtub-related death occurred in the absence of adult supervision but with another sibling (2 to 7 years of age) present.[8] Parents must be reminded that young children should never be left alone in the bathtub and that older preschoolers are incapable of adequately supervising a younger sibling during a bath.

The Consumer Product Safety Commission (CPSC) estimates that as many as one infant per week drowns in a bucket. These buckets are usually about 14 in high or about half the height of a top-heavy crawling toddler. Even partially filled buckets weigh more than an infant does and, therefore, do not tip over when the infant falls in. The severity of the injury may be increased by toxic materials contained in the buckets. African-American children and boys are at increased risk for these injuries. Parents should be counseled that any large container, bucket, or bathtub should be emptied immediately after use.[9]

Supporting rings, consisting of a ring with three or four legs with suction cups that attach to the bottom of the tub, have been popular for use while infants are bathed. These devices give parents a false sense of security, leading to injuries and drowning deaths from infants being left unattended (see TIPP slip by the American Academy of Pediatrics (AAP) on home water hazards for young children, Resources section).

10.2.2 Preschoolers and Swimming Pools

Backyard swimming pools and spas represent the greatest risk to preschoolers, particularly young preschoolers, 18 to 30 months of age. Of the 600 annual drowning deaths of children from birth to 5 years of age, more than 300 occur in residential swimming pools. Annually, approximately 2300 nonfatal injuries sustained in residential pools occur in this age group.

Boys suffering submersion injuries outnumber girls by about two to one. Almost 70% of these children drowned in their own backyard pools, and another 20% drowned in a relative's pool. Three fourths of the time they were being supervised by one or both parents, but the children were not expected to be in the pool area. Seventy percent were not wearing swimming clothes, almost half were last seen in the home, and most were "missing" for less than 5 minutes. Half of the time the parent was supervising two or more children, and almost always the parent was engaged in routine household chores.[10] The risk of drowning is three to five times greater during the first 6 months of exposure to a swimming pool than in later periods (see TIPP slip on pool safety for children, Resources section).

Although parental supervision should always be emphasized, it is unlikely that this alone will substantially change the drowning rate for this age group. Most parents believe that they are adequately supervising a child who is out of sight for less than 5 minutes. Families who have frequent access to a backyard pool (their own or one belonging to a neighbor or close relative) should be encouraged to place fencing around all four sides of the pool or spa (or they should encourage the same from neighbors and relatives) (Fig 10.2, p 222). Evidence supports fencing as effective in reducing the risk of drowning.[11] Fences should be at least 48-in high. Spacing between the slats should not exceed 4 in. If chain link fence is used, the diamond-shaped openings should not exceed 1¾ in. Gates must be self-closing and self-latching. Ideally gates should open away from the pool so an unlatched gate closes if a toddler leans against it from outside the pool area. If families

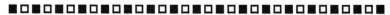
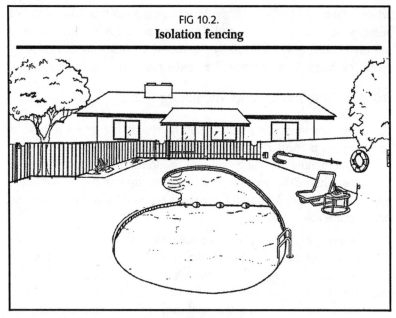

FIG 10.2.
Isolation fencing

Courtesy of the Tucson, Arizona Drowning Prevention Committee.

have already installed a fence, maintenance of the fence, and especially of the gate, must be emphasized. No part of the house with windows or doors should form part of this barrier.

Although fencing is the only barrier documented as effective, other barriers may be added as additional layers of protection. Pool safety covers have received the most support. The American Society for Testing and Materials has issued an automatic pool safety cover standard. Families who have a pool safety cover must be reminded to close the cover completely after each pool use. Floating solar covers should be specifically excluded. To children, they seem to be safe surfaces, but children may sink beneath the cover and not be visible. Adults have also drowned beneath these covers because they have been unable to break out from underneath them. Other barriers, such as door alarms, automatic door closers for hinged and sliding doors, or pool alarms may be used. None of these measures, however, have been documented to decrease the risk of drowning, and *no* barrier is effective unless it is consistently maintained and used appropriately.

Two aspects of prehospital care of children injured by submersion are closely linked to survival and outcome: duration of submersion and duration of resuscitation.[1] Duration of submersion is associated with steadily increasing risk. Children found within 1 to 2 minutes have a uniformly good outcome, and children submersed less than 5 minutes generally recover. Children submersed for longer than 10 minutes often die or sustain severe neurologic impairment.[12]

Outcome is also affected by the immediate performance of cardiopulmonary resuscitation (CPR) or rescue breathing (the breathing part only of CPR) at the scene before the arrival of emergency personnel.[13] All families with young children should be encouraged to become certified in CPR and should know how to access local emergency medical services. A poolside phone is essential.

The issue of swimming lessons to help prevent drowning of young children remains controversial.[6,14] While there is little dispute that children can be taught various swimming skills, no documentation exists that these skills can prevent drowning. Some experts have concern that increased familiarity with the pool environment may make children too comfortable around water or that acquisition of swimming skills by children may make parents less vigilant supervisors. It is unreasonable to expect children who have learned to swim to the side of the pool to use that skill when they have unintentionally entered a pool, possibly fully clothed and experiencing fear and confusion. Until more definitive work is done on this important question, the AAP does not recommend organized swimming lessons for children younger than 3 years as a prevention strategy for drowning.

10.2.3 School-age Children

School-age children are much more likely to drown in natural bodies of water than in backyard swimming pools. Nonpool drownings are linearly and inversely related to socioeconomic status.[4] African-American children are twice as likely to drown as white children, and boys are three times as likely to drown as girls.[15] Children with seizure disorders are also more likely to suffer injury from immersion and to drown.[16]

Prevention efforts in the school-age group should be focused on learning to swim and on appropriate water safety rules, such as never swimming alone and always wearing a personal flotation device (PFD) when boating.

Personal flotation devices should be approved by the US Coast Guard. The Coast Guard rates PFDs as types 1 to 4. Type 1 jackets float most effectively but are available in only two sizes and do not usually fit small children. Type 2 jackets are available in a variety of sizes, are designed to float the person face up, and are the best type available for most children. Type 3 jackets are more appropriate for older children who are engaged in water sports such as skiing, during which they will be continuously observed and could be rescued quickly. Type 4 preservers are only cushions and should not be considered adequate protection for children or adults (see TIPP slip on life jackets and life preservers, Resources section).

Local conditions such as thinning ice or seasonal waterfalls may increase the risk of drowning to older children and should be reviewed with parents and children.

School-age children with epilepsy deserve special discussion. Their risk of drowning is 4 to 10 times that of children without epilepsy. Supervision and appropriate family rules become the preventive strategies of choice. Baths, especially unsupervised baths, pose substantial risks to older children with seizure disorders. Such children should be encouraged to shower if their need for privacy precludes supervised bathing. Swimming can be enjoyed safely if supervision is adequate and the supervisor is able to rescue the child should a seizure occur while the child is in the pool.[16]

10.2.4 Adolescents and Risk Taking

After preschoolers, adolescents and young adults (15 to 24 years of age) have the second highest rates of drowning. The drownings also occur primarily in natural bodies of water, as they do among school-age children, but male preponderance becomes even more striking with drowning among boys exceeding drowning among girls by six to one. Alcohol use is associated with as many as half of these drownings.[4]

Teenagers drown not only during swimming activity, but also when they are engaged in other water activities such as boating, sailing, waterskiing, or using jet skis. Morbidity and mortality are somewhat analogous to adolescent traffic injuries because of their association with

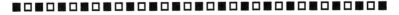

risk-taking behavior, use of alcohol, and failure to use protective equipment (ie, PFDs). Use of alcohol is associated with one third to two thirds of all recreational boating fatalities. Of drownings among older adolescent boys, 40% to 50% are believed to be alcohol-related.[4] A small study of injuries while jet-skiing revealed that most injured riders were teenagers with little actual training in the use of these watercraft. Case reports suggest that most serious injuries occur from collisions with swimmers, other watercraft, or structures such as piers or docks.[17]

Diving-related injury first becomes an issue during adolescence. Injuries to males outnumber injuries to females, and alcohol is associated with 50% of these injuries. Diving injuries occur in natural bodies of water about half of the time and in shallow water (<4-ft deep) 70% of the time. Therefore diving in any above-ground pool should be prohibited. This rule should be enforced with younger children so they do not assume that when they are older they can safely dive into shallow water. Diving injuries account for one of eight spinal cord injuries, with half of those injuries resulting in quadriplegia.

A summary of age-appropriate counseling topics and handouts from TIPP is presented in Table 10.1.

TABLE 10.1. Age-Appropriate Counseling Guidelines for Water Safety Education*			
Age, y	**Drowning Site**	**Strategies**	**TIPP Handouts**
Infants, Birth–1	Bathtub, bucket	*Adult* supervision, empty bathtub and bucket	Home Water Hazards for Young Children
Preschool children, 1–5	Swimming pool	Four-sided fencing, supervision, cardiopulmonary resuscitation	Pool Safety for Children
School-age children, 5–12	Swimming pool, natural bodies of water	Swimming lessons, "pool rules," personal flotation devices	Water Safety for Your School-age Child Life Jackets and Life Preservers
Adolescents, >12	Natural bodies of water, diving injury	Personal flotation devices, no alcohol, jump feet first the first time they enter the water	Life Jackets and Life Preservers

*Adapted from the AAP *Physician's Resource Guide.*

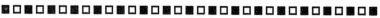
10.2.5 Hot Tubs, Spas, and Whirlpools

Although there are few statistics on injuries from hot tubs, spas, and whirlpools, reports of unfortunate incidents serve to highlight the hazards of these facilities. Pregnant women and young children should not use a hot tub, spa, or whirlpool before consulting with a physician.

Hyperthermia/heat stress

Children, especially those who have not reached puberty, are at increased risk of heat stress in hot tubs. Prolonged elevation of body temperature in the 104° to 105°F range may lead to heart or brain damage, heat stroke, and death. The likelihood of a heat stress situation could be increased if one entered the hot tub in a dehydrated condition or consumed food or alcohol prior to entering the hot tub, reducing the blood flow to the heart and brain. Children will more quickly become hyperthermic in a hot tub because their ratio of surface area to body mass is greater than that of adults.[18]

Risk to fetus

Pregnant women should be aware that the use of hot tubs presents risks to the fetus. Animal experiments have documented hyperthermic teratogenesis. A recent study found that seven out of 63 women who may have suffered hyperthermia from a hot bath during the first month of pregnancy had babies with birth defects.[18] The first trimester appears to be the greatest period of risk for neural tube and central nervous system injury.

Skin infections

Skin infections are another potential hazard associated with hot tub, spa, and/or whirlpool use. Folliculitis, inflammation of hair follicles, is probably the most common infection associated with hot tub use. *Pseudomonas aeruginosa,* one bacteria that causes this ailment, may collect in hot tubs and whirlpools when chlorine levels are not maintained adequately.[18] Local skin, as well as systemic toxicity, may occur.

Drownings

The main hazard from hot tubs and spas is the same as that from pools — drowning. Since 1980, more than 700 deaths in hot tubs and spas have been reported to the CPSC. About one third of those were drownings of children under age 5.[19] Drownings have occurred when young children have fallen into unprotected hot tubs. Adults have drowned in hot tubs as a result of the heat, usually because they have taken sedative drugs or have been drinking alcohol. Adolescents would have the same risks.

Hair entanglement

Since 1978, 48 incidents (including 13 deaths) have been reported to the CPSC in which hair was sucked into the suction fitting of a spa, hot tub, or whirlpool, causing the victim's head to be held under water. Hair becomes entangled in the drain cover as the water and hair are drawn through the drain. The CPSC helped develop a voluntary standard for drain covers to reduce the risk of hair entrapment. Consumers should be sure they have new drain covers that meet this standard. Never allow a child to play in a way that could permit his or her hair to come near the drain cover. If the drain cover is missing or broken, shut down the spa until the cover is replaced.[19]

Body part entrapment

Since 1980, 18 incidents have been reported to the CPSC in which body parts have been entrapped by the strong suction of the drain of pools, wading pools, spas, and hot tubs. Of these, 10 entrapments have resulted in disembowelment and 5 persons have died. The CPSC helped develop a standard requiring dome-shaped drain outlets and two outlets for each pump to reduce the powerful suction if the drain is blocked.

Hot tub temperatures

The CPSC knows of several deaths from extremely hot water (approximately 110°F) in a spa. High temperatures can cause drowsiness, which may lead to unconsciousness and drowning. In addition, raised body temperature can lead to heat stroke and death. In 1987, the CPSC helped develop requirements for temperature controls to make sure that spa water temperatures do not exceed 104°F. For the safety of children, it is extremely important that the water in a hot tub be kept at the right temperature. (For comparison, the usual bath water temperature for a child is approximately 101°F).

Safety recommendations

The CPSC and the Centers for Disease Control and Prevention offer the following safety precautions:

- Always use a locked safety cover when the spa is not in use.
- Always supervise children in and around tubs and spas.
- Make sure the spa has dual drains and drain covers required by current safety standards.
- Have a professional check the spa regularly to ensure its safe working condition and that drain covers are not cracked or missing.
- Know where the cutoff switch for the pump is so that it can be turned off in an emergency.
- Be aware that drinking alcohol or taking sedatives before or during spa use could lead to drowning.
- Maintain the water temperature at 104°F or lower.

Summary

While young children should not be allowed to use hot tubs, spas, and whirlpools, their use can be pleasantly relaxing for older children and adolescents if the simple precautions previously outlined are followed.

10.3 Advocacy

In addition to office-based counseling (summarized in Table 10.2, p 229), pediatricians can help prevent drowning by promoting the following community interventions.

- Encourage local and state health departments to collect accurate data about drownings and near-drownings so local trends and prevention efforts can be evaluated.
- Ensure that local emergency medical services are adequately prepared to treat childhood drowning.
- Promote regulations requiring adequately trained lifeguards at public or private recreational swimming areas.
- Promote programs aimed at increasing the number of families who are trained in CPR.
- Promote efforts that limit access to alcohol by teenagers and boat operators.

TABLE 10.2.
Water Safety Counseling Guidelines for Parents and Other Caregivers*

For Infants and Preschoolers
- Never leave young children alone in bathtubs. Never rely on supporting rings. Do not rely on an older sibling for supervision of an infant or preschooler.
- Do not leave infants or toddlers unattended in the bathroom. Infants can drown in toilets.
- Provide constant and direct supervision of young children around swimming pools, wading pools, ponds, and all natural bodies of water.
- Never expect swimming instruction to eliminate the risk of drowning in children.
- Supervise children in the water even if they are wearing flotation devices; these devices are not substitutes for constant supervision.
- To substantially lower a child's risk of drowning in a residential swimming pool, install a four-sided isolation fence. Use AAP or CPSC guidelines regarding fencing dimensions, construction, and gates.
- Never leave pool covers partially in place, because children can become trapped beneath them. Pool covers are not a substitute for fencing.
- Keep tables and chairs away from pool fences to prevent children from climbing over the fence into the pool.
- Keep toys and tricycles away from the pool area so they are not an attraction to the pool.
- Remove and secure the steps to above-ground pools whenever they are not in use.
- Learn CPR and keep rescue equipment at poolside, including a life preserver, shepherd's crook, and cordless telephone.
- Never leave infants or children unattended around 5-gallon buckets containing even a small amount of liquid. Empty buckets when not in use.
- Instruct baby-sitters fully about pool, bathtub, and bucket safety.

For School-age Children
- Ensure that children learn to swim from qualified instructors who incorporate safety training into the program.
- Ensure that all recreational swimming is supervised by a lifeguard or an adult. Knowing how to swim is not a license to swim alone.
- Learn CPR and keep appropriate safety equipment at the poolside (see previous section of the Table).
- Ensure that Coast Guard–approved PFDs are worn for all recreational boating, water-skiing, and other water sports.
- Avoid drowning risks associated with cold weather recreational activities (eg, walking or ice skating on thin ice) on ponds and other bodies of partially frozen water.
- Review diving safety, as discussed for teenagers in the next section of the Table, as older children learn to dive.
- Ensure that children never go down a pool slide head first.

For Teenagers
- Review safety issues for school-age children, as appropriate.
- Advise teenagers not to swim alone.
- Recognize the dangers of alcohol or other drug use in association with boating and other aquatic recreational activities.
- Understand the seriousness and irreversibility of spinal cord injury from diving into shallow water.

TABLE 10.2. Water Safety Counseling Guidelines for Parents and Other Caregivers,* continued
For Teenagers, continued • Never allow teenagers to dive into above-ground pools. • Diving should be done only from the end of the diving board, never from the sides, or from the side of the pool. Teenagers should enter pools feet first. • Advise teenagers not to dive into unfamiliar bodies of water or into any water where diving is not specifically approved or sanctioned. They should never dive from piers or docks. • Ensure that teenagers learn CPR, and encourage inclusion of CPR training in high school.

*AAP indicates American Academy of Pediatrics; CPSC, Consumer Product Safety Commission; CPR, cardiopulmonary resuscitation; PFD, personal flotation device.

• Encourage the use of PFDs and their availability at local beaches.

• Promote legislation mandating "isolation" fencing that surrounds all four sides of backyard swimming pools and spas. (A model pool legislation packet is available from the AAP.) A related strategy is to seek the adoption of language in the uniform building code that mandates fencing.

10.4 Resources

1. American Academy of Pediatrics
   141 Northwest Point Blvd
   PO Box 927
   Elk Grove Village, IL 60009-0927
   800-433-9016

   Ask for the "Physician's Resource Guide for Water Safety Education," which includes the AAP policy statement and its model legislation for pool enclosures. TIPP materials and a comprehensive state legislation packet on pool barriers are also available.

2. American Red Cross
   2025 E St, NW
   Washington, DC 20006
   202-728-6531

Materials about infant and preschool aquatic programs, class-room safety instruction, and other water safety instruction issues are available.

3. Consumer Product Safety Commission
Office of Information and Public Affairs
Washington, DC 20207
301-504-0580

Several educational materials aimed at pool owners, including guide-lines for barrier fencing and safe practices, are available.

4. YMCA of the United States
101 N Wacker Dr
Chicago, IL 60606
800-USA-YMCA

Ask for information about organized swimming instruction for chil-dren younger than 5 years of age.

References

1. Kallas HJ, O'Rourke PP. Drowning and immersion injuries in children. *Curr Opin Pediatr.* 1993;5:295–302

2. National Safety Council. *Accident Facts.* Itasca, IL: National Safety Council; 1995

3. Waller AE, Baker SP, Szocka A. Childhood injury deaths: national analysis and geo-graphic variation. *Am J Public Health.* 1989;79:310–315

4. Wintemute GJ. Childhood drowning and near-drowning in the United States. *Am J Dis Child.* 1990;144:663–669

5. Rice DP, Mackenzie EJ, and Associates. *Cost of Injury in the United States: A Report to Congress.* San Francisco, CA: Institute for Health & Aging, University of California and Injury Prevention Center, and The Johns Hopkins University; 1989

6. American Academy of Pediatrics, Committee on Injury and Poison Prevention. Drowning in infants, children, and adolescents. *Pediatrics.* 1993;92:292–294

7. Baker SP, Waller AE. *Childhood Injury: State-by-State Mortality* Facts. Baltimore, MD: The Johns Hopkins Injury Prevention Center; 1989

8. Jensen L, Williams SD, Thurman DJ, Keller PA. Submersion injuries in children younger than 5 years in urban Utah. *West J Med.* 1992;157:641–644

9. Mann NC, Weller SC, Rauchschwalbe R. Bucket-related drownings in the United States, 1984-1990. *Pediatrics.* 1992;89:1091–1093

10. Present P. *Child Drowning Study: A Report on the Epidemiology of Drownings in Residential Pools to Children Under Age Five.* Washington, DC: US Consumer Product Safety Commission; 1987

11. Pitt WR, Balanda KP. Childhood drowning and near-drowning in Brisbane: the contribution of domestic pools. *Med J Aust.* 1991;154:661–665

12. Quan L, Kinder D. Pediatric submersions: pre-hospital predictors of outcome. *Pediatrics.* 1992;90:909–913

13. Kyriacou DN, Arcinue EL, Peek C, Kraus JF. Effect of immediate resuscitation on children with submersion injury. *Pediatrics.* 1994;94:137–142

14. Pearn JH. Current controversies in child accident prevention: an analysis of some areas of dispute in the prevention of child trauma. *Aust N Z J Med.* 1985;15:782–787

15. Baker SP, O'Neill B, Ginsburg MJ, Li G. *The Injury Fact Book.* 2nd ed. New York, NY: Oxford University Press; 1992

16. Diekema DS, Quan L, Holt VL. Epilepsy as a risk factor for submersion injury in children. *Pediatrics.* 1993;91:612–616

17. Gomez G, Martin LC, Castro MR. Nautical accidents. *Surg Clin North Am.* 1991; 71:419–432

18. Duda, M. The medical risks and benefits of sauna, steam bath, and whirlpool use. *Phys Sports Med.* 1987;15:170–182

19. US Consumer Product Safety Commission. *Consumer Product Safety Alert: Spas, Hot Tubs, and Whirlpools.* Washington, DC: US Consumer Product Safety Commission; 1996

CHAPTER 11

Fires and Burns

Burns in children are among the most devastating of all injuries. Patients with severe burns require prolonged hospitalization for pain control and wound care, fluid and nutritional balance, prevention and treatment of infection, multiple skin grafts, and psychological care. Many of these problems endure through a lengthy period of rehabilitation. Most burns from flames, scalds, and contact with other thermal energy sources are preventable.

Fires and burns are the third most common cause of unintentional injury death — after motor vehicle and falls — causing more than 5000 deaths annually. More than 1000 of these deaths occur in children younger than 15 years. Each year, more than 50 000 acute hospital admissions result from the more than 1.25 million burn injuries.[1,2] Approximately 23 000 of these admissions are in burn-center hospitals.[2] In 1993, approximately 238 000 people were treated in hospital emergency departments for thermal (151 000), electrical (6100), scald (77 700), and other (2900 unspecified) burns related to consumer products.[3] Most of the approximately 284 000 to 441 000 additional injuries from burns treated in emergency departments are scalds resulting from food and beverage spills.[4,5]

In 1985, Rice et al[6] estimated lifetime direct morbidity and mortality costs of all injuries from fires and burns at $3.8 billion annually. More recent figures, using a different methodology, estimate the economic loss from fire-related fatal and nonfatal unintentional injury at $8.2 billion in 1995.[7] If lost quality of life is included in the calculations, this figure more than doubles. Yet another calculation estimates the cost of 1993 deaths and injuries from fires at $15.5 billion, based on a willingness-to-pay approach to risk valuation.[8]

Among children younger than 1 year, fire- and burn-related deaths follow nonfirearm homicide and motor vehicle crashes as a leading cause of injury death. Between ages 1 and 9 years, deaths from fire and burn injury are second only to those from motor vehicle injury.[9]

Although scalds make up a higher percentage of hospital admissions than burns from fires,[10,11] the fatality rate of those hospitalized from fires (12% in the first hospitalization) far exceeds that of other hospitalized patients with burns (3%).[10]

Examination of trends from 1971 to 1991 shows a decline of approximately 50% in the rates of both fire- and burn-related deaths and also in acute hospital admissions for burn injury. These changes are most likely because of an increase in public fire and burn safety education, more widespread use of smoke detectors, stronger building and fire codes and standards, safer consumer products and workplaces, and expansion in the network of burn treatment centers. Changes in our societal lifestyle, such as declines in smoking and alcohol abuse, as well as changes in home cooking practices, have also contributed to this reduced incidence. The decrease in hospitalizations for burn injury may, in part, also result from a treatment shift from the inpatient to the outpatient setting.[2]

The type of injury from a fire or burn is generally related to the age and developmental level of the child: infants may be scalded from drinking liquids heated in a microwave or by being bathed in water that is too hot; toddlers may spill hot liquids or food or touch hot surfaces or electrical wiring; preschool and early school-age children may play with matches or cigarette lighters; and adolescents, who are frequently high-risk takers, may be susceptible to almost all the same kinds of hazards encountered by adults.

Although burns may also be caused by ultraviolet and ionizing radiation, electricity, and chemicals, this chapter deals with injuries and deaths related to residential fires, scalds, and heat and flame from a variety of consumer products including fireworks, smoking materials, matches, cigarette lighters, wearing apparel, cooking equipment, home heating devices, faulty wiring, and flammable liquids.

11.1 Residential Fires

11.1.1 Scope of the Problem

In 1993, an estimated 470 000 residential structure fires resulted in 3825 nonfirefighter deaths, 22 000 injuries, and $4.8 billion in property loss.[12] These fires accounted for about 75% of all structure fires, 83% of deaths, and 74% of injuries. The major equipment types involved in these fires were cooking (24%) and heating (18%). During 1980 to 1993, estimated residential structure fires decreased about 38% and deaths decreased about 30%, while injuries increased by 7%.

11.1.2 Risk Factors

Death rates relative to population are the highest among preschool children and the elderly.[1] Home fires result in more than 90% of all unintentional fire- and burn-related deaths in children younger than 15 years.[13] Young children may have difficulty escaping from burning buildings, even though a smoke detector may be sounding. The majority of these home fire-related deaths among children occur as a result of smoke inhalation, rather than directly from burns.[14] Overall, toxic gas effects from smoke inhalation outnumber burns as a cause of deaths from fires by roughly 3 to 1.[15]

Across all ages, the male to female ratio is approximately 1.5 to 1 for deaths from home fires. The ratio is only 1.3 to 1 for children but is slightly higher for preschool children (younger than age 6). The rate of deaths from home fires for preschool children is double, relative to population, of all age groups combined, whereas the death rate for school-age children is less than 60% of the rate for all ages. Part of the difference is due to children playing with fire, usually matches or lighters, which accounts for more than one third of all deaths from home fires in preschool children.[16] African-Americans and Native Americans die at more than twice the rate of whites from residential fires. Differences in the fire death ratio based on race appear to primarily reflect the high death rates associated with poverty or lower levels of education, both of which typically show up as stronger risk factors (in a statistical sense) than race.[17,18]

Higher rates of residential fire deaths occur in the southeast, compared with lower rates in the western part of the United States. The higher southeastern rates correlate with a larger fraction of the population living in poverty, especially in rural areas, which have by far the highest fire death ratio by size of community. Milder winters lead to more use of portable space heaters and space heating among the rural poor in the southeast, which is a factor in the higher death rates, though not nearly so much so since the early 1980s.[18,19]

Deaths from fires occur disproportionately in the winter months when heating systems and lighting systems are most utilized. Deaths from home fires are associated with high blood alcohol concentrations in half of adult victims. A common scenario involves an intoxicated adult falling asleep on a chair or bed, dropping a lighted cigarette, which may smolder for several hours undetected before a fire erupts, killing people at night while they sleep as toxic fumes overcome them.

The major causes of fatal home fires, based on 1993 data, begin with cigarettes and other lighted tobacco products, resulting in 26% of fatal home fires. Incendiary or suspicious fires — arson or suspected arson — accounted for 20%. Upholstered furniture (17%) and mattresses and bedding (17%) often, but not always, involved smoking materials as heat sources. Fires from heating equipment fires caused 14% of fatal home fires. Children playing with fire accounted for 11% of deaths from home fires and more than one third of the deaths of preschool children.[20]

11.1.3 Intervention Strategies and Prevention Messages

Deaths and injuries from residential fires may be mitigated by a variety of interventions including those related to the safe use of the consumer products discussed in the following sections: 11.4 — smoking materials; 11.5 — matches; 11.6 — cigarette lighters; 11.8 — cooking equipment; and 11.9 — home heating devices.

Intervention strategies for all of these are discussed here:

1. Small children should never be left home alone and should be under close adult supervision whenever possible.
2. Smoke detectors should be installed and functioning in the hallway near each sleeping area and on each level of the home, including the basement. They should be placed on the ceiling or 6 to 12 in below the ceiling on the wall. Smoke detectors are the first line of defense in a fire, alerting one in time to escape a fire. It is estimated that the presence of a smoke detector cuts the risk of dying in a home fire almost in half.[21] All smoke detectors should bear the label of an independent testing laboratory. Detectors with a flashing light in addition to a sound alarm should be installed in households with hearing-impaired or deaf individuals, including one inside their bedroom. Smoke detectors should be tested monthly. At any given time, it is estimated that one fifth of the smoke detectors in homes are not

working — primarily because batteries are dead or missing. Batteries should be replaced at least once a year, or more frequently if they make a "chirping" sound; never "borrow" the batteries for other uses. The smoke detector should be unobstructed, should be kept clean, and should not be painted.

3. Exit Drills in the Home (EDITH)[21]: An escape plan should be in place with at least two exits from each part of the house, especially the bedrooms. The escape plan should be practiced at least every 6 months, being sure that windows and doors can unlock and open quickly, and that everyone knows to leave immediately, without gathering clothing or valuables; then the fire department can be called from a neighbor's house. The plan should be known by, and rehearsed with, all care providers.

If the home has an upper level, a noncombustible fire escape ladder should be available. If no escape ladder is available, and if more than two stories from the ground, persons should not jump, but rather wait for the fire department.

A pre-designated meeting place should be established outside the home. If someone is trapped, the rescue should be left to the trained firefighter; never return to a burning building. Children should be taught that firefighters are "good strangers" and never to hide from them if there is a fire.

A special escape plan should be provided for small children, the elderly, and individuals with disabilities, which meets their needs for lifting, breathing, etc. Good escape planning should include alerting the fire department in advance to the presence in a household of one or more individuals who may have difficulty escaping. If possible, the sleeping area of such an individual should be on the ground floor for easier egress. Neighbors of hearing-impaired children who cannot speak should be taught sign language for "fire."

4. In the event of a fire, the closed door should be tested for heat and should not be opened if heat or smoke is present.

Occupants of a burning home should crawl low on their hands and knees under the smoke and toxic gases. The cleanest air is 12 to 24 in above the floor. All doors should be closed as the occupants leave each room to keep the fire from spreading.

Apartment dwellers should not use an elevator in a fire because the elevator may stop at a burning floor. Apartment dwellers should know where the nearest alarm box is, so that other tenants can be warned.

5. If clothes begin to burn, the person should **stop, drop, and roll** to smother the flames.

6. Cool a burn immediately with cool running water. When cool, apply a clean dry dressing; do not coat the burn with butter or greasy ointments.

7. Adults, adolescents, and older children should use a fire extinguisher only if they know how to use it properly, the fire is small and self-contained, and they have a clear escape route available. If a fire is not in a very early stage, they should not use the fire extinguisher; rather, get the family out of the home and call the fire department. The best fire extinguishers are multipurpose (A:B:C) dry chemical extinguishers, which are effective in all three classes of fires: class A fires involve ordinary combustibles such as paper or wood; class B fires involve flammable or combustible liquids; and class C fires involve electric equipment. One extinguisher should be located in the kitchen, in the path of exit travel, so that an escape route exists if the fire cannot be controlled. A second extinguisher should be located in a workshop. It is important that adults and adolescents in the family know how to use the extinguisher quickly. Extinguishers should be checked at least once a month by looking at the pressure gauge and removing the extinguisher from the mounted bracket, to be sure this can be done easily. A recharging service company should be used for repair or recharging the extinguisher after each use.

The extinguisher should be aimed at the base of the fire, using a sweeping motion. Persons should leave the fire if they feel in danger. It is best to call or have someone else call the fire department *before* trying to fight the fire.

8. Automatic fire sprinkler systems are affordable and practical for many homes. They respond to high heat automatically and spray water on the fire. Only those sprinklers near the fire discharge when the system is activated, and they produce less water damage than fire department hoses. They also reduce the amount of smoke and toxic gases present. It is estimated that they decrease the risk of death in a fire by one third to two thirds.[21]

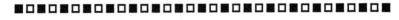
9. Baby-sitters should be shown around the house or the apartment, instructed about escape routes in the event of a fire, instructed not to smoke, given emergency numbers, and instructed to leave immediately with the child or children and call the fire department from a neighbor's house in case of a fire.

Educational messages about the prevention of fires and burns are part of the work of the National Fire Protection Association (NFPA), the US Fire Administration, the US Consumer Product Safety Commission (CPSC), and other organizations. The NFPA *Learn Not to Burn* curriculum is designed for school-age children and their families, and a *Learn Not to Burn* preschool program has recently been developed.

Some of the prevention messages in these and other educational programs include the following:

1. Do not smoke. If you smoke, avoid smoking indoors. If you smoke indoors, never smoke in bed.

2. If disposable butane lighters are present in the home, only those with child-resistant features should be available. These should be kept out of the view of young children and should not be of bright color or shiny finish if possible. Never use a lighter as a source of amusement for children. It may encourage them to think of lighters as a toy and try to light one on their own. Although children as young as 2 years old are capable of operating lighters, most children who start fires by playing with matches or lighters are at least 3 years old. These children are curious about fires but do not understand the danger. When children start a fire, they may leave the scene without telling anyone about the fire.

   Lighters and matches should be kept high and out of the reach and view of children, preferably in a locked cabinet. Matches should be kept in a child-resistant container. Children should be taught not to play with lighters, matches, or other ignition sources, and to tell a grown-up when they find them.

3. Food should not be left cooking unattended on the stove. Do not cook late at night, because you may be more likely to fall asleep. Cooking areas should be kept clear of combustibles. Wear short or tight-fitting sleeves while cooking; loose clothing could catch fire.

   Never throw water on a grease fire; rather, smother the flames with a pot lid or larger pan, using an oven mitt to protect your hand and arm. Turn off the burner. Keep the lid firmly in place until the pan is completely cooled — lifting the lid will introduce oxygen and may cause the flames to reignite. For a fire in an oven, close the oven door to smother the fire and turn the oven off. Call the fire department if the flames do not go out quickly.

4. Heating devices should be kept at least 3 ft from curtains, furniture, or other objects that can burn, as well as far from flammable liquids. Portable space heaters should not be left on when persons leave home or go to sleep because dangerous levels of carbon monoxide may build up or uncontrolled burning could cause a fire; keep children and pets away from them. Fireplaces should be covered with a metal or tempered-glass screen to keep sparks from dropping into the room. Chimneys and fireplaces should be inspected for cracks, obstructions, and creosote accumulations; heating systems should also be inspected annually.

5. Electrical circuits and extension cords should not be overloaded. Blown fuses should be replaced with fuses of the proper size, and frayed or cracked electrical cords should also be replaced. Extension cords should not be run under carpets or across doorways. Lighting equipment should have good wiring and proper size bulbs. Electrical outlets should be properly grounded. Televisions, stereos, and radios should have enough air space around them to prevent overheating.

6. Use flashlights in emergencies, rather than candles. If candles are used, be sure holders are in good condition and securely standing. If candles are used on window sills, be sure that drapes or curtains are very securely fastened to the window frame, well away from the candle. Never leave candles burning when you leave a room for more than a few moments.

7. Flammable liquids are involved in hundreds of fatal home fires each year. These include gasoline, acetone, turpentine, alcohol, benzene, charcoal lighter fluid, paint and lacquer thinner, and contact cements. They produce invisible vapors that may travel unnoticed to a distant ignition source, such as a spark or a pilot light.

Never smoke around flammable liquids, and do not store or use them near heat or ignition sources such as gas water heaters. (Gas water heaters are safer if elevated above the ground, in order to raise the pilot light.) Store them outside of the home, out of the reach of children, and use a nonglass, properly labeled, and tightly closed safety can. Some spray-can products are combustible liquids held under pressure. Oily rags should be hung outside to dry or should be stored in a tightly-sealed metal container.

8. Whenever possible, homes should be furnished and finished with fire-resistant or fire-retardant materials. When buying upholstered furniture, one should look for the gold tag designating compliance with the Upholstered Furniture Action Council's Voluntary Action Program. This furniture has increased resistance to ignition by cigarettes. Furniture fabrics with nylon, polyester, acrylic, and olefin generally resist cigarette ignition better than rayon or cotton.

Walls should be made of gypsum or other noncombustible wallboards. Wall paneling, ceiling tiles, and insulation should be labeled as fire retardant or should have reduced flame-spread characteristics.

11.1.4 Recommendations for Pediatricians

1. As part of office anticipatory guidance, parents should be counseled about fire and burn prevention including adequate supervision of children, use of smoke detectors, fire escape plans, safe behavior in fires, initial treatment of burns, and other fire- and burn-prevention messages discussed in section 11.1.3.

2. Pediatricians can join with other community members to support the following activities:

   • Encouraging adolescents and adults not to smoke

   • Working with media to increase public awareness of burn injury and prevention

   • Working with fire departments and local schools to provide comprehensive fire and burn prevention education to students and their families

   • Working with fire departments and other community agencies to distribute smoke detectors in giveaway programs targeted to areas at high risk for fires[22,23]

   • Supporting the lowering of insurance premiums for sprinkler-protected buildings

   • Establishing or maintaining an adequate fire-response system

   • Helping to sustain the network of burn centers that treat children.

3. Pediatricians should be involved with legislation and regulation to accomplish the following:

- Decrease the use of cigarettes and other smoking materials and/or promote the substitution of fire safe cigarettes — those with a lower propensity to start fires (section 11.4.3).
- Work to improve building codes that require smoke detectors and sprinkler systems in all new dwellings and retrofit multiple-family rental units. Building codes related to well-lighted egress, wiring, appliances, heating devices, and sprinklers may also have an impact on fire reduction.
- Consider mandating a minimum age under which a child cannot be left alone without adult supervision.

11.2 Scald Burns

Scald burns occur as a result of contact with hot liquid or steam and represent a significant hazard. Most scald burns occur indoors from contact with hot food and drink or from hot tap water.

11.2.1 Scope of the Problem

Scalds from hot liquids are the major cause of nonfatal burn-related emergency department visits and hospitalization.[11] The Shriner's Burn Institute in Boston reported that 82% of admitted patients younger than 5 years had scald burns, and 60% of these occurred in the kitchen, frequently when children tipped over containers on the stove, counters, or tables.

In 1993, an estimated 77 700 emergency department visits occurred as a result of hot water and product-related scald burns.[3] Products most frequently associated with these injuries included cookware, tableware, ranges, and coffeemakers. Approximately 40% occurred in children younger than 15 years. The hospitalization rate of those with scald burns was 70% higher than those with thermal (contact and flame) burns.[3] Many of the additional 284 000 to 441 000 nonproduct-related burn injuries seen in emergency departments may be related to scald burns from spilling hot food and beverages.

Each year approximately 34 deaths occur and 3800 to 5100 injuries are seen in emergency departments as a result of scalding from hot tap water; 28% of these injuries required hospitalization.[3,24-26] (An unknown additional portion of the 22 300 emergency department visits attributed to hot water by the CPSC represent tap water scalds, in cases where the heating source could not be identified.[3]) In general, these burns are more severe than most other scald burns, because they often involve a relatively large burn surface area and immersion measured in seconds or minutes rather than a spill, which runs off immediately. In one study, the mean body burn surface area was 20.2% (range, 1% to 99%) for 33 hospitalized patients.[27]

11.2.2 Risk Factors

Children who are the most frequent victims of scald burns are younger than 5 years (usually 6 months to 3 years); males (54%) slightly outnumber females. Most of these burns result from spilling hot food, a beverage such as coffee or tea, or a cooking pan with hot water or soup.

Tap water scald injuries occur most frequently in the bathtub or shower, but may also occur in the kitchen or bathroom sink. Most victims are children younger than 5 years (typically between 6 months and 3 years). Others at risk for injury include the elderly and those with physical or mental disability.[27,28] These three risk groups account for almost 90% of those burned by hot tap water.[27] These individuals have in common a decreased perception of danger, less control over their environment, and slower reaction time to a burn situation. Similar prevention approaches could therefore be used to protect all three groups.[27–30] Before 1980, manufacturers preset electric water heaters at 150°F and gas water heaters at 140°F. Average home water temperatures were approximately 142°F.[28] At these temperatures, a full-thickness (deep second- or third-degree burn) would occur in an adult in 2 to 5 seconds.[31] Children probably require one third to one fourth of that time to burn.[32] The installed water heater was an unsafe product when set at those temperatures.

A variety of other types of scald burns have been reported in specific risk groups. Infants have experienced mouth and splash burns as a result of nursing bottles and baby food jars being warmed in microwave ovens.[33–35] The container may feel cool to the touch while the contents are dangerously hot. (Other types of unintentional and abusive burn injury involving microwave ovens have been described.[36]) Scald burns may also occur when chemical hot packs are used during the rewarming of hypothermic patients.[37] Scald burns related to the use of hot water vaporizers for respiratory illness have been reported, both from contact with the steam and from tipping over the vaporizer.[38]

11.2.3 Intervention Strategies

In the late 1970s and early 1980s, members of the American Academy of Pediatrics (AAP) addressed the issue of tap water scald prevention. Office counseling about the danger of hot tap water was introduced through The Injury Prevention Program (TIPP) at the 2-month to 4-year health supervision visits. Epidemiologic studies were done to define the problem better.[27,28] Patients were instructed to test the maximum temperature of the hot water at the tap and, if high, to turn down the water heater thermostat until the desired temperature of 120° to 130°F (49° to 54°C) was achieved. This one-time action would presumably passively protect all members of the household, because at these temperatures, a contact time of 30 seconds to 10 minutes is needed for an adult to receive a full-thickness burn.[31] In-office and public education programs were also studied.[29,39,40]

Members of the AAP worked to pass local and state legislation requiring that water heaters be preset by manufacturers at a safe (120° to 130°F) temperature and display appropriate warning labels prior to sale in that community or state. Because of these efforts and the threat of litigation, water heater manufacturers agreed in the late 1980s to a voluntary standard of presetting all electric water heater thermostats at 120°F in the factory and changing the detent position (the thermostat setting used by the installer) of all gas water heaters to 120°F.[41] Five years after passage of a 1983 Washington State law for water heaters to be preset at 120°F, and after extensive educational efforts, approximately 80% of homes in Seattle had a maximum hot water temperature less than 130°F, compared with only 20% in 1977.[42] Furthermore, the admission rate for children with these burns dropped by more than 50%, with most of the decrease occurring among unintentional burns; the proportion of abusive burns increased from 31% to 47%.

Other efforts to prevent tap water scald burns have focused on promoting the use of antiscald devices on faucets. These devices automatically shut off the hot water when the water temperature flowing through the faucet is higher than a safe temperature. In many localities, building codes require these devices on the bathtub faucets of new homes; however, this requirement does not protect the child being bathed in the kitchen or bathroom sink. Furthermore, campaigns to retrofit faucets in existing apartments and homes have not been widespread, primarily because of expense and inconvenience.

11.2.4 Recommendations for Pediatricians

1. Through in-office TIPP counseling and anticipatory guidance, parents should be reminded of the following points:

Children should not be held while carrying or drinking hot liquids. Parents should not leave cups or dishes of hot liquids near the edge of a table, counter, or stove, or where they can be pulled down using a tablecloth, a cord from an electrical appliance, or an outward-turned pot handle. Parents should not have children in the kitchen while cooking.

To reduce the chances of a severe mouth burn, parents should be discouraged from heating bottles of formula or milk in a microwave. Warmed liquids should be mixed well and tested for suitability of the temperature before they are fed to infants or young children.

Parents should be instructed that, when using a vaporizer for an upper respiratory illness, a cool-mist vaporizer is preferable to avoid burns. Also, parents who are instructed to use the "steamy hot-shower mist" in treating croup should be aware that direct contact with the hot water is dangerous.

Parents should be encouraged to check their maximum hot water temperature at the faucet, by running the hot water into a cup for several minutes, at a time when little hot water was used during the previous hour. A candy or meat thermometer, or a liquid-crystal device designed for that purpose,[29,30] should be used to test the water. If the maximum hot water temperature is found to exceed 120°F, the water heater thermostat should be lowered, and the testing procedure should be repeated on the following day. A setting of 120°F provides adequate hot water for most household uses.

Parents should also be reminded never to leave infants or small children alone in the tub or alone in the bathroom for any reason, since many burns result from children turning the hot water onto themselves or onto a sibling. (Also children can drown.) The bath water should always be checked before a child enters or is placed into a bathtub or shower, especially when away from home, such as in a hotel. (If you or a parent notice dangerously hot water in a hotel, report it to the management; this effort may save another guest from a severe burn.) The hot water should be turned off before the cold, to avoid hot water dripping on the child and to allow the metal faucet to cool.

2. Work with utility companies in your area to have them notify customers, at least once a year through billing inserts, that hot tap water can be dangerous, and that lowering the water heater thermostat not only provides passive protection from burn injury, but also results in substantial energy savings.

3. Work with the media and apartment owners in the area to assure that landlords are aware of the danger of hot tap water, and that they set hot water heater thermostats for tenants so that the maximum delivered hot water temperature is not greater than 120°F, and that they prevent tenants from having access to the water heater thermostat, in order to avoid litigation in the event of a burn. Landlords should also be encouraged to retrofit kitchen and bathroom faucets with antiscald devices.

4. Work with legislators and building code authorities to assure that all new homes and apartments have antiscald devices on bathroom and kitchen faucets. All public housing should be retrofitted with these devices.

5. Pediatric training should include recognition and reporting of intentional burn injury patterns, such as those from cigarettes and from scalds.[24,25]

11.3 Fireworks-Related Injury

In 1966, the Child Protection Act imposed a ban on exploding fireworks containing more than 130 mg (2 grains) of exploding powder. This regulation restricted sales of cherry bombs, aerial bombs, M-80 salutes, and other fireworks more than 1.5 in in length and 0.5 in in diameter, as well as mail order kits to build such fireworks. In 1973, the CPSC was given responsibility for regulation of fireworks under the Federal Hazardous Substance Act. In response to a proposal to ban all fireworks for personal use regardless of size or class, the CPSC enacted a temporary ban in 1974, pending further hearings. Opposition to the ban came from individuals and from the pyrotechnic industry, and the ban was rescinded in the same year. In 1976, a new set of regulations was developed and remains in force. These regulations banned from interstate commerce firecrackers containing more than 50 mg of powder. The regulations also established performance requirements, such as fuse burn time limits and requirements to prevent blow-out and tip-over for fireworks devices; also, cautionary labeling requirements were established for all types of fireworks devices. In 1991, the CPSC banned reloadable tube aerial shell fireworks devices with shells with an outer diameter larger than 1.75 in, and many importers agreed to refrain from importing these devices during 1990; few if any were expected to be imported after 1991.[43,44]

The CPSC has classified fireworks by the amount of explosive "black powder" in the fireworks, as well as the size:

Class A fireworks are composed of solid explosives containing more than 50 mg of gun powder. This group includes detonators such as blasting caps, solid explosives such as TNT and dynamite, and liquids that explode on impact.

Class B fireworks also contain more than 50 mg of gun powder but function by rapid combustion rather than detonation. This class includes large firecrackers, cherry bombs, M-80s, and aerial fireworks that are used in licensed public displays.

Under federal statutes, fireworks in class A and B are illegal for sale to the general public; however, class B fireworks can sometimes be obtained by mail order through several companies in the United States.

Class C fireworks (consumer fireworks) are the most frequent cause of fireworks-related injuries seen by the health care professional. Federal law permits class C fireworks, which must contain 50 mg (0.77 grains) or less of explosive material, to be sold to the public. Allowable class C devices include fountains and candles that shoot out sparks or flaming balls, rockets with sticks (called "bottle rockets," because they are often placed in a soda bottle for ignition), other rockets, sparklers, and smoke devices. Class C fireworks are allowed for sale because the CPSC believed that quality control and mandatory labeling requirements would provide protection of the public. Within class C, states and local authorities further regulate their sale. Some states ban the sale and use of all common fireworks; others regulate some, but not all, class C fireworks; and still others allow the sale and personal use of all class C fireworks.

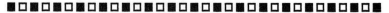
11.3.1 Scope of the Problem

Although only a small number of people die each year as a direct result of injuries caused by fireworks or the fires they cause,[7] data from the CPSC National Electronic Injury Surveillance System show that since 1990, an estimated 12 000 fireworks-related injuries have been seen in emergency departments annually in the United States. Approximately 9000 of these injuries were seen between June 23 and July 23, surrounding the Independence Day celebrations. About 8% of the holiday-period injuries were serious enough to require hospitalization — about double the percentage of hospitalization for all consumer product-related injuries.[44] Fire departments responded to more than 30 000 fires started by fireworks in 1993, resulting in $21 million in property damage.[45]

11.3.2 Risk Factors

Although the severity of fireworks-related injuries seems to be related to the content of explosive powder in the device, the most frequent causes of these injuries are class C fireworks, presumably containing no more than 50 mg of powder.[44] Approximately 30% of the fireworks-related injuries that occurred during the 1994 holiday period involved class A and class B fireworks (they have been banned from sale to consumers for many years) and about 56% involved other fireworks sold to the public, most frequently rockets, Roman candles, and sparklers. The remaining incidents included homemade fireworks (6%), devices used in public displays (4%), and others (3%). (Small paper-cased firecrackers, 1- to 1.5-in long and 0.25 in in diameter, were associated with an estimated 7% of the injuries.)

In spite of the required labeling ("Use only under adult supervision"), more than one third of the injuries (38%) were to children younger than 15 years. Together, children and teenagers accounted for 58% of the injuries.

The estimated hospital emergency department–treated injuries associated with fireworks during the July 4, 1994, study period occurred at a rate of 3.6/100 000 US population. Children 10 to 14 years old had a higher injury rate, 10.8/100 000 population, and those 5 to 9 years old were injured at a rate of 4.7/100 000 population; 73% of all injuries reported were to males, and injuries among males younger than 20 years accounted for 44% of all reported injuries.

When the age of the victim and the relation to fireworks type are examined, injuries to children younger than 5 years were most frequently associated with sparklers. Sparklers contain pyrotechnic mixtures that can reach temperatures 1000° to 2000°F at the tip and may cause serious burns to the skin, corneal abrasions, and ignition of clothing.[43,46] In children 5 to 14 years of age, a wide variety of devices was involved, including large illegal firecrackers, rockets, and Roman candles. Most of the preschool-age children were injured by fireworks ignited by someone else. Of the estimated 550 children younger than 5 years who were injured, 130 were reportedly struck by exploding particles when fireworks ignited by someone else landed near them. On the other hand, older children were more likely to have been the users of fireworks.

Hand and finger injuries were the most commonly reported and accounted for 35% of all injuries; approximately two thirds of these injuries were burns. Crushes, fractures, and amputations were involved in the remainder of the cases. The more serious injuries generally involved class B fireworks; most people were injured while holding them. Head injuries (excluding the eye) were the second most commonly reported injury, accounting for 29% of the total. Approximately 74% of these injuries were burns, 16% lacerations, and 2% fractures. Many resulted from malfunctions, including tip-overs, short fuse burn time, erratic flight paths, long fuse burn times, and delayed operation.

Eye injuries accounted for 16% of the total. In some studies, approximately one third of fireworks-related eye injuries result in permanent loss of vision.[43] Half of the eye injuries and an even higher percentage of those resulting in permanent blindness or enucleation are caused by bottle rockets.

Firecrackers also produce extremely high sound levels that may result in hearing loss.[47] At a distance of 3 m, the sound level was measured in the range of 130 to 190 dB using eight different firecrackers. The damage risk level for adults is 130 dB peak sound level. Approximately 4% to 5% of young children had significant sensorineural hearing loss 2 days after exposure to a loud sound, and approximately 3% of these children had an average 30-dB loss 3 months after exposure.

Although deadly fireworks devices were banned by the Child Protection Act of 1966, cherry bombs containing 2 g of flash powder and M-80s containing as much as 40 to 50 g of flash powder are still illegally manufactured and continue to pose a threat. Living in a state where fireworks are banned altogether does not ensure safety. Any person with a serious desire to use fireworks can visit a nearby state that allows sale or can purchase them from mail-order companies.

11.3.3 Intervention Strategies

Intervention strategies involve primarily education and enforcement. Children should be taught at an early age that fireworks are dangerous explosive devices and that they should not pick them up, but rather inform an adult if they find them. Sparklers burn at high temperatures and are not toys.

Laws relating to the manufacture, distribution, sale, and use of fireworks at the federal level and the state level should be enforced. The most effective intervention is to ban all use of fireworks with the exception of public displays, where injuries rarely occur.

11.3.4 Recommendations for Pediatricians

The AAP recommends the following actions for pediatricians[48]:

1. Encourage accurate reporting of fireworks-related injuries, death, and fires. (Perhaps a toll-free hotline could be set up to report instances of fireworks trauma to a central unit, especially around the July 4 holiday. The data obtained could be used to promote further fireworks control measures.)

2. Become familiar with the state laws regarding class C fireworks and work to prohibit sales to the general public, including those by mail order, of all fireworks, even the presently legal class C "safe and sane" devices. Ideally this would be done on a federal level, either by federal law or by CPSC regulations. Sales to professional pyrotechnicians for the purpose of creating public displays should be exempted; however, it may be necessary to initiate a licensing mechanism for such purchasers. International import of class C devices for private use should also be banned.

3. The AAP should work with national government agencies to achieve a federal ban on all fireworks for private use. The model state fireworks law proposed by the NFPA should be supported. Individual pediatricians and state chapters should work to increase the number of communities and states that ban fireworks (except for public, sanctioned displays).

4. Pediatricians should educate parents and community leaders about the dangers of the so-called safe and sane (class C) fireworks. Parents should be encouraged to attend public fireworks displays rather than to purchase fireworks for home use. When families want to have home fireworks despite the well-documented risks involved, children should never be allowed to ignite them, nor should they be around any devices without adult supervision. Anyone using fireworks should wear safety glasses. Also, pediatricians should emphasize the heightened danger of fireworks use by persons who have been consuming alcoholic beverages.

11.4 Smoking Materials

The term "smoking materials" does not refer to matches or lighters (discussed in sections 11.5 and 11.6), but only to lighted tobacco products, such as cigarettes, cigars, or pipes.

11.4.1 Scope of the Problem

Smoking materials are the leading cause of deaths from fire in the United States, accounting for 22% of all deaths from fires and 26% of all deaths from residential fires in 1993. In that year, 1029 deaths, 3446 injuries, and $391 million in direct property damage resulted from smoking-material fires. Although the highest death, injury, and dollar losses occur in structural fires, 70% of fires begun by smoking materials are "outdoor and other," and 5% are vehicular.[49]

In 1993, an estimated 6600 cigarette-related burns were seen in emergency departments, and 800 of these patients were admitted to the hospital; 54.7% were children younger than 15 years.[3] A study group estimated the total direct cost of cigarette-ignited fire deaths, injuries, and property damage in 1990 at approximately $4 billion (in 1992 dollars).[50]

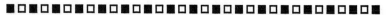
11.4.2 Risk Factors

Three fourths (77%) of residential fires caused by smoking material and 65% of the associated deaths in 1993 resulted from abandonment or careless disposal of smoking materials. Other misuses (such as impairment from alcohol or other drug use, and falling asleep with a lit cigarette, cigar, or pipe) raise this figure to 90% to 95% for fires and deaths. Almost all fires and deaths caused by smoking material involve cigarettes, with cigars and pipes representing no more than 3% combined. Bedding, mattresses, and upholstered furniture are most commonly ignited in residential fires, although trash is most frequently involved in nonresidential fires.[49]

Although cigarette-related deaths are normally associated with those old enough to smoke, nearly 100 children younger than 10 years die each year from fires caused by smoking materials. Children 10 years old and older have the lowest rates, probably because this group has a low percentage of smokers, a low percentage of intoxication, and is more capable of escaping fire than younger children. The death rate then rises steadily with age, and people age 85 years or older are at highest risk.[16]

11.4.3 Intervention Strategies

Although smoking cessation efforts often emphasize the health risks of smoking, the high incidence of fires, injury, and death should also be emphasized in these programs. In addition, fire safety public education programs that focus on careless behavior are also essential. Specifically, messages about the dangers of smoking in bed, smoking when impaired by drugs or alcohol, and smoking around high-risk groups such as the very young, the very old, and the physically handicapped should be emphasized.

During the 1970s and early 1980s, attention was turned toward modifying mattresses and upholstered furniture to use materials more resistant to ignition from cigarettes. Although a reduction has occurred in the number of fires involving these products, they remain the leading items ignited in smoking-material structure fires. The products are now more resistant to ignition by smoking materials, but, in some cases, they may produce more toxic smoke or burn faster once ignited.

More recently, attention has shifted from the products ignited to the smoking material itself. The Cigarette Safety Act of 1984 established a technical study group to study the feasibility of developing cigarettes and little cigars that would be less likely to start fires. In 1987, the group reported that it was technically feasible to develop a cigarette with decreased propensity to ignite other items.[51] The characteristics that resulted in less likelihood of a cigarette to ignite furniture or mattresses were reduced circumference, lower density tobacco, the presence of a filter, and less-porous reduced-citrate paper. The report estimated that in 1986 through 1996, 15 000 lives, 46 000 injuries, and $2.4 billion in property damage would have been saved through prevention of 230 000 cigarette-related fires.

The Fire Safe Cigarette Act of 1990 required the National Institute of Standards and Technology and the CPSC to investigate cigarette ignition propensity and to develop a standardized method for testing cigarettes for their propensity to ignite other items. A final report on these activities was issued by the CPSC and presented to Congress in August 1993. It concluded that it is practicable to develop a fire-safe cigarette and recommended additional technical study. In February 1994, a new bill, the Fire Safe Cigarette Act of 1994, was introduced to require that the CPSC issue a safety standard for cigarettes, but the bill has not been enacted. In the absence of federal legislation, state legislators who provided much of the initial impetus for fire-safe cigarette legislation are again considering the option of state-level action. Litigation related to the alleged withholding of fire-safe cigarette technology from the marketplace may also lead to progress in this area.[52]

11.4.4 Recommendations for Pediatricians

Recommendations are included under residential fires (section 11.1.4). Also pediatricians should strongly support state and federal legislation that would lead to the production and substitution of fire-safe cigarettes for those currently being sold.

11.5 Matches

Preschool children have a risk of death from fire that is more than twice the risk for all age groups combined, and the leading cause of those fires is related to "child play." Children who are too young to understand the consequences of their hazardous actions are described as "playing" if a fire results. Matches and lighters are the most common heat sources resulting in fire from child play.[53] The leading items first ignited in child play-related home fires include bedding and mattresses, upholstered furniture, and clothing; these account for two thirds (66%) of deaths, where the first-ignited item is known. Trash is also a leading cause of incidents of fire but not for deaths.

Fatal home fires caused by child play tend to start in the bedroom or living room, which together account for 83% of fatal fires where the area of origin is known. Most children who play with fire use rooms where they normally go for their activities and where they are often left alone to play.

11.5.1 Scope of the Problem

During 1989 to 1993, children playing with matches caused a mean annual incidence of 9560 home fires, 131 deaths, 812 injuries, and $87 million of direct property damages.[53] Matches account for 32% to 43% of all child play-related home fires, deaths, injuries, and property damage where the heat source was known. Adding lighters increases this figure to 78% to 84%.

In 1993, an estimated 2300 match-related burns were seen in emergency departments; 400 of these patients were admitted to the hospital; 36.1% involved children younger than 15 years.[3]

11.5.2 Risk Factors

Limited information is available about the age of the person who starts a match-related fire. Of approximately 100 match fires in the home caused by child play investigated by the CPSC, 43% of fires, resulting in 35% of deaths and 37% of injuries, were started by children younger than 5 years. (For lighters the corresponding numbers were 73%, 93%, and 83%, respectively.)[54]

Most of the fatal *victims* of home fires involving child play are preschoolers; 76% are younger than 6 years. Often victims are younger than the children who start the fires. Educational interventions and product redesign must target preschoolers and probably need to be effective to ages as young as 3-year-olds. Caregivers need to be educated, too, and are critically important because of the limits on education possible with 3-year-olds.

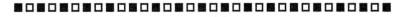
11.5.3 Intervention Strategies

Mass media programs on the danger of matches and lighters are best designed for parents and caregivers of preschoolers. Parents must be encouraged to supervise children and to keep matches and lighters out of reach and out of sight.

Labels on matches should remind adults about the dangers of small children playing with fire, and attention should be given to increasing the resistance of children to the use of matches.

11.5.4 Recommendations for Pediatricians

Recommendations are included under residential fires (section 11.1.4).

11.6 Cigarette Lighters

11.6.1 Scope of the Problem

During 1989 to 1993, children playing with lighters caused a mean annual incidence of 8050 home fires, 162 deaths, 1268 injuries, and $99.2 million of direct property damages.[53] Approximately 30 million households own one or more working lighters.[55] Lighters are frequently used for purposes other than lighting smoking materials and may often be left within a child's reach.

In 1993, an estimated 4300 cigarette lighter–related burns were seen in emergency departments; 400 of these patients were admitted to the hospital; 45.3% involved children younger than 15 years.[3]

11.6.2 Risk Factors

A fire caused by child play is more likely to result in death if the ignition source is a lighter (15.4 deaths per 1000 fires) rather than a match (9.5 deaths per 1000 fires). Field studies have shown that the median age of the lighter operators in fatal fires was 4.2 years, and the median age of the victims (usually siblings) was 2.6 years.[56] They also found that adults did not consider the lighters to be hazards and had kept them in open view in two thirds of the incidents. Also, children as young as 2 years demonstrated that they could operate the lighters.

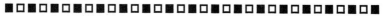
11.6.3 Intervention Strategies

In 1988, the CPSC declared an intent to establish regulations requiring that lighters be child resistant. A CPSC data analysis resulted in a relative risk of 31.0 for lighters compared with matches for death caused by children playing with these ignition sources (expressed in terms of annual sales of disposable lighters and matchbooks, assuming 2500 lights per lighter and 20 matches per matchbook).

The CPSC recently set a mandatory safety standard that requires disposable butane lighters, inexpensive refillable lighters, and certain novelty lighters to be child-resistant. The standard covers novelty lighters that may be attractive to children — the types that play music, have flashing lights, or resemble toys. The standard became effective in July 1994 and applies to more than 95% of the 600 million lighters purchased in the United States each year. Before 1994 manufacturers were not required to have child-resistant features on their lighters. It is estimated that 85% of children ages 2½ to 4½ years will be unable to operate lighters that meet the standard.

11.6.4 Recommendations for Pediatricians

Recommendations are included under residential fires (section 11.1.4).

11.7 Wearing Apparel

11.7.1 Scope of the Problem

Each year more than 200 clothing-related fire deaths are reported. In 1993, 5000 emergency department visits for clothing-related burns occurred, of which 1000 required hospitalization. The severity of these burns is typically high, with hospital stays often longer than 1 month.

11.7.2 Risk Factors

Although about three fourths of the deaths occur in the over-65-year age group, one third of the serious burns occur in children younger than 15 years.[3,57]

Many fabrics burn easily, especially fuzzy, napped-surface, lightweight, and loose-woven, or loose-fitting fabrics. Fabrics made of cotton, cotton/

polyester blends, rayon, and acrylic are relatively easy to ignite, and they burn fast. Small flames from matches, cigarette lighters, and candles are the major source of ignition, followed by ranges, open fires, and space heaters.[57] Pajamas, nightgowns, and robes are most commonly ignited.

Halloween is a special time when children experience fabric-related burns. Costumes made with flimsy materials and outfits with big, baggy sleeves or billowing skirts may come in contact with jack-o'-lanterns, candles, or other sources of ignition.

11.7.3 Intervention Strategies

Sturdy fabrics should be selected with a smooth, tight weave, such as denim and wool, which are less likely to burn quickly. Fabrics such as 100% polyester, nylon, wool, and silk should be purchased. They are difficult to ignite and tend to self-extinguish.

Sleepwear for children should be labeled with fire-retardant information. Cleaning instructions should be followed to retain this flame-resistant property. If a garment can be easily removed if it catches fire, injuries may be less severe.

The CPSC recommends that when Halloween costumes are purchased or made, masks, beards, and wigs should be labeled "flame-resistant."[58] Although this label does not assure that these items will not catch fire, it does indicate that the items will resist burning and should extinguish quickly when removed from the ignition source. Snug-fitting costumes should be used and candlelit jack-o'-lanterns should be kept away from landings and doorsteps where costumes could brush against the flame. Indoor jack-o'-lanterns should be kept away from curtains, decorations, and other furnishings that could be ignited.

11.7.4 Recommendations for Pediatricians

1. Parents should be encouraged to select apparel made in the manner described in section 11.7.3; loose-fitting, cotton, non–flame resistant clothing should not be substituted for sleepwear.
2. Parents can also be counseled to teach their children about the stop, drop, and roll method of extinguishing clothing fires and the use of cool water in the first aid treatment of a burn.

11.8 Cooking Equipment

11.8.1 Scope of the Problem

Cooking equipment is the leading cause of home fires reported to US fire departments.[59] In 1993, cooking equipment was associated with 111 100 fires, 334 deaths, 5664 injuries, and $452 million of direct property damage. In recent years, 70 to 80 deaths and more than 400 injuries per year occur in children younger than 18 years. When unreported fires are included, an estimated 12 344 000 fires occur. These fires account for a total of 642 000 injuries and illnesses that are not reported to fire departments. Although the number of reported fires has declined by 18.4% since 1980, the number of injuries has increased by 25.9%.

Between 1989 and 1993, an annual average of 138 000 reported fires began in the kitchen, and more than two thirds of the kitchen fires involved cooking. The range (the stove plus the oven) accounts for at least 83% of home cooking fire losses.

Cooking ranges and ovens accounted for more than 22 000 burns seen in emergency departments in 1993, resulting in more than 700 hospitalizations from the emergency department.[3]

11.8.2 Risk Factors

Males have a higher rate of home cooking-fire deaths than females by nearly one third.

Unattended cooking is the leading cause of home cooking-equipment fires and is associated with falling asleep or inadequate control of a cooking process involving an open flame. Though 73% of those injured were awake and unimpaired, only 22% of the fatal victims were awake and unimpaired. More than half of those injured were engaged in fighting the fire; thus, they possibly underestimated the danger of the fire.

Forgetting to turn off equipment and placing combustibles too close to a heat source also play a causal role. Usually the fires start with cooking materials, but they may also start with wall coverings, cabinets, gas fuel, wire insulation, or curtains. Although gas-fueled stoves are associated with a higher rate of death, relative to usage, electric stoves have higher rates of injury, fire, and property damage.

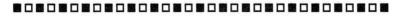
11.8.3 Intervention Strategies

Because most cooking-related fires result from leaving items that are cooking unattended, individuals should be closely attentive when cooking. Material that can be ignited, particularly grease, pot holders, plastic utensils, and other non–cooking equipment, should not be left in or around cooking equipment. Wear short or close-fitting sleeves while cooking; loose, easily ignited clothing is a serious fire risk.

Cooking equipment such as ovens or stoves should not be used to heat the kitchen or the home. Cooking late at night should be avoided, since persons may be more likely to fall asleep. Parents should make sure that smoke detectors are working to decrease the risk of death if a fire should break out.

Contact burns in children often occur from touching cooking or heating equipment or hot electrical appliances. Parents must periodically inspect the kitchen and other areas of the home for these hazards. Teach parents to enforce a "kid-free zone" to keep children at least 3 ft away from the stove at all times. Candy and cookies should not be stored above a stove, because children may try to climb on the cooking equipment to get to them.

Since more than half of injuries related to fires from cooking occur while attempting to control fires, the public should be educated about how to fight common cooking fires, how to operate a fire extinguisher, and how to know when not to fight a fire.

11.8.4 Recommendations for Pediatricians

From in-office anticipatory guidance, parents should be made aware of the intervention strategies for prevention of cooking-related burns (sections 11.1.3 and 11.8.3).

11.9 Home Heating Devices

The term "home heating device" refers to portable or built-in kerosene or oil heaters, coal- or wood-burning stoves, gas or liquid-propane (LP) gas heaters, electric heaters, floor furnaces (built into the floor), home radiators, fireplaces, as well as to central heating and water heaters. These devices may cause injury and death from fire, from contact burns, and from carbon monoxide poisoning and other indoor air pollution resulting from improper venting or incomplete combustion.

11.9.1 Scope of the Problem

In the 1970s, the number of home heating-related fires rose, probably as a result of high oil prices and increased use of wood stoves, fireplaces, and portable kerosene heaters. In recent years, the number of these fires has fallen; however, 84 100 home heating-related fires still occurred in 1993, resulting in 524 deaths, 2450 injuries, and $589.7 million in direct property damage; these are figures reported to fire departments and include only a small proportion of the total number of heating-related burns.[19]

In 1993, an estimated 17 800 people were seen in emergency departments for burns from heaters and radiators; approximately 75% were children younger than 15 years.[3] One thousand of these individuals were hospitalized. An additional 600 children had furnace-related burns.

11.9.2 Risk Factors

The problem of fires related to home heating primarily stems from portable and space heaters, which account for three fourths of all home heating-related fires and deaths. These devices have a higher rate of death per million households using them than do central heating units (furnaces) or water heaters. Portable and other space heaters provide much opportunity for error by people using them (installation, maintenance, fueling, operation, and placement of items around them). Room gas heaters and portable kerosene heaters have the highest death rates from fire relative to the number of households using them. Room gas heaters are also associated with more than 100 deaths per year due to carbon monoxide poisoning. Wood stoves and fireplaces with inserts also rank high in death rates from fire relative to usage and have the highest rate of property damage relative to households using them.

Fires related to home heating often are caused by the following: lack of regular cleaning, leading to highly flammable creosote buildup in wood-burning devices and associated chimneys and connectors; failing to give space heaters space, by installing heaters too close to combustibles; basic flaws in construction of wood-burning heating equipment; and fueling errors, such as refueling indoors or spilling fuel while moving the heater.

Death rates from fire related to home heating are especially high in poor, rural areas. These devices are often overtaxed by heating unreasonably large areas. Home heating safety may have cost implications that will not be affordable for low-income households.

Unvented gas and kerosene space heaters may produce significant levels of carbon monoxide, nitrogen dioxide, and respirable particulates, some of which may contain carcinogenic compounds.

11.9.3 Intervention Strategies

Heating devices should have a guard around the flame or heating coil, in order to keep children, pets, and clothing away from the heat source. Heaters should be tested and labeled by an independent testing laboratory. Manufacturers' instructions should be carefully followed, especially instructions about ventilation. Installation and maintenance should be checked by local building or fire officials where required or possible.

Portable kerosene heaters must be refueled outdoors, away from flame and other heat sources, when the heater is cool, and only with the type of kerosene specified by the manufacturer for that device; never use gasoline in a kerosene heater.

Space heaters should be placed on the floor and never on furniture. Space heaters need space. With very few exceptions, home heating devices need a 36-in clearance from combustibles.

Wood and coal stoves, fireplaces, chimneys, and chimney connectors need to be inspected annually by a professional and cleaned as often as inspections indicate.

Remove ashes only when cool and store them in a metal container. An approved floor board should be used under the stove.

Fireplaces should have a metal or heat-tempered glass screen, and only seasoned wood should be burned.

Central heating systems are associated with the lowest fire risk. Nevertheless, they should be inspected annually by a qualified professional, and combustible materials should not be stored near them.

Areas around heating devices should be free of papers and trash.

Homes burning any fuel for heat should have carbon monoxide detectors appropriately installed.

11.9.4 Recommendations for Pediatricians

From in-office anticipatory guidance, parents should be made aware of the intervention strategies for prevention of cooking-related burns (sections 11.1.3 and 11.9.3).

11.10 Resources

1. National Center for Health Statistics
   6525 Belcrest Rd
   Hyattsville, MD 20782
   301-436-8500

   Information regarding deaths from fires and burns, hospital discharges, hospital emergency and outpatient department visits, physician office visits, and household interviews may be obtained.

2. US Consumer Product Safety Commission
   Office of Information and Public Affairs
   Washington DC 20207
   301-504-0580

   The CPSC has information about product-related fire and burn injuries that result in hospital emergency department visits. These data are from the National Electronic Injury Surveillance System (NEISS) that samples visits from 100 of the 6100 hospital emergency departments in the United States.

   CPSC also collects data on fire- and burn-related deaths. These data are from death certificates, medical examiner and coroner reports, newspaper clippings, consumer complaints, and other sources.

3. US Fire Administration
   11825 S Seton Ave
   Emmitsburg, MD 21727
   301-447-1358

   USFA uses fire department data from 41 states to publish periodic reports in the National Fire Incident Reporting System.

4. American Burn Association
   Jeffrey R. Saffle, MD, Secretary
   Department of Surgery
   University of Utah
   50 N Medical Dr
   Salt Lake City, UT 84132
   800-548-2876

   The new American Burn Association registry contains reports regarding approximately 20 000 acute burn admissions to those of the nation's 130 burn centers that now participate. This registry will soon be part of the American College of Surgeons trauma registry.

5. National Fire Protection Association
   1 Batterymarch Park
   Quincy, MA 02269-9101
   617-770-3000

   NFPA is an international nonprofit membership organization dedicated to reducing the burden of fire on the quality of life. It publishes the *Learn Not to Burn* curriculum and other consumer and professional educational materials, as well as consensus model codes and standards and other annual statistical reports using data from fire departments to estimate the number, cause, and cost of fires and the number of civilian and firefighter deaths and injuries.

References

1. Baker SP, O'Neill B, Ginsburg M, Li G. *The Injury Fact Book.* 2nd ed. New York, NY: Oxford University Press; 1992

2. Brigham PA, McLoughlin E. Burn incidence and medical care use in the United States: estimates, trends, and data sources. *J Burn Care Rehabil.* 1996;17:95–107

3. Harwood B. Common products that cause uncommonly severe burn injuries. *NFPA J.* 1996;90:79–83

4. Burt CW. Injury-related visits to hospital emergency departments: United States, 1992. Advance data from vital and health statistics; Hyattsville, MD: National Center for Health Statistics. 1995;261:1–20

5. Burt CW. Injury-related visits to hospital emergency departments: United States, 1993. Advance data from vital and health statistics; Hyattsville, MD: National Center for Health Statistics. 1996;271:1,15

6. Rice DP, MacKenzie EJ and Associates. *Cost of Injury in the United States: A Report to Congress,* 1989. San Francisco, CA: Institute for Health & Aging, University of California San Francisco and Injury Prevention Center, The Johns Hopkins University; 1989

7. National Safety Council. *Accident Facts.* 1995 ed. Itasca, IL: National Safety Council; 1995

8. Hall JR Jr. The total cost of fire in the United States. Quincy, MA: National Fire Protection Association, Fire Analysis and Research Division; 1995

9. National Center for Health Statistics. *Mortality Tapes.* Hyattsville, MD: US Public Health Service; 1992

10. Feck GA, Baptiste MS. The epidemiology of burn injury in New York. *Public Health Rep.* 1979;94:312–318

11. Katcher ML, Delventhal SJ. Burn injuries in Wisconsin: epidemiology and prevention. *Wis Med J.* 1982;81:25–28

12. Karter M Jr. Fire loss in the United States in 1993. *NFPA J.* 1994;88:57–60

13. Baker SP, Fingerhut LA, Higgins L, Chen LH, Braver ER. *Injury to Children and Teenagers: State-by-State Mortality Facts.* Baltimore, MD: The Johns Hopkins Center for Injury Research and Policy; 1996

14. Robinson MD, Seward PN. Hazardous chemical exposure in children. *Pediatr Emerg Care.* 1987;3:179–183

15. Hall JR Jr. Burns, toxic gases, and other hazards associated with fires. Quincy, MA: National Fire Protection Association, Fire Analysis and Research Division; December 1996

16. Slayton DM, Miller AL. Patterns of fire casualties in home fires by age and sex, 1989–93. Quincy, MA: National Fire Protection Association, Fire Analysis and Research Division; September 1995

17. Mierley MC, Baker SP. Fatal house fires in an urban population. *JAMA.* 1983;249: 1466–1468

18. Hall JR Jr. US fire patterns by state. Quincy, MA: National Fire Protection Association, Fire Analysis and Research Division; 1995

19. Hall JR Jr. US home heating fire patterns and trends through 1993. Quincy, MA: National Fire Protection Association, Fire Analysis and Research Division; October 1995

20. Hall JR Jr. The US fire problem overview report through 1994: leading causes and other patterns and trends. Quincy, MA: National Fire Protection Association, Fire Analysis and Research Division; April 1996

21. National Fire Protection Association. *Fire in Your Home: Prevention & Survival.* NFPA No. SPP-52D. Quincy, MA: National Fire Protection Association; 1993

22. Gorman RL, Charney E, Holtzman NA, Roberts KB. A successful city-wide smoke detector giveaway program. *Pediatrics.* 1985;75:14–18

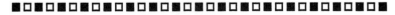
23. Shaw KN, McCormick MC, Kustra SL, Ruddy RM, Casey RD. Correlates of reported smoke detector usage in an inner-city population: participants in a smoke detector give-away program. *Am J Public Health.* 1988;78:650–653

24. Ayoub C, Pfeifer D. Burns as a manifestation of child abuse and neglect. *Am J Dis Child.* 1979;133:910–914

25. Feldman KW. Child abuse by burning. In Kempe CH, Helfer RE, eds. *The Battered Child,* ed 3. Chicago, IL: University of Chicago Press; 147–162

26. US Consumer Product Safety Commission. *Tap Water Scalds Alert.* Washington, DC: US Consumer Product Safety Commission; 1996

27. Katcher ML. Scald burns from hot tap water. *JAMA.* 1981;246:1219–1222

28. Feldman KW, Schaller TS, Feldman JA, McMillon M. Tap water scald burns in children. *Pediatrics.* 1978;62:1–7

29. Katcher ML. Prevention of tap water scald burns: evaluation of a multi-media injury control program. *Am J Public Health.* 1987;77:1195–1197

30. Katcher ML, Landry GL, Shapiro MM. Liquid-crystal thermometer use in pediatric office counseling about tap water burn prevention. *Pediatrics.* 1989;83:766–771

31. Moritz AR, Henriques FC Jr. Studies of thermal injury, II: the relative importance of time and surface temperature in the causation of cutaneous burns. *Am J Pathol.* 1947;23:695–720

32. Feldman KW. Help needed on hot water burns. *Pediatrics.* 1983;71:145–146

33. Puczynski M, Rademaker D, Gatson RL. Burn injury related to the improper use of a microwave oven. *Pediatrics.* 1983;72:714–715

34. Sando WC, Gallagher KJ, Rodgers RL. Risk factors for microwave scald injuries in infants. *J Pediatr.* 1984;105:864–867

35. Hibbard RA, Blevins R. Palatal burn due to bottle warming in a microwave oven. *Pediatrics.* 1988;82:382–384

36. Alexander RC, Surrell JA, Cohle SD. Microwave oven burns to children: an unusual manifestation of child abuse. *Pediatrics.* 1987;79:255–260

37. Feldman KW, Morray JP, Schaller RT. Thermal injury caused by hot pack application in hypothermic children. *Am J Emerg Med.* 1985;3:38–41

38. Colombo JL, Hopkins RL, Waring WW. Steam vaporizer injuries. *Pediatrics.* 1981; 67:661–663

39. Thomas KA, Hassanein RS, Christophersen ER. Evaluation of group well-child care for improving burn prevention practices in the home. *Pediatrics.* 1984;74:879–882

40. Webne S, Kaplan BJ, Shaw M. Pediatric burn prevention: an evaluation of the efficacy of a strategy to reduce tap water temperature in a population at risk for scalds. *J Dev Behav Pediatr.* 1989;10:187–191

41. Katcher ML. Efforts to prevent burns from hot tap water. In Bergman AB, ed. *Political Approaches to Injury Control at the State Level.* Seattle, WA: University of Washington Press; 1992;69–78

42. Erdmann TC, Feldman KW, Rivara FP, Heimbach DM, Wall HA. Tap water burn prevention: the effect of legislation. *Pediatrics.* 1991;88:572–577

43. Wilson RS. Ocular fireworks injuries and blindness: an analysis of 154 cases and a three-state survey comparing the effectiveness of model law regulation. *Ophthalmology.* 1982;89:291–297

44. Kelly SL. Fireworks injuries, 1994. Bethesda, MD: US Consumer Product Safety Commission, Directorate of Epidemiology; December 1994

45. Hall JR Jr. US fireworks injuries remain high. *NFPA J.* 1995;99:61–66

46. Berger LR, Kalishman S, Rivara FP. Injuries from fireworks. *Pediatrics.* 1985; 75:877–882

47. Gupta D, Vishwakarma SK. Toy weapons and firecrackers: a source of hearing loss. *Laryngoscope.* 1989;99:330–334

48. American Academy of Pediatrics, Committee on Injury and Poison Prevention. Children and fireworks. *Pediatrics.* 1991;88:652–653

49. Stewart LJ. The US smoking-material fire problem through 1992: the role of lighted tobacco products in fire. Quincy, MA: National Fire Protection Association, Fire Analysis and Research Division; October 1996

50. Ray DR, Zamula WW, Miller TR, et al. Societal costs of cigarette fires. Washington, DC: US Consumer Product Safety Commission; August 1993

51. Technical Study Group on Cigarette and Little Cigar Fire Safety. Toward a less fire-prone cigarette. Final report. Washington DC: US Consumer Product Safety Commission; 1987

52. Brigham PA, McGuire A. Progress toward a fire-safe cigarette. *J Public Health Policy* 1995;16:433–439

53. Hall JR Jr. Children playing with fire: US experience, 1980–1992. Quincy, MA: National Fire Protection Association, Fire Analysis and Research Division; 1995

54. Smith L. Responses to ANPR comments on a standard for child-resistant cigarette lighters. Washington, DC: US Consumer Product Commission; 1990

55. Consumer Product Safety Alert. Child-resistant lighters protect young children. Washington, DC: US Consumer Product Safety Commission; July 1994

56. Harwood B. Fire hazards involving children playing with cigarette lighters. Washington, DC: US Consumer Product Safety Commission; 1987

57. US Consumer Product Safety Commission. *Your Home Fire Safety Checklist.* Washington, DC: US Consumer Product Safety Commission; 1994

58. Consumer Product Safety Alert. Halloween safety. Washington, DC: US Consumer Product Safety Commission; 1993

59. Hall JR Jr. US home cooking fire patterns and trends through 1993. Quincy, MA: National Fire Protection Association, Fire Analysis and Research Division; October 1995

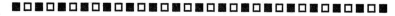

Suggested Readings

McLoughlin E, Crawford JD. Burns. *Pediatr Clin North Am.* 1985;32:61–75

McLoughlin E, McGuire A. The causes, cost, and prevention of childhood burn injuries. *Am J Dis Child.* 1990;144:677–683

Wilson MH, Baker SP, Teret SP, et al. *Saving Children: A Guide to Injury Prevention.* New York, NY: Oxford University Press; 1991;85–99

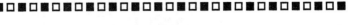

CHAPTER 12

Firearms

12.1 Scope of the Problem

Firearm-related trauma in the United States has become a leading cause of death during childhood and adolescence. In 1992, almost 38 000 Americans died from gunshot wounds; 5379 were younger than 20 years, a 61% increase for this age group since 1986 (Table 12.1). In 1990, 12.6% of the deaths of 10- to 14-year-old children and 26.6% of the deaths of 15- to 19-year-old adolescents were due to firearm-related injuries. National data indicate that Americans of all ages suffer nonfatal firearm injuries at a rate 2.6 times that of fatal injuries.[1] From birth through age 24 years, the rate of nonfatal injuries is 4 times that of fatal shootings (Table 12.2, p 270). Firearm-related deaths exceed motor vehicle–related deaths in several states and will soon be the leading cause of traumatic death in the United States should current trends continue.[2] Other developed countries do not have the level of firearm-related death and disability found in the United States.[3] Gunshot wounds are so common in the United States that they must be considered an epidemic.

In the American Academy of Pediatrics (AAP) Periodic Survey No. 25 (September 1994), 19% of practicing pediatricians reported that they

TABLE 12.1.
Firearm-Related Fatalities Among Children and Adolescents From Birth to 19 Years of Age*

	1986	1988	1990	1992	1993
Homicide	1505	1944	2874	3362	3661
Suicide	1292	1386	1476	1426	1460
Unintentional	469	543	541	501	526
Undetermined	72	91	66	90	104
Total	3338	3964	4957	5379	5751

*From the National Center for Health Statistics.

TABLE 12.2.
Fatal and Nonfatal Firearm Injuries, June 1, 1992
Through May 31, 1993

Age, y	Nonfatal	Fatal	Ratio (Nonfatal to Fatal)
0-14	3768	895	4.2
15-24	43 382	10 506	4.1
25-34	27 420	9056	3.0
35-44	15 528	6239	2.5
≥45	8680	11 053	0.8

*Adapted from Annest et al.[1]

had treated or served as a consultant for firearm-related injuries during the previous year. In one pediatric resident continuity clinic serving a population with 85% Medicaid enrollment, approximately 4% of families surveyed (during a study of safety-related behavior) said they had a gun at home (report available from AAP Department of Research). A study of families attending pediatric practices found that 37% of households had a gun; 17% had a handgun — often kept loaded and accessible.[4]

Firearm-related deaths begin in infancy, increase throughout childhood, and peak during the teenage and young adult years. Deaths caused by shooting are categorized as homicide, suicide, or unintentional. Overall, suicide is more common than homicide, but homicide predominates until the fourth decade of life. Unintentional deaths have varied little over the past decade, accounting for about 500 childhood deaths annually (Table 12.1). Because the United States has not established a national system to track injuries (as opposed to deaths), less is known about trends in nonfatal shootings.

A variety of weapons are involved: nonpowder firearms (pellet guns and BB guns), handguns (pistols and revolvers), and long guns (rifles and shotguns). The "gun habit" begins at an early age when young children play with toy guns.[5] Older children and adolescents have access to nonpowder firearms. More than 25 000 injuries are related to these weapons each year, predominantly among children 5 to 14 years old.[6] Powder firearm-related injuries become a major cause of death and injury by age 15 years. Handguns account for the bulk of the trauma inflicted by powder firearms, both fatal and nonfatal. Efforts to understand and terminate the firearm injury epidemic must focus on the central role of the handgun.

Adolescents have experienced an astounding increase in death from firearm-related injuries since the 1980s — a 154% increase in the 15- to 19-year-old age group. Police data for Chicago, Ill, from 1985 to 1993 demonstrate substantial increases in fatal and nonfatal firearm assaults (officially called aggravated battery, implying some type of injury related to being struck by the gun or a bullet) against children and teenagers.[7] In fact, the nonfatal assault rate among 16-year-old black males in Chicago exceeded 3700/100 000 in 1992; thus, 3.7% of 16-year-old African-American males were assaulted with a firearm.

Guns are apparently easily available to adolescents: 34% of high school juniors surveyed in Seattle, Wash (1990 to 1991), and 61% surveyed in Chicago (1993 to 1994) said they had easy access to guns. Gun ownership was claimed by 6% of adolescents in Seattle and 11.5% in Chicago; many asserted they had shot at another person. A 1993 Harris poll of students in grades 6 through 12 reported 59% who thought they had easy access to a gun and 39% who said they knew someone who had been shot.

The costs of treating pediatric patients for gunshot wounds are not fully understood. A review of Connecticut hospital discharge data determined the average hospital costs to be $8000, whereas a study by the National Association of Children's Hospitals and Related Institutions found the average hospital bill to be more than $14 000.[8,9] Losses to society are great, and have increased in recent years, especially when measured as years of productive life lost before age 65 years, which for firearm-related deaths now total more than 1 million annually in the United States.[10] (A child or young adult who dies of any cause loses more years of productivity than an older adult.) The costs of rehabilitation and psychological trauma have not been systematically measured, but are large. The burden on the families and friends of persons injured or killed by firearms is long lasting but difficult to measure.

12.2 Risk Factors

Firearms are ubiquitous in the United States. About half of all homes harbor a firearm[11]: this totals more than 200 million guns of which approximately 60 million are handguns. No one is exempt from firearm-related injury, but certain factors are associated with increased risk of death and injury.

12.2.1 Gun Ownership

Gun ownership is a risk factor for firearm-related death in the home.[12] Although personal and home security are often cited as reasons for having a firearm in the home, a gun is far less likely to kill an intruder than a family member or an acquaintance. According to one analysis, a gun in the home is 37 times more likely to be used in a suicide and nearly five times more likely to be used in a criminal homicide than in self-defense.[12] Homicide is about three times more common in homes with guns than in those without guns. Illicit drug use and a history of domestic violence increase the risk.[13] The risk of suicide is increased fivefold in homes with a gun.[14]

Although the scope of the firearm injury problem is unique to the United States, the risks related to firearms in the home are not. Internationally, significant correlations exist between rates of firearm-owning households and rates of all homicide (r=.658), all suicide (r=.515), homicide with a gun (r=.746), and suicide with a gun (r=.900).[15] The international experience with private ownership of guns lends credence to the concept that firearm accessibility contributes heavily to firearm-related trauma.

12.2.2 Demography

Males are at greater risk than females for fatal or nonfatal gunshot wounds. African-Americans are more likely to be shot than are whites or Hispanics. For adolescents and young adults, the gender and race or ethnicity differences seem to be consistent with a higher rate of injuries from assaults among males and African-Americans.[1] Increases in firearm-related homicides (and probably injuries) over the past decade may be related to increases in rates of assault, as documented in Chicago through age 16. Therefore, the easy access to guns reported by adolescents must be taken seriously. Teenage assault with firearms in urban areas often affects acquaintances and may be associated with membership in a street gang. Urban gun violence and homicide among youth is also associated with the drug trafficking prevalent in many inner-city neighborhoods. Assault with a gun is more common in communities with lower median household income and with more households with income below the federal poverty level.[7] Several studies have demonstrated that socioeconomic status (ie, poverty) is more important than race as a risk factor; race may be a proxy for poverty, especially in inner cities.

Young children are the usual victims of unintentional shootings. Most shoot themselves or are shot by a child of similar age at one of their homes, with a gun found in the home. Handguns found in the bedroom are often the firearm used in these unintentional shootings. Hunting-related unintentional injuries are more common in persons younger than 20 years than they are in older people (when grouped by 10-year age increments); 25% of self-inflicted unintentional hunting injuries occur among children and teenagers. Adolescents who experience hunting-related gunshot wounds are often unsupervised.

Teenagers are at particular risk of suicide because they can be moody, impulsive, and immature, susceptible to peer group influence, and may experiment with alcohol and other drugs that impair judgment. Among white male adolescents, suicide by using a firearm is more common than is homicide committed with a firearm. Teenage suicide is highly associated with access to handguns (odds ratio=9.4 compared with no access); the risk is greatest for those without evidence of psychological problems who have a loaded handgun at home (odds ratio=32.3).[16] When a gun is used, a suicide attempt is likely to be successful; there are 3.3 fatalities for every nonfatal suicide attempt with a gun.

12.3 Intervention Strategies

Successful intervention strategies must rely on the known risk factors for firearm-related injuries and the developmental correlates of the children at risk. Pediatricians may be asked to guide schools and communities because of their expertise as child safety advocates. Strategies commonly considered include stricter laws and punishment of individuals who misuse guns ("getting tough on violent crime"), gun control initiatives, education programs on firearm safety, school-based conflict resolution programs, public education campaigns, and clinical counseling. Christoffel[17] has described a range of legislative and regulatory options available to decrease firearm-related trauma (Table 12.3, p 274).

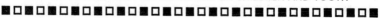
TABLE 12.3.
Options for Legislating and Regulating Guns*

Enforce existing laws

Increase regulation under existing laws

Owner liability for use of guns by a child

Required gun safety education in schools

Increased sales taxes on guns and ammunition

Firearm registration and licensure

Background checks on persons who want to purchase a gun

Modify ammunition

Modify guns

Ban assault weapons

Ban handguns where children are present

Ban handguns

Regulate ownership and use of long guns (ie, rifles and shotguns)

Regulate construction of toy guns

Regulate nonpowder firearms

Regulate new products as they reach the market (eg, armor-piercing bullets and plastic handguns)

Omnibus firearm safety legislation

*Based on Christoffel.[17]

12.3.1 The Public Health Approach

The public health approach to firearm-related injuries identifies and measures the agent(s) of morbidity and mortality and seeks solutions that *prevent* injury.[18] From the public health perspective, crime is not the central issue, although violent injuries are recognized as important. Firearms are the tools that turn violent confrontations deadly; what may have been a bloody nose or a laceration becomes a brain injury inflicted by a bullet. Interventions are devised to address the effects of the epidemic and then evaluated. There is no single intervention; many are available. Individual and public education can be evaluated. Conflict resolution curricula can be considered. Guns may be modified so it is more difficult to fire them. Laws and regulations addressing guns as hazardous consumer products, gun owner responsibility, or restricting some types of ammunition and guns are interventions that have been considered.

The public health approach identifies the handgun and its ammunition as the principal vector of the kinetic energy causing injury and death. This approach seeks to protect *everyone* from injury. Programs that only address unintentional injury or only punish gun misusers are incomplete solutions. The risks and benefits of handgun ownership can be measured quantitatively.

This comprehensive approach is reminiscent of the efforts to decrease the use of cigarettes, the vectors of chemicals that result in cancer and heart disease. Similarly, it may take many years to convince Americans of the health risks of handgun ownership. As health professionals with great opportunity to influence family behavior and child health, pediatricians can participate in this public health effort in the clinical, research, and policy arenas.

12.3.2 Punishment of Individuals Who Misuse Guns

On the surface, it would seem that punishing individuals who misuse or improperly store firearms would be a highly effective approach. Although punishment is appropriate, we must recognize that the United States has more prisons and more people in prison than most other nations, yet it has the highest rate of firearm-related homicide in the world. Tough laws have not appeared to have diminished firearm-related injuries and deaths. It is not clear whether toughening laws and prison sentences further, though politically attractive, will have an appreciable effect on reducing firearm morbidity and mortality. This approach does not address suicide or unintentional injury.

12.3.3 Gun Control

Controlling ownership of firearms is an emotionally and politically charged topic. In contrast to punishment, this strategy attempts to influence the use of firearms before someone is injured. All too often, crime, violence, property protection, and personal injury are debated as if they were inseparable. However, *violence* is not the same as *crime,* and not all crime is violent. Handguns can turn violent confrontations deadly, even when there was no criminal intent at the outset. Gun control can be considered a means to decrease *injuries,* quite separate from its possible utility as a way to reduce crime or violence in our society.

A patchwork of local, state, and national laws limits the effectiveness of gun control laws and makes it difficult to demonstrate the effectiveness of these laws, although there is some published evidence of their benefit.[19] Because handguns are the firearms most often used to injure or kill, the emphasis should be on *handgun* control, and ways to limit all types of injuries — homicide (and nonfatal firearm assault), suicide, and unintentional injuries — should be sought. Restricting access to handguns may be a means to protect everyone.

12.3.4 Firearm Education

There is much disagreement over the role of firearm education efforts as part of an overall strategy to reduce firearm injuries. Part of the problem is that efforts to teach children safe behaviors around guns have not been adequately evaluated. Some gun owner groups have advocated gun education as *an alternative* to reducing gun ownership in environments where children live and play. Public health advocates have argued that the role of education is limited because the youngest children in need of protection (in this and other areas of injury prevention) may fail to recall safety information and use it correctly. Older children and teenagers may fail to heed warnings during play, while showing off, or during stressful times. Pediatricians should help assure that organized educational efforts directed at children and adolescents have an evaluation component to demonstate their effectiveness. Likewise, they should assure that such programs not be instituted as a *replacement* for the AAP-approved passive protection strategy of *reducing availability* of firearms in environments with children and adolescents.

Among those who have chosen to use guns for hunting or sport, proper safety education by a qualified instructor — ideally involving both child and parent — is an important component of safe use and practice. Such training (and demonstrated competence) should be required for those who plan to use firearms for recreational use. Programs should emphasize safe locked storage of firearms, separate storage of ammunition, abstinence from alcohol use, and never treating a firearm in a casual fashion (eg, no horseplay, joking, boasting).

12.3.5 School-Based Conflict Resolution Programs

(See also chapter 8.3.)

Conflict resolution programs have been suggested as a way to decrease the occurrence of violence among youth. If successful, these programs may indirectly protect children from intentional firearm-related injuries, but to date, evidence for their effectiveness is lacking. Many school districts have adopted programs at considerable expense and without plans to evaluate their long-term efficacy in reduction of violence or the number of injuries. As with all educational programs, pediatricians should help assure that further evaluation of school-based conflict resolution programs occurs before promoting widespread implementation.

12.3.6 Public Education

Public education campaigns can be used to enlighten the general public (and public officials) about the problem of firearm-related injuries and deaths. The goals of a campaign and the messages used must be carefully considered: a campaign aimed at passing a new law should be different from one intended for mothers living in high-risk neighborhoods. Pediatricians can bring science to public education campaigns, especially pertaining to the public health aspects of handgun injuries.

12.3.7 Clinical Counseling

Programs are available for use by pediatricians in their practices to counsel families about violence or about firearms; adequate evaluations of efficacy are virtually nonexistent. The STOP (Steps to Prevent Firearm Injury) Program, a joint effort of the AAP and the Center to Prevent Handgun Violence, may be evaluated in the future. The STOP Program emphasizes that it is safest to keep guns, especially handguns, out of children's homes, but if a family has a gun it should be unloaded and kept in a locked cabinet or drawer. Bullets should be locked in a separate place. The STOP Program materials seem to be easy to use, but currently the efficacy of the program is unknown.

12.4 Associated Problems

12.4.1 Toy Guns

(See also chapter 15.4.5.)

Toy guns that fire projectiles injure about 400 children each year, may contribute to antisocial behavior, and may be a source of training for use of real firearms. More than half of those injured are younger than 5 years; 90% are younger than 15 years, and approximately 70% are boys. Most injuries involve the face or eyes. In addition to the injury caused by the impact of projectiles, projectiles pose a risk of aspiration. In 1981, the US Consumer Product Safety Commission (CPSC) estimated the direct costs of injuries from toy guns to be $640 000 per year. The health care savings available from redesign of these toys would offset the cost of the redesign. The CPSC has authority to regulate these products.[5]

An important consideration is the realistic appearance of some toy guns. Especially in dark or shadowy circumstances, the toy may be perceived as a real weapon. Police officers have mistaken children with toy guns for criminal suspects brandishing real guns, with dire consequences. Toy guns manufactured with brightly colored parts (to distinguish them from real guns) are still mistaken for real guns in dim light.

12.4.2 Nonpowder Firearms

Nonpowder firearms (also called air guns, air rifles, BB guns, and pellet guns) caused more than 30 000 injuries during 1992 and 1993 in the United States, with an inpatient admission rate of about 6.5%.[1] Severe eye injuries have long been associated with nonpowder firearms, but fatal chest, head, neck, and face injuries also occur. Most injuries involve boys younger than 15 years; more than 80% are younger than 25 years.[6]

Parents should recognize that nonpowder firearms are *firearms*, not toys. They are designed to resemble powder guns. Some have muzzle velocities greater than 700 ft/sec; impact at 130 ft/sec can penetrate the eye and 350 to 370 ft/sec can penetrate skin and bone. The CPSC has not regulated these nonpowder firearms because of concern that regulations might impair their utility. The AAP has called for regulation of nonpowder firearms.[20]

12.5 Recommendations

12.5.1 The Pediatrician's Role

Pediatricians should bear witness to the injury and death caused by handguns in their communities. They should counsel families about the danger of keeping firearms, especially handguns, in their homes. They may also address the issues related to toy guns and the dangers of nonpowder firearms. Pediatricians should become involved in local efforts to curb violence and violent injury, but they must insist that an evaluation component be included in all programs so resources are not wasted and ineffective programs are not perpetuated.

Pediatricians and pediatric organizations may become involved with the HELP (Handgun Epidemic Lowering Plan) Network of Concerned Professionals. The HELP Network emphasizes a public health approach and the role of health professionals' expertise in curbing the handgun epidemic.

Pediatricians should provide office-based anticipatory guidance about firearm-related injuries. Some practitioners believe that all the children at risk are in practices other than their own, but many pediatricians have personally cared for patients who have been shot.[21] While parents may not agree to remove a gun from the home, most families are willing to follow advice about safe storage of firearms, and most parents who do not own a gun would accept a pediatrician's advice not to purchase one.[22] For health care providers seeking guidance for office-based counseling, including sample dialogue, the STOP Program is a helpful resource (see Resources section).

When discussing firearm-related injuries with families, friends, policy makers, print and broadcast reporters, and other physicians, pediatricians can make the following points:

- The risks of handgun ownership outweigh the benefits. Handguns are much more likely to result in harm to the owner, a family member, or an acquaintance, than they are to serve to protect against an intruder.

- Firearm-related injuries are the leading cause of traumatic death in the second decade of life, surpassing even vehicle occupant fatalities.
- Handguns are involved in most firearm-related injuries and deaths.
- The best protection for children and teenagers is to keep firearms — especially handguns — out of their homes and extended environments.
- If it is necessary to have a handgun, it should be unloaded and stored in a locked cabinet or drawer. Ammunition should be locked in an area separate from the gun.
- Injury prevention efforts must address homicide, suicide, and unintentional shootings.
- The effectiveness of educational programs for young audiences should be evaluated before widespread adoption.

12.5.2 AAP Policy

The AAP urges pediatricians and other health care providers to emphasize the importance of removing guns from high-risk homes — those where alcohol or other drug abuse is likely or present and homes with adolescent boys. Likewise, high-risk youth — victims of previous gun violence, with a history of domestic or peer violence, those who are depressed or who have attempted suicide, or have a history of carrying weapons — require special intervention and often referral to community-based social support services.

The AAP supports legislation and regulations to limit the availability of handguns in environments where children work and play and efforts to reduce the romanticization of gun use in the popular media. Pediatricians are urged to support broad-based community coalitions to reduce firearm-related injuries and deaths. These and other recommendations are in published AAP policy statements.[11,23] A model legislative bill, the Protection of Children from Handguns Act, is available from the AAP Division of State Government Affairs.

■□■□■□■□■□■□■□■□■□■□■□■□■□■□■□■□■

12.6 Resources

1. American Academy of Pediatrics
   141 Northwest Point Blvd
   PO Box 927
   Elk Grove Village, IL 60009-0927
   800-433-9016

   "Silence the Violence" is an AAP speaker's kit available to members.
   Policy statements and model legislation are also available.

2. EAST Violence Prevention Task Force
   Eastern Association for the Surgery of Trauma
   Hospital of the University of Pennsylvania
   3400 Spruce St
   Philadelphia, PA, 19140
   215-662-7320

   "America's Uncivil War: Slides on the Epidemic of Firearm Violence"
   is a set of slides and a monograph. EAST also provides an annotated
   bibliography.

3. East Boston Neighborhood Health Center
   10 Gove St
   East Boston, MA 02128

   Ask for the "Guide to Violence Prevention and Treatment."

4. HELP Network of Concerned Professionals
   Children's Memorial Hospital
   2300 Children's Plaza
   Box 88
   Chicago, IL 60614
   312-880-3826

5. Physicians for Social Responsibility
   Chicago Chapter
   59 E Van Buren St, Suite 807
   Chicago, IL 60605
   312- 663-1777

   "Firearm Violence: Community Diagnosis and Treatment" is a slide
   set with an accompanying speaker's manual.

6. STOP Program
Center to Prevent Handgun Violence
1225 Eye St, NW, Suite 1100
Washington, DC 20005
202- 289-7319

This educational packet, appropriate for in-office use, was developed jointly with the AAP.

References

1. Annest JL, Mercy JA, Gibson DR, Ryan GW. National estimates of nonfatal firearm-related injuries: beyond the tip of the iceberg. *JAMA*. 1995;273:1749–1754

2. Deaths resulting from firearm- and motor-vehicle-related injuries: United States, 1968–1991. *MMWR Morb Mortal Wkly Rep*. 1994;43:37–42

3. Fingerhut LA, Kleinman JC. International and interstate comparisons of homicide among young males. *JAMA*. 1990;263:3292–3295

4. Senturia YD, Christoffel KK, Donovan M. Children's household exposure to guns: a pediatric practice-based survey. *Pediatrics*. 1994;93:469–475

5. Tanz RR, Christoffel KK, Sagerman S. Are toy guns too dangerous? *Pediatrics*. 1985; 75:265–268

6. Christoffel KK, Tanz R, Sagerman S, Hahn Y. Childhood injuries caused by nonpowder firearms. *Am J Dis Child*. 1984;138:557–561

7. Powell EC, Tanz RR. Assaulting our urban children. *Arch Pediatr Adolesc Med*. 1994;148(suppl):61

8. Zavoski RW, Lapidus GD, Lerer TJ, Banco LI. A population-based study of severe firearm injury among children and youth. *Pediatrics*. 1995;96:278–282

9. Allen I. *Financial Impact on Inpatient Resources in Children's Hospitals Caused by Firearm Injuries: FY 1991*. Alexandria, VA: National Association of Children's Hospitals and Related Institutions; 1993

10. Firearm-related years of potential life lost before age 65 years: United States, 1980–1991. *MMWR Morb Mortal Wkly Rep*. 1994;43:609–611

11. American Academy of Pediatrics, Committee on Injury and Poison Prevention. Firearm injuries affecting the pediatric population. *Pediatrics*. 1992;89:788–790

12. Kellermann A, Reay DT. Protection or peril? an analysis of firearm-related deaths in the home. *N Engl J Med*. 1986;314:1557–1560

13. Kellermann AL, Rivara FP, Rushforth NB, et al. Gun ownership as a risk factor for homicide in the home. *N Engl J Med*. 1993;329:1084–1091

14. Kellermann AL, Rivara FP, Somes G, et al. Suicide in the home in relation to gun ownership. *N Engl J Med*. 1992;327:467–472

15. Killias M. International correlations between gun ownership and rates of homicide and suicide. *Can Med Assoc J.* 1993;148:1721–1725

16. Brent DA, Perper JA, Moritz G, et al. Firearms and adolescent suicide: a community case-control study. *Am J Dis Child.* 1993;147:1066–1071

17. Christoffel KK. Toward reducing pediatric injuries from firearms: charting a legislative and regulatory course. *Pediatrics.* 1991;88:294–305

18. Kellermann AL, Lee RK, Mercy JA, Banton J. The epidemiologic basis for the prevention of firearm injuries. *Annu Rev Public Health.* 1991;12:17–40

19. Sloan JH, Kellermann AL, Reay DT, et al. Handgun regulations, crime, assaults, and homicide: a tale of two cities. *N Engl J Med.* 1988;319:1256–1262

20. American Academy of Pediatrics, Committee on Accident and Poison Prevention. Injuries related to toy firearms. *Pediatrics.* 1987;79:473–474

21. Webster DW, Wilson ME, Duggan AK, Pakula LC. Firearm injury prevention counseling: a study of pediatricians' beliefs and practices. *Pediatrics.* 1992;89:902–907

22. Webster DW, Wilson ME, Duggan AK, Pakula LC. Parents' beliefs about preventing gun injuries to children. *Pediatrics.* 1992;89:908–914

23. American Academy of Pediatrics, Committee on Adolescence. Firearms and adolescents. *Pediatrics.* 1992;89:784–787

Suggested Readings

Violence and the public's health. *Health Aff (Millwood).* 1993;12

Rand MR. *Guns and Crime: Handgun Victimization, Firearm Self-Defense, and Firearm Theft. Crime Data Brief.* Washington, DC: US Department of Justice, Office of Justice Programs, Bureau of Justice Statistics; 1994. Publication NCJ-147003

Stringham P, Spivak H. What pediatric primary care clinicians can do when confronting aggressive youth. *Bull NY Acad Med.* 1994;71:1–18

CHAPTER 13

Mechanical Airway Obstruction: Choking, Strangulation, and Suffocation

13.1 Scope and Definitions

Choking is respiratory distress that results from an unsuccessful attempt at swallowing. It is typically caused by the attempted ingestion of food that is not properly chewed, or from a small object that is swallowed when mistaken for food. The term is used to describe an internal event leading to respiratory distress and is distinguished from an external event, such as *strangulation* or *suffocation.*

A choking episode can have four outcomes. After some initial distress, the food or object may be successfully swallowed without subsequent obstruction or problem. The food or object may be expelled by coughing or vomiting. The food or foreign object may remain lodged in the esophagus, usually at the upper esophageal sphincter (cricopharyngeus muscle). Finally, the material may lodge within the child's airway (larynx, trachea, or bronchi), which is *aspiration.* Aspiration can be fatal if there is complete blockage of the pharynx, larynx, or trachea.

Asphyxiation is the term used to describe airway obstruction from aspiration or strangulation that results in cerebral anoxia or death.[1]

Entrapment is the condition of being enclosed or confined in a closed space, which can lead to injury or death from asphyxiation, such as in a refrigerator or in a grain elevator.

In the United States, unintentional death by mechanical airway obstruction (by choking, strangulation, suffocation, or entrapment) results in about 700 deaths each year to children and adolescents. Half of these deaths occur in the first year of life and three quarters occur in children younger than 5 years. It is the leading cause of unintentional injuries that result in death in the first year of life and is exceeded only by motor vehicles, drowning, and fires as causes of unintentional injuries that result in death to preschoolers.

Death may also be caused *intentionally* by mechanical obstruction of the airway, either externally or internally. The National Center for Health Statistics recorded 134 homicides by suffocation to children and adolescents (from birth to 19 years of age) for 1992, 35 of which were in the first year of life. The actual number of victims of fatal child abuse by suffocation may be considerably higher (see chapter 8.1). Suffocation (including hanging) is a popular method of suicide in adolescents and is responsible for more than 400 deaths each year in the second decade of life (see chapter 8.2).

13.2. Epidemiology

Death from mechanical airway obstruction is most common in the first year of life. The age distribution of deaths from mechanical asphyxiation is given in Table 13.1, p 287.

Death from asphyxiation, either from choking or from suffocation, is more common in males than in females — even in the first year of life. In children, food and nonfood items are responsible for approximately equal numbers of deaths from choking.[2]

Nonfatal events of mechanical airway obstruction are much more common than deaths. Aspiration is seen with some frequency beginning around 10 months of age and continues to increase in frequency into the preschool years. Foods and coins are the most common causes of nonfatal choking, although any small household objects, including pieces of toys, can be involved. Balls (and other small spherically shaped objects) and deflated balloons, which tend to conform to and occlude the airway, are commonly implicated as causes of death.[3]

Unintentional strangulation typically results from clothing or a string around a child's neck that becomes caught on furniture or some other object. Other consumer products implicated in strangulations include window blind cords and the lids of toy chests.[2] Entrapment and asphyx-

TABLE 13.1.
Unintentional Pediatric Deaths From Airway Obstruction
United States, 1992*

Age, y	Aspiration	Suffocation	Total
<1	103	229	332
1	51	43	94
2	27	21	48
3	13	12	25
4	4	7	11
5-9	23	35	58
10-14	16	61	77
15-19	21	46	67
Total	258	454	712

*Data from the National Center for Health Statistics. Aspiration (E911, E912) indicates inhalation or ingestion of food or other object causing obstruction of respiration; suffocation (E913), any unintentional external mechanical cause of suffocation, including hanging, plastic bags, strangulation, or confinement in a closed space. Homicides and suicides are excluded from the data.

iation can occur in unsafe crib environments — in decorative cutouts in the headboards, between the crib frame and an ill-fitting mattress, or between crib bars that are too widely spaced. Suffocation can occur if children have access to plastic bags; those made of thin plastic and used for dry cleaning and garbage are a particular hazard. Entrapment can also occur in household items such as refrigerators, ice chests, and clothes dryers.

13.3 Risk Factors for Choking

13.3.1 Children Who Are Prone to Choking

Safe swallowing is difficult for young children for reasons of anatomy, experience, and judgment. The sequence of eruption of the deciduous (primary) teeth between 6 and 36 months of age makes children vulnerable to choking. The incisors (biting teeth) erupt before the molars (chewing teeth), which may not be completely erupted until near the third birthday.

This vulnerability to choking caused by the sequence of tooth eruption is amplified by the child's lack of experience and cognitive skills to avoid choking. The ability of a child to know and remember to chew hard or chunky foods well is not automatic by a certain age, but comes with time and experience. The same is true for remembering to eat slowly. Great individual variability exists in the timing of the eruption of teeth as well as in the behavioral aspects of chewing and swallowing, in swallowing coordination, and in sound judgment about how well to chew. Nevertheless, foods that require considerable chewing prior to swallowing are generally handled less well by the child younger than 3 years than by an older child.

Considerable variation also exists in the maturity of the swallowing mechanism in children of the same age. Children who have difficulty swallowing (who frequently choke on food) should be fed cautiously and should be introduced more slowly to foods that are more difficult to chew and swallow. Likewise, children with certain behavioral characteristics may increase their risk of choking as do those who put "everything" in their mouths and those who impulsively eat fast. Children with developmental disabilities may need special food preparation and special attention around mealtime to prevent them from choking.

13.3.2 Foods That Are Choking Hazards

Because no federal regulations exist regarding foods that are given to children, physician guidance is critical. Foods that require careful chewing are best avoided.

The foods that most frequently cause death or injury are hot dogs, sausages, grapes, carrots, peanuts, or other seeds from fruits or vegetables, such as watermelon.[4] Peanuts contain oils that are particularly irritating to the lungs of young children and have been shown to result in permanent alteration of ventilation and perfusion (Table 13.2, p 289).

13.3.3 Situations Likely to Lead to Choking

There are clearly some situations that are likely to lead to choking on food. Eating while rushed, running, laughing, or while in other ways being distracted is likely to increase the risk of choking.

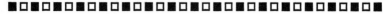
```
┌─────────────────────────────────────────────────────────┐
│                       TABLE 13.2.                          │
│            Hazardous Foods for Young Children*             │
│───────────────────────────────────────────────────────── │
│                  Hot dogs and sausages                     │
│                  Chunks of meat                            │
│                  Grapes, raisins                           │
│                  Apple chunks                              │
│                  Nuts, peanuts, popcorn                    │
│                  Watermelon seeds                          │
│                  Raw carrots                               │
│                  Hard candy                                │
└─────────────────────────────────────────────────────────┘
```

*Children younger than 4 years should avoid these foods. (This list is not all-inclusive.)

The likelihood of choking therefore depends on four variables: (1) the behavior characteristics of the child, (2) the maturity of the swallowing mechanism of the child, (3) the type of food being eaten, and (4) the eating situation.

Risk factors for choking on nonedible objects are similar to those for choking on foods. Children up to about 4 years of age manifest "mouthing" behaviors and explore their environment orally. Some children, however, show mouthing as an exaggerated behavior or temperamental quality. For these children, almost every object in the environment is tasted and, if attractive to them or mistaken for food, swallowing may be attempted. Such children are also at risk for choking.

13.3.4 Objects That Are Choking Hazards

Any object small enough to fit in a child's mouth is a potential choking hazard. Of particular concern are objects that are small enough to fit in the mouth and, because of their size and shape, can lodge in the upper esophagus or in the airway causing respiratory compromise either by external compression of the airway or as an obstructive plug. Sometimes the composition of the ingested object or the aspirated object itself increases the hazard and concern, such as small disk batteries that leak corrosive alkali.

Small metallic currency is the most common foreign object that causes injuries to children worldwide. Coins, particularly pennies, are the right size and shape to lodge in the upper esophagus. (Disk-shaped objects are less likely to lodge in the airway.)

Other small objects that may be ingested include parts of toys intended for older children, jewelry, arts and crafts items, small pieces of hardware, and office supplies such as paper clips and the plastic caps on ballpoint pens. Small rubber balls and marbles are a particular hazard because of their size, shape, and ubiquity.

13.4 Intervention Strategies

13.4.1 Education

Parents should be educated about prevention of choking, suffocation, and strangulation according to their child's developmental stage. For the newborn, cribs may pose a suffocation hazard. Parents should be informed that older cribs may have improperly spaced slats (greater than 2⅜-in gaps), poorly fitting mattresses, decorative cutouts in the headboard, or corner posts that can catch clothing. The use of crib gyms or decorations that hang across the crib is an unsafe practice. By 4 to 5 months of age, infants can pull themselves up on their hands and knees where they may entangle their necks in cords or ribbons (see chapter 4.1 for parent checklist items on crib safety).

Parents should not use makeshift pacifiers and rattles. Ordinary latex feeding nipples may break apart and cause choking.[5] Homemade rattles are likewise hazardous. Such makeshift products do not meet the federal standards for size and integrity that govern the manufacture of rattles and pacifiers in the United States.

Choking from common household products is best discussed with parents at or before the 6-month health maintenance visit. At around 4 months of age, infants are able to bring objects to their mouths. By 6 months of age, infants have developed the fine motor dexterity to pick up small objects and put them in their mouths. At this age, a home survey for small household objects and toys that belong to older siblings is important. Objects such as marbles, small rubber balls, and latex balloons should be mentioned specifically as hazards because they are frequently implicated in injury events and can be fatal for infants because of their size and shape. Balloons should not be available to children younger than 8 years because they may chew on deflated balloons or hold them over their mouths. With a gasp, the thin latex can be drawn into a child's airway where it is nearly impossible to dislodge.[6]

Safe foods should also be discussed at the 6-month visit. This topic can be integrated into physician counseling about finger foods. Parent education brochures available from the American Academy of Pediatrics (AAP) can be helpful. Although lists of foods that commonly cause choking are useful, parents may also benefit from an understanding of the principles behind such lists. Appropriate foods are those that crumble or quickly dissolve in the mouth, as opposed to those that are round and firm.[4] Infants should be fed solid foods only by adults, and only when sitting upright. Parents should be encouraged to take a basic life support course or at least know the emergency measures for a choking infant (see Table 13.3 as well as the AAP brochure, "Choking Prevention and First Aid for Infants and Children: Guidelines for Parents").[7]

In the second half of the child's first year of life, emerging mobility is an additional risk for choking. Children approaching their first birthdays may pull themselves up to a stand at toy chests with heavy hinged lids. These lids have fallen on the heads of a number of children, strangling them.[8] Toy boxes are best without lids. Likewise, newly mobile children may reach for and place looped blind and drapery cords around their necks. Such cords should be well out of reach. A better alternative is to cut the looped cords and attach to the ends either a "breakaway" tassel or two separate tassels. (Consumer brochures describing safe modification of looped window covering cords are available from the Window Covering Safety Council; 800-506-4636.)

TABLE 13.3.
Choking Prevention Guidelines for Parents

- Keep foods known to be a choking hazard from children until 4 y of age
- Ensure that children eat while sitting at the table; children should never walk, run, or play with food in their mouths
- Prepare and cut food for young children and teach them to chew their food well
- Supervise mealtime for young children; many choking events occur when older brothers or sisters offer unsafe foods to a younger child
- Avoid toys with small parts and keep other small household items out of reach of young children

Parents should be warned to keep plastic bags away from children. Discarded dry cleaning bags should be immediately removed from the house.

13.4.2 Enforcement of Safety Regulations

Promulgation and enforcement of product safety regulations by the Consumer Product Safety Commission have lead to substantial reductions in the number of choking and strangulation events in the United States during the past 20 years (see Appendix G). Like most regulatory efforts, however, they have their limitations. For example, the small parts standard prohibits small parts on toys or consumer products intended for children younger than 3 years.[9] The standard utilizes a test device called the small parts test fixture (SPTF) (Fig 13.1), which is a "truncated cylinder" $1\frac{1}{4}$ in in diameter that has a sloping floor, giving the cylinder a depth that ranges from 1 to $2\frac{1}{4}$ in. Any toy or part of a toy that completely fits within this unusually shaped container must be labeled for use only by children older than 3 years. The appropriateness of this

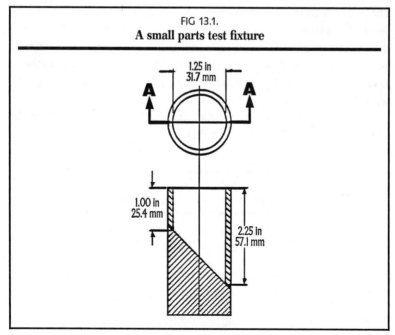

FIG 13.1.
A small parts test fixture

1.25 in
31.7 mm

A   A

1.00 in
25.4 mm

2.25 in
57.1 mm

A small parts test fixture may be obtained from Discovery Toys (800-426-4777), Toys to Grow On (213-603-8890), and other mail-order sources.

standard in screening out objects that can lead to *nonfatal* choking is suggested by a recent study of approximately 140 injury-causing foreign bodies that revealed that more than 99% of identifiable foreign bodies fit within the cylinder.[10] The SPTF may not be as effective, however, in screening out objects whose ingestion results in death, and stricter federal consumer guidelines may be warranted.

An analysis of 355 objects causing deaths in children suggested that spherical objects should be at least 4.44 cm in diameter, and linear objects should be at least 7.62 cm in length to prevent fatal choking. This conclusion is based empirically on the shapes and sizes of the objects that have caused fatalities. A stricter standard would screen out objects that can reach the posterior pharynx where the involuntary phase of swallowing is initiated.[11]

Concern has been raised that the labeling on toys with small parts, although it informs parents that the toys are not intended for children younger than 3 years, does not explain *why* the toy is inappropriate. Parents therefore often assume that labeling is informational, relating to the child's educational level rather than to safety.[12,13] The standard also exempts balloons, the product most frequently implicated in the choking deaths of children.[6]

A rule issued by the Consumer Product Safety Commission effective August 1995 corrects some of these deficiencies. Packaging for toys with small parts, small balls (with diameters $<1\,3/4$ in), and marbles contain the label:

> ## CHOKING HAZARD   Small parts.
> ## Not for children under 3 years.

Packages of balloons now contain the warning label:

> ## CHOKING HAZARD   Children under 8 years
> ## can choke or suffocate on unin ated or
> ## broken balloons. Adult supervision required.

13.4.3 Engineering

As a result of federal safety regulations, many products intended for use by young children are engineered such that choking or strangulation is unlikely or impossible, for example, one-piece pacifiers that do not fit within a child's mouth, toys with no small detachable parts, and cribs with closely spaced slats and tight-fitting mattresses. Many opportunities for engineering improvements remain in everyday products to further lessen the likelihood of mechanical airway obstruction. All cords on window shades and blinds could be made either without loops or with breakaway loops. Toy boxes can be made without heavy hinged lids, and children's hooded clothing could be manufactured without drawstrings. (This latter design defect has led to injury or death of a number of children when the drawstring has been caught on playground equipment, fences, or cribs.)

13.4.4 Clinical Aspects of Foreign Body Ingestion

To prevent complications of foreign body ingestion, the physician must recognize the variability of presentation and develop appropriate management.

Parents who have witnessed a choking episode frequently bring their child to the physician or emergency department for evaluation. Most of these children — probably more than 90% — fortunately have vomited the matter or completed swallowing the object by the time of evaluation and are discharged from the hospital and instructed to return only if symptoms develop. Children who have persistent signs and symptoms — airway distress, cyanosis, apnea, or drooling — must be managed emergently. Physicians should recognize, however, that in possibly half the cases, signs and symptoms may initially be completely absent when a foreign body remains lodged in the airway or esophagus.

Aspiration or ingestion events that are not witnessed are often challenging to correctly diagnose because symptoms may be completely absent for weeks or months and, when present, may mimic asthma or cause drooling, fever, pneumonia, or weight loss rather than choking or respiratory distress. The longer the time interval between the event and a correct diagnosis, the more frequent the complications and the more difficult the diagnosis, the determination of the exact location of the object, evaluation, extraction, and subsequent hospital course.

Radiologic evaluation is helpful but can be imprecise. Foreign bodies in the airway are generally not radiopaque, and findings of hyperaeration and atelectasis can occur in healthy infant lungs. In a recent study,[14] chest films have been shown to have a sensitivity of only 65%. Airway fluoroscopy is more sensitive because subtle areas of atelectasis can be observed dynamically. If the child is not in distress and dysphasia is noted, airway fluoroscopy can be performed in conjunction with a barium swallow to evaluate the esophagus.

Computed tomography (CT) is not routinely used to diagnose airway or esophageal foreign bodies. The images obtained with CT are useful only when a localized area of tissue reaction is confirmed – generally a late finding when pulmonary and esophageal foreign bodies are present. The early presentations of children who have choked on food or foreign bodies characteristically lack localizing symptoms or signs because the tissue has had little time to react. Magnetic resonance imaging has similar limitations and is impractical for the vast majority of choking events.

Physical examination is important when it is abnormal. The presence of wheezing that is new or localized is critical. The localized absence of breath sounds on auscultation of the lung is likewise important.

When there is a constellation of symptoms, physical signs, and an abnormal – or sometimes even normal – radiologic evaluation, consultation with specialists who perform bronchoscopy (otolaryngologists, pulmonologists, and pediatric surgeons) is important. Bronchoscopy can be considered and should be performed either immediately or when close follow-up detects a persistent medical problem.

Close supervision of children following a choking episode must be emphasized to the parents or other caregivers. Asymptomatic children may become symptomatic after a quiescent period.

13.5 Recommendations for the Pediatrician

13.5.1 Office-Based Counseling

As discussed in the previous section on education, the physician should provide anticipatory guidance based on the child's age and developmental stage. Parents of newborns require information on safe sleeping environments to prevent entrapment and suffocation. As children become mobile and develop fine motor skills, information about small parts and household fixtures and products with strings and cords should be discussed. Likewise, information about food safety should precede the introduction of finger foods. Pediatricians should incorporate this information into routine discussions of child development and their more general counseling about injury prevention.

13.5.2 Advocacy

Preemptive measures to protect young children from hazards in their environment have been a goal of the AAP, and success has been achieved during the last 2 decades by working with governmental agencies such as the Consumer Product Safety Commission and through educational material provided through TIPP (The Injury Prevention Program). Significant progress in the prevention of injuries from choking and suffocation can be seen in government standards for cribs, pacifiers, rattles, and small parts.

13.6 Resources

1. US Consumer Product Safety Commission
   Washington, DC 20207
   800-638 2772
   301-504-0990

   The CPSC provides information on prevention of choking, suffocation, strangulation, and entrapment associated with household and consumer products.

2. The Danny Foundation
   3160-F Danville Blvd
   PO Box 680
   Alamo, CA 94507
   800-83 DANNY

   The foundation provides a variety of educational materials on crib safety.

References

1. Black RE, Johnson DG, Matlak ME. Bronchoscopic removal of aspirated foreign bodies in children. *J Pediatr Surg.* 1994;29:682–684

2. Baker SP, O'Neill B, Karpf RS. *The Injury Fact Book.* Lexington, MA: Lexington Books; 1984

3. Reilly JS, Walter MA. Consumer product aspiration and ingestion in children: analysis of emergency room reports to the National Electronic Injury Surveillance System. *Ann Otol Rhinol Laryngol.* 1992;101:739–741

4. Harris CS, Baker SP, Smith GA, Harris RM. Childhood asphyxiation by food: a national analysis and overview. *JAMA.* 1984;251:2231–2235

5. Millunchick EW, McArtor RD. Fatal aspiration of a makeshift pacifier. *Pediatrics.* 1986;77:369–370

6. Ryan CA, Yacoub W, Paton T, Avard D. Childhood deaths from toy balloons. *Am J Dis Child.* 1990;144:1221–1224

7. American Academy of Pediatrics. *Choking Prevention and First Aid for Infants and Children* [pamphlet]. Elk Grove Village, IL: American Academy of Pediatrics; 1988

8. Singer WD, Luther L. Trauma from toy boxes. *J Pediatr.* 1982;100:242–243

9. Small Parts Regulations under the Federal Hazardous Substances Act. 16 CFR Part 1501. *Federal Register.* June 7, 1988;53:20885

10. Reilly JS, Walter MA, Beste D, et al. Size/shape analysis of aerodigestive foreign bodies in children: a multi-institutional study. *Am J Otolaryngol.* 1995;16:190–193

11. Rimell FL, Thome A Jr, Stool S, Reilly JS, et al. Characteristics of objects causing choking in children. *JAMA.* 1995;274:1763–1766

12. Widome MD. Pediatric injury prevention for the practitioner. *Curr Probl Pediatr.* 1991; 21:428–468

13. Langlois JA, Wallen BA, Teret SP, Bailey LA, Hershey JH, Peeler MO. The impact of specific toy warning labels. *JAMA.* 1991;265:2848–2850

14. Svedstrom E, Puhakka J, Kero P. How accurate is chest radiography in the diagnosis of tracheobronchial foreign bodies in children? *Pediatr Radiol.* 1989;19:520–522

■□■□■□■□■□■□■□■□■□■□■□■□■□■□■□■□■

CHAPTER 14

Product Safety

Almost 5000 children die every year and thousands more are injured
by unsafe products, by the unsafe operation of products, and by the
unanticipated or unplanned for use of products by children. In an era
of consumerism, parents are eager to identify allies to assist them in
making purchases that are not only cost conscious but safe. The pediatrician has a unique opportunity to educate parents about products
that pose hazards to children and provide counseling on the levels of
necessary supervision for others. Fortunately the practitioner also has
allies in protecting children against product-related injuries. Publications
from organizations such as the Consumer Federation of America are a
rich source of information for the public and pediatricians.[1]

The Consumer Product Safety Act of 1972 established the Consumer
Product Safety Commission (CPSC) (see Appendix G). This independent
regulatory agency of US government has been charged to protect consumers from unreasonable risks of injury associated with consumer
products. To accomplish this mission, the Commission uses many information sources to determine which products are injuring children. More
than 15000 products fall within the Commission's jurisdiction. Sources
examined include death certificates, medical examiners' reports, data
on fires from the National Fire Incident Reporting System, voluntary
reporting by consumers of product-related problems, reports from
lawyers, and news clippings. In addition, since the inception of the
Commission, data from an emergency department monitoring system
have been utilized to keep track of products that are associated with
injuries to children. The current system includes 100 representative
emergency departments in the United States and includes 11 children's
hospitals. The National Electronic Injury Surveillance System (NEISS)
provides approximately 335 000 product-related injury reports each
year. This system provides four levels of data: surveillance of emergency
department injuries; special information documented from emergency
department visits; follow-up interviews of injured persons; and even
comprehensive on-site investigations with the injured person and other
witnesses. Armed with this information, the CPSC has the authority to
set mandatory standards, ban a product, order recalls of unsafe prod-

ucts, or institute labeling requirements. In addition, under the provisions of the Administrative Procedure Act, any individual or agency has the right to petition the Commission to initiate a proceeding to issue regulations under any of the statutes administered by the Commission. The American Academy of Pediatrics has pursued this avenue to protect children's health on a variety of product-related issues. The regulatory approach to prevention of injury fits well into the philosophy of a "passive" approach to disease prevention at the community level.

Only a portion of product-related injuries reported to the Commission involve children's products and are covered elsewhere in this manual. The remainder of this chapter deals with widely used products that can pose a risk to children's health whether or not they are products specifically intended for use by children.

14.1 Appliance and Picnic Cooler Entrapment

Since October 1958, the Federal Refrigerator Safety Act has required that refrigerators can be opened from the inside. Since then, manufacturers of other appliances also have voluntarily redesigned their products to provide safety doors or interlock devices that help prevent entrapment. Nevertheless, a variety of containers may pose a hazard to children in the home. In California between 1960 and 1981, 124 children died of entrapment in containers in the home such as refrigerators, washers and dryers, and toy boxes. In past years, the CPSC also received reports of numerous deaths from suffocation involving children, most of whom were preschool age, who crawled inside latch-type freezers, washers or dryers, picnic coolers, ice boxes in campers, and old-style latch-type refrigerators. In all cases, the CPSC reported that the doors could not be easily pushed open from the inside. Circumstances surrounding the events disclosed that the children were often playing "hide-and-seek" and used the appliance or chest as a hiding place. The tight-fitting gasket on most of the appliances cut off air to the child. This, along with the insulated construction of the appliance, also prevented the child's screams from being heard. Deaths occurred not only in abandoned appliances but also in any area of the home, yard, or vehicle where these containers are normally used.

Parents should be advised to identify containers that may potentially entrap their child. The CPSC recommends that:

- The surest approach to childproof old refrigerators and other appliances is to remove the door completely, which in most cases only requires use of a screwdriver. (It is unlawful in most jurisdictions to discard old refrigerators without first removing the door.) If the door will not come off, remove or disable the latch completely so it cannot lock. A third alternative is to fasten the door shut so it cannot be opened. (A chain and padlock can be used if the chain can be secured through the handles so it will not slide off. Strong filament tape wrapped around the appliance several times may be used temporarily but may deteriorate over time and need replacement.)

- Keep children away from old refrigerators, freezers, dryers, or coolers still in use. Instruct children not to play inside these appliances. Keep the door to the utility room locked.

- If a child is missing, appliances and picnic coolers should be among the first places checked (the swimming pool should always be checked first). A few minutes may save a child's life.

The number of deaths due to entrapment is declining, possibly as a result of the design change in units manufactured since 1958. However, the standard specifies a maximum of 15 lb of internal pressure necessary to open the door, which is often beyond the capabilities of the children who are trapped. In addition, a child who is trapped may become disoriented and not know to push the door. Consequently preventive measures are still required to minimize the risk of injury.[2]

14.2 Button Batteries

Batteries can pose a hazard to children. Button batteries used to power watches, calculators, cameras, hearing aides, and games are swallowed by 500 to 800 children annually. Children also place these batteries in their ears and nose. Injury may be caused by electrolyte leakage from the battery, mercury toxicity, and pressure necrosis. Complications arising from button batteries include malignant otitis externa with tympanic membrane and ossicle necrosis, nasal septum perforation or nasal meatus stenosis, esophageal impaction and tissue necrosis, bowel perforation, and elevation of blood mercury levels. Fortunately, if the battery does not become impacted in the esophagus, the majority pass through the body without difficulty. Preventive strategies include having manufacturers provide more securely fastened, child-resistant battery compartments on devices intended for use by children.[3] In one series of ingestions of button batteries from hearing aids, one third of the batteries were removed by a child from his or her own hearing aid. Button batteries must not be easily retrievable from the trash by children.

14.3 Bunk Beds

Bunk beds have been associated with fatalities when they are stacked and when they are used as single beds. Young children have died when they were trapped between the bed and the wall; when their bunk bed mattress and mattress foundation collapsed while they were playing on or under the beds, and when they were trapped between the guard rail and exposed edge of the mattress or bed frame.[4] Each year more than 34 000 children are treated in emergency departments for injuries related to bunk beds. Most of the injuries resulted from falls, often from the top bunk or ladder. Injuries occurred during sleep and play. Most injuries related to bunk beds involve the head; in one study 9% of all injuries required hospital admission — all as a result of falls from the top bed. Most injuries can be prevented if the following advice is adhered to:

- Never allow children younger than 6 years on the upper bunk.
- Close the space between the lower edge of the guard rail and the upper edge of the bed frame to $3\frac{1}{2}$ in or less.
- For older children, use guardrails on both sides of the bed. Always keep the guardrails in place on the top bunk. Children roll over during sleep and may fall out of bed. For younger children, use guardrails on both sides of the beds for the twin bed configuration (even if the beds are up against the wall).
- If the child has a medical disorder that increases the risk for falling, the top bunk bed should not be used.
- Regularly check the mattress supports to ensure against dislodgement or wear. Do this even if the bunk beds are used as twin beds. Regularly check the ladder to ensure that it is secured to the bed frame and will not slip when used. Replace loose or missing rungs on the ladder.
- Ensure that the area around the bed is free of breakable objects or sharp toys and furniture or other potential hazards. Children have fallen upon glass, furniture, or toys. One child was injured by a ceiling fan blade when climbing into the top bunk.

- Make sure the mattress is the correct length. A regular-sized mattress on a twin extra-long bed creates a gap where a child could become entrapped.
- Children in bunk beds need proper supervision. Bunk beds are not for rough play. Young children are frequently injured when they fall from the top bunk. Advise children to use the ladder and not other furniture to climb in and out of the top bunk.
- A night light in the bedroom lessens the risk of injury should the child need to climb down from the top bunk during the night. Ensure that the night light is not in contact with any flammable fabrics or objects.

Purchasing Points:

- The purchase of second-hand bunk beds is not recommended.
- Parents should look for beds that comply with the ASTM voluntary standard for bunk beds that have two guardrails.
- Parents should consider buying a second set of guardrails from the retailer or manufacturer for the bottom or second twin bed.

14.4 Bean Bag Pillows or Infant Cushions

Infant bean bag cushions have been banned by the federal government. As of January 24, 1992, 35 infant deaths from suffocation were linked to bean bags. During April and July 1990, all manufacturers of these cushions voluntarily agreed to a recall and stopped production. In July 1992, production of bean bag cushions was banned. Bean bag cushions are typically 24 in long and 12 in wide. They have a soft fabric covering and are loosely filled with plastic foam beads or plastic pellets. The cushion can suffocate a baby because it conforms closely to the contour of the baby's face when the baby lies face-down. It has been postulated that suffocation occurs from rebreathing high percentages of expired air from within the cushion.[5] These cushions, which were promoted for use by infants younger than 1 year, were manufactured by at least 12 different companies, and almost 1 million of these cushions have been sold nationwide.

If these cushions cannot be returned to the manufacturer for a refund, they should be destroyed so there is no chance that they may be used by a person who may be unaware of the risk of suffocation.

14.5 The Barbecue Grill

The barbecue grill poses a variety of hazards to children. Younger children may fall onto hot grills left on the ground. Children may also step on hot coals or fall onto hot coals left on the ground or buried in shallow sand pits.[6] The burns may be full thickness (deep second or third degree burns) and require hospitalization. A second hazard is associated with the use of accelerants such as methyl hydrate, lighter fluid, and gasoline to enhance ignition. The first portion of the flammable liquid contacting the heat ignites instantly and the ignition "flashes back" along the remainder of the fluid while it is still in the air. This airborne proportion of the accelerant explodes, and burning droplets can be showered a distance of many feet. Burns can range from partial-thickness "flash" burns to more serious full-thickness burns and may involve ignition of clothing as well. Finally, carbon monoxide poisoning has occurred as a result of grill use. In an effort to complete the cooking despite inclement weather, grills have been brought indoors. Grills have also been used as heaters by people who are unaware of the lethality of the products of combustion generated by a charcoal grill in an enclosed space.

The following measures should lessen the number of injuries associated with barbecue grill use:

- Children near barbecue grills should be closely supervised at all times.
- Accelerants should only be used prior to igniting the coals, never during or after ignition.
- Grills should never be brought indoors or into poorly ventilated spaces.

14.6 Garage Door Openers

According to the CPSC, between 1982 and May 1995, at least 58 children between 2 and 14 years of age were trapped and killed under automatic garage door openers. The CPSC also reports that children have suffered brain damage or other serious injuries, including pelvic fractures, facial lacerations, and proptosis and diplopia secondary to traumatic displacement of orbital fat, when the closing door failed to stop and reverse direction.

A voluntary 1982 ANSI/UL standard (325–192) calls for a variety of safety features not found on earlier model garage door openers. Most openers manufactured since 1982 have a "quick-release" mechanism that permits the opener to be detached from the door. During closing, a properly operating garage door will stop and reverse when it touches an object. This can be checked by placing a 2-in wooden block on the floor of the garage in the door's path. If the door does not properly reverse on striking the block, the unit should be disengaged until repaired or replaced. Some older model openers stop but do not reverse the closing door when it touches an object. As well, some openers have a device intended to reverse the closing door when it strikes an object, but for reasons related to age, incorrect installation, or lack of maintenance, they may not be safe enough to prevent entrapment of a child. These openers cannot be adjusted or repaired to provide the automatic reversing feature found on later devices. Therefore, to add protection against entrapment, the CPSC recommends an optional automatic "electric eye" installed near floor level to reverse a closing door automatically whenever an object crosses the door's path. Companies that install garage door openers can install these safety devices.

Consumers should inspect automatic garage doors every 30 days to verify the system is functioning properly. Hardware and fittings should be checked to keep the door on track at all times. Should a hazard exist, the door opener should be disconnected as specified in the owner's manual, and the door should be opened and closed manually until repaired or replaced. Parents should be informed about the differences between residential and commercial doors such as those found in apartments and commercial buildings. Although the same safety advice applies to both types of doors, many garage doors in current commercial operation do not meet modern safety regulations and are more dangerous than residential garage doors.

Children should not be allowed to play in areas where automatic garage doors are in operation. For residential garage door openers, the wall switch in the garage that controls the door should be positioned as high as practical to restrict its use by children. Remote control door operating devices should be kept locked in the car and away from children. Parents must discuss with their children the dangers associated with garage doors as part of driveway and home safety.[7]

14.7 Hair Dryers

There are tens of millions of hair dryers in the United States. These appliances pose a threat of electrocution when used near water. Since 1977, the CPSC has documented more than 130 deaths in children younger than 10 years. Typically, electrocution occurs when a child turns on a hair dryer in the bathtub or a hair dryer inadvertently falls into the water.

Since October 1987, manufacturers have adopted a voluntary standard that protects against electrocution if the appliance comes into contact with the water when the switch is in the "off" position. However, such protection is not provided if the switch is in the "on" position. Effective January 1991, a new voluntary standard for hand-held hair dryers provides protection against electrocution if the switch is in either position.

Despite this technological innovation, millions of hair dryers currently on the market will cause electrocution if they fall into water. Old hair dryers do not need to be discarded. Rather, a ground-fault circuit interrupter (GFCI) should be installed by a qualified professional in the circuit where the hair dryer is normally plugged in. This device, which is built into the wiring of new shock-resistant hair dryers, protects against electrocution or severe electrical shock injuries. All appliances plugged into the outlet are similarly secure against electrical discharge from water immersion. The GFCI protection can be a receptacle replacement or a portable GFCI that may be used in other circuits in the home. In the event that an appliance falls into water, the GFCI interrupts the flow of electricity.

The GFCI devices described are also strongly recommended for outdoor receptacles, generally for those used for outdoor equipment such as electric lawn mowers, hedge trimmers, and other devices requiring electrical power that could come in contact with water.

When replacing a hand-held hair dryer, parents should select a product that has a built-in miniature shock protector, which should be described on the packaging. The hair dryers can be identified by their rectangular-shaped plugs with a "re-set" button at the end of the cord. Caregivers must check the package for confirmation of safety by an independent testing laboratory.

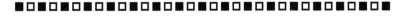
General safety precautions for hair dryers include the following:

- Do not leave a hair dryer plugged in. Disconnect the hair dryer when it is not in use.

- If a hair dryer is used near a sink, make sure the sink is drained of water before plugging in the hair dryer.

- If a hair dryer is dropped into water while the plug is still attached to an outlet, unplug the cord first before touching the dryer or the water.

- Do not use hair dryers that have been submerged in water until they have been inspected by an appliance service center.

- Keep hair dryers out of the reach of young children. Hair dryers have been associated with contact burns. Dryers are capable of delivering air heated to 129°F after 2 minutes of use.

- Do not use hair dryers to dry a child's skin or to treat diaper rash because they can cause serious burns.[8]

- Never poke hair pins or wires through the grillwork protecting the element of the hair dryer.

14.8 Infant Carriers

There are primarily two types of infant carriers designed to be strapped to an adult — one that is soft and forms a pocket for the infant and is carried in the front, and one that resembles a backpack with a frame that is carried on the back. The front carriers are more suited for younger infants and the backpack is preferred for children older than 5 or 6 months, when their neck muscles are sufficiently strong to handle minor jolts and jarring.

Infant carriers should never be used to transport children in an automobile. Even if the adult is using the seat belt, the carrier straps are not sufficient to hold the child in the event of a crash, and the seat belt itself could inflict significant injury.

When a front carrier is being evaluated for purchase, parents are advised to choose a model that easily unlatches. Straps should be wide enough to carry the child's weight comfortably. If more than one parent is going to be using the carrier, the straps should easily adjust. The carrier should be easy to take off and put on without assistance. The carrier should support the child's head and shoulders well. When seated in the carrier, children should have their legs spread apart, with good support under the backs of their legs, and their knees should be lower than their buttocks.

Children who have reached a weight of approximately 15 lb and are 6 months of age can be carried in a backpack-style carrier. In addition to the characteristics identified for a front carrier, the back carrier should be lightweight, have padding over the metal frame, and have smooth edges. Models with a shoulder harness are recommended. The carrier should have a restraining strap so that it can hold a child who tries to climb out or push out. Parents should try out the different models they are considering and purchase a backpack that matches their child's current weight and size. Parents often prefer purchasing a carrier that has a stand. However, if the carrier seat is used as a stand, it must have a wide sturdy base for stability and nonskid feet to prevent slipping. Stand-supporting devices should lock securely. Caregivers should never a leave a child in a carrier on a table, couch, chair, or elevated surface. The floor is the safest place for a carrier with a stand.

14.9 Jewelry

Jewelry often poses an aspiration hazard to young children.[9] Necklaces caught on parts of cribs or playpens have strangled infants. Toy jewelry that fails the small parts test (see section 15.4.1) for toys should not be given to children younger than 3 years. (Concern about the risk of aspiration of small plastic beads prompted the elimination of the beaded name bracelet identification used years ago by many hospitals.) Children who have their ears pierced as early as the neonatal period possibly as part of a cultural or family tradition, are at risk of both aspiration and ingestion of the earrings. If the infant or child has pierced ears, the earrings should have a locking back or a screw back to reduce the possibility of aspiration. The wearing of finger rings, which poses a similar risk of aspiration, should be discouraged.

Among some adolescents, nose piercing has become popular. At least one case of aspiration of the back of the nose ring has been documented. Any jewelry that involves body piercing can be associated with infection or scarring. Adolescents and their parents are often unaware of these risks.

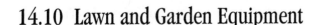
14.10 Lawn and Garden Equipment

Ride-on lawn mowers and garden tractors are associated with significant numbers of childhood injuries. The frequency and seriousness of ride-on mower injuries were not widely appreciated before a hazard analysis was published by the CPSC in 1988.[10] The CPSC estimates that there are about 7 million such vehicles in use. Recent (1994) data from the CPSC's NEISS suggest that about 5000 pediatric injuries are treated annually in US emergency departments. Common mechanisms of injury to children include falling or darting into the path of the mower, falling off of a riding mower and being run over, or being hit by flying objects propelled by the mower's blades.

Injuries tend to be serious, resulting in hospitalization twice as frequently as with consumer products in general. Limb amputations are frequently reported.[11] About 15 children are killed each year by ride-on lawn mowers and garden tractors.

Prevention strategies with regard to ride-on mowers have been outlined by the American Academy of Pediatrics.[12] Parents should be educated about the frequency and seriousness of ride-on mower injuries. An important message is to suggest that young children be kept indoors when the lawn is being mowed, and that children should never be permitted to ride as passengers on lawn mowers. It is unsafe and inappropriate to allow children and young adolescents (up to age 14 years) to operate ride-on mowers. In light of the complexity of these machines and their ability to cause injury, all novice operators would benefit from a period of safety training and supervised instruction prior to their use. Various aspects of product design also need improvement, which may have an impact on injury rates.

Injury can occur frequently from nonriding lawn mowers as well. In addition to the injuries caused by turning blades and projectiles, including broken blades, kicked up by the lawn mower, burns have been recorded as a result of a gas tank explosion during refilling and contact with hot lawn mower mufflers. Children have been hurt at distances of many yards from material thrown by the lawn mower. The blade spins at up to 3000 revolutions per minute.

Nylon line lawn trimmers and motorized lawn edgers have also caused significant injury. Children have been hurt as far as 30 ft away from the lawn trimmers. Eyes have been perforated by pieces of nylon line as well as projectiles kicked up by the trimmers. The CPSC noted a significant increase in these injuries as the numbers of trimmers in use increased. As with lawn mowers, lawn edgers can propel objects at speeds that can equal or exceed those of a bullet. A variety of projectile injuries have been reported with these power tools.

Children should be kept indoors and supervised when outdoor power equipment is being used. Individuals must be alert and turn mowers off if children are in the mowing area. Extra care must be practiced when backing up or approaching corners, shrubs, and trees. Children should never be allowed to operate a ride-on mower or garden tractor, even if supervised. As a general precaution, adults should clear the mowing area of objects that can be picked up and thrown by blades such as toys, wires, and other debris.

Generally, children assisting in gardening should dress appropriately for the task. Long pants and long-sleeved shirts provide protection from thrown objects. Close-fitting clothes should be worn to prevent them from getting caught in a motorized part. Sturdy shoes with a slip-resistant rubber soles should be worn. Eye protection should be worn at all times, and heavy gloves should be used when changing, sharpening, or cleaning blades. Hearing protection may be considered when using noisy motor-driven equipment. Power tools need to be turned off and made inoperable if they must be left unattended, which reduces their chance of use by children. Electrical power tools should not be used in wet or damp conditions. The likelihood of an electrical shock is reduced by the use of a ground fault circuit interrupter.

14.11 Lawn Darts

According to the CPSC, lawn darts were responsible for approximately 6700 injuries between January 1978 and December 1987. Three quarters of the persons injured were children younger than 15 years, and at least three children have been killed by lawn darts. In December 1988, the sale of lawn darts was banned by the CPSC. Families who own these darts should discard them or, preferably, destroy them. The darts are typically 12 in long with a heavy metal or weighted plastic point at one end and three plastic fins on a rod at the other end. While the tip may not be sharp enough to be obviously dangerous, the darts, when grasped by the rod and thrown underhand toward a target, can easily fracture bones and cause serious injuries, including eye loss. It is estimated that many sets of these dangerous darts still exist in American garages and basements. Pediatricians should ask parents whether they own these darts because they are in an ideal position to counsel parents about a completely preventable injury.[13]

14.12 Pacifiers

Pacifiers have been regulated by the CPSC since 1977. The legislation stipulates that pacifiers must be strong enough not to separate into small pieces, to prevent the infant from choking or suffocating. Pacifier guards or shields also must be large enough and firm enough to prevent the pacifier from being drawn entirely into an infant's mouth. They must have ventilation holes to make it possible for the infant to breathe if the pacifier shield enters the mouth. Merchants cannot sell pacifiers with a ribbon, string, cord, or yarn attached, and the pacifier must be labeled with the following statement:

> **WARNING — DO NOT TIE PACIFIER AROUND CHILD'S NECK AS IT PRESENTS A STRANGULATION DANGER.**

Despite these standards, the CPSC receives reports of infants who have strangled on pacifier cords or ribbons tied around their necks. Pacifier cords also have caught on crib corner posts, crib toys and gyms, pieces of furniture, and even doorknobs. If parents keep the pacifier on a cord, the cord should attach to the infant's clothing rather than hang around the infant's neck and should be no more than 7 in long to reduce the possibility of strangulation.

Pacifier nipples are constructed of three different substances: vinyl, silicone, or latex rubber. The CPSC reports that, while some pacifiers still contain a chemical that causes cancer in animals (di [2-ethylhexyl] phthalate), the levels are so low as not to pose a risk to children. Rubber pacifiers contain minute amounts of nitrosamines, which have caused cancer in animals and are suspected in some human cancers.

The CPSC recommends that pacifier nipples, as well as bottle nipples, be regularly inspected and discarded if there is any change in the texture, tears appear, or there are holes or evidence of weakening. Pacifiers deteriorate with age and exposure to food and sunlight.

Despite the attention to detail in the construction of pacifiers, their use should be supervised. Children may lodge the pacifier shield in their mouths when they turn the pacifier sideways.

A pacifier should never be fastened around an infant's neck; nor should any other object such as a medallion be tied by a cord, ribbon, or yarn around an infant's neck.

Deaths have been reported when makeshift pacifiers have been improvised by parents and hospital staff for newborns.[14] This practice is to be avoided. Smaller pacifiers are available for this age group. Finally, candy pacifiers, which resemble a soother, do not have the same resistance to separation as noncandy pacifiers and can separate and pose a potential aspiration hazard to younger children.

14.13 Shopping Cart Injuries

Each year in the United States, an estimated 25 000 children younger than 15 years are treated in an emergency department for shopping cart injuries.[15] The vast majority (84%) involve children younger than 5 years. More than 600 of these injuries resulted in hospitalization. The majority of injuries treated in the emergency department are to the head and neck, most commonly from children falling out of the cart and the cart tipping over.[16] Children often fall out of the cart when they are standing in the basket. Tip-overs more frequently occur with younger children.

Risk of injury appears to be related to riding in the basket (particularly the older child) or riding in the seat without a seat restraint. Many shopping carts are not equipped with seat restraints, and those that are equipped with restraints are often not used. Lack of supervision is a contributing factor because it may be difficult for parents who are preoccupied with shopping to supervise several children.

Several preventive strategies have been suggested. Parents should not place children in the baskets of carts, where they can stand and fall out. Placing young children in the seats of shopping carts is a good option if a seat belt is available. This, however, does not prevent injury if the cart tips over. The shopping carts themselves should be redesigned to widen their wheelbase and lower the center of gravity to afford greater stability.

Parents should avoid long shopping trips with young children and shopping when their children are tired or hungry. Grocery stores may be encouraged to provide child care for parents during shopping. Parents may also find other child care arrangements if shopping trips prove to be "behaviorally difficult" times. Shopping trips with two parents may improve levels of child supervision.

14.14 Waterbeds

From 1988 through 1994, the CPSC received reports of 115 deaths of infants younger than 1 year that involved waterbeds. The mechanism usually responsible for death is suffocation, when an infant either rolls or moves to the edge of the mattress and becomes wedged between the mattress and bed frame or bed frame and wall and cannot breathe. In other situations, infants or children, asleep in the face-down position, suffocate when their nose and mouth become trapped in the depression caused by the weight of their head and body. The obvious preventive strategy is to ensure that parents and caregivers never leave infants on adult or youth beds with water mattresses. As well, waterbed mattresses should have warning labels about the dangers of leaving infants asleep or unattended on water mattresses and the associated risk of suffocation. Children with special health care needs who have difficulty in moving from the face-down prone position should not be left unattended or put to bed on a waterbed mattress.

14.15 Workshop Tools

Children are often drawn to people working with electrical tools in a home workshop. To avoid having children imitate what they see in the workshop, which could result in tragedy, small tools should be locked in cupboards and the work room itself should be locked and inaccessible to young children.

Children should not be in the area where power tools are being used. Risks include contact from cutting or drilling edges, debris that can cause eye injury, and loud noise that can damage hearing.

Around the age of 11 or 12 years, it is appropriate to gradually intro-duce children to the workshop and its tools. Power tools should be only introduced after the mastery of less dangerous nonpower tools. Children should be taught about the applications and limitations of tools as well specific hazards associated with their use. Parents should demon-strate how to avoid electrical shock by preventing body contact with grounded surfaces. Tool guards must be kept in place during operation. The work area should be kept clean; cluttered floors and benches invite mishaps. Power tools should never be used in wet or damp locations or exposed to rain. Good illumination of the work area is crucial to avoid injury. Older children should eventually learn to use the right tool for the right task. They need to appreciate that tools should not be forced during use, which increases the risk of injury. Loose clothing and jewelry should not be worn, to prevent them from getting caught in moving parts. Long hair should be tied back with a protective hair covering. Safety glasses or goggles must be used with all tools. Children should be taught to use an ergonomically correct approach and to keep proper footing and balance at all times while operating power tools. Parents should demonstrate that tools must be disconnected before bits, blades, and cutters are changed. Safety devices on saws or other power tools should not be disabled. Finally, fatigue and use of medications and alcohol or other drugs can adversely influence the operation of workshop tools.

14.16 Resources

1. Consumer Product Safety Commission
   Division of Hazard and Injury Data Systems/EHDS
   Washington, DC 20207
   800-638-8095
   800-909-0924 (fax)
   amcdonal@cpsc.gov (e-mail)

   Health care providers can file product-related injuries or unsafe products on these toll-free lines.

2. Consumer Product Safety Commission Hotline
   800-638-2772
   800-638-8270 (TTY number for speech- or hearing-impaired)
   info@cpsc.gov (e-mail)

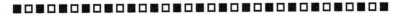
Health care providers can encourage patients and their parents to report product-related injuries or unsafe products on this hotline. The hotline is also an invaluable resource for obtaining information about product recalls or consumer alerts and CPSC safety publications.

3. CPSC
Publications List
Washington, DC 20207

Send a postcard to this address to get a list of the CPSC publications available.

CPSC web site and gopher site
http://www.cpsc.gov
cpsc.gov

Use this Internet and gopher site to obtain product recall information through the Internet.

CPSC
Fax-On-Demand Service (FODS)
301-504-0051 (fax)

Catalogs of available documents can be ordered by using the handset of a fax machine to dial this number and following instructions for using this service.

References

1. Gillis J, Fise MER. *The Childwise Catalog: A Consumer Guide to Buying the Safest and Best Products for Your Child. Newborn Through Age 5*, 3rd ed. New York, NY: HarperCollins; 1993

2. Kraus JF. Effectiveness of measures to prevent unintentional deaths of infants and children from suffocation and strangulation. *Public Health Rep.* 1985;100:231–240

3. Litovitz T, Schmitz BF. Ingestion of cylindrical and button batteries: an analysis of 2382 cases. *Pediatrics.* 1992;89:747–757

4. Selbst SM, Baker MD, Shames M. Bunk bed injuries. *Am J Dis Child.* 1990;144: 721–723

5. Kemp JS, Thach BT. Sudden death in infants sleeping on polystyrene-filled cushions. *N Engl J Med.* 1991;324:1858–1864

6. Wiebe RA, Yamamoto LG. Charcoal burns. *Pediatrics.* 1986;77:773–774

7. Blair GK, MacNab AJ, Smith D. Garage door injuries in children. *Can Med Assoc J.* 1992;147:1187–1189

8. Deans L, Slater H, Goldfarb IW. Bad advice; bad burn: a new problem in burn prevention. *J Burn Care Rehabil.* 1990;11:563–564

9. Becker PG, Turow J. Earring aspiration and other jewelry hazards. *Pediatrics.* 1986; 78:494–496

10. Smith EVT. *Hazard Analysis: Ride-on Mowers.* Washington, DC: US Consumer Product Safety Commission; May 1988

11. Alonso JE, Sanchez FL. Lawn mower injuries in children: a preventable impairment. *J Pediatr Orthop.* 1995;15:83–89

12. American Academy of Pediatrics, Committee on Accident and Poison Prevention. Ride-on mower injuries in children. *Pediatrics.* 1990;86:141–143

13. Sotiropoulos SV, Jackson MA, Tremblay GF, Burry VF, Olson LC. Childhood lawn dart injuries: summary of 75 patients and patient report. *Am J Dis Child.* 1990; 144:980–982

14. Millunchick EW, McArtor RD. Fatal aspiration of a makeshift pacifier. *Pediatrics.* 1986;77:369–370

15. Smith GA, Dietrich AM, Garcia T, Shields BJ. Epidemiology of shopping cart–related injuries to children: an analysis of national data for 1990 to 1992. *Arch Pediatr Adolesc Med.* 1995;149:1207–1210

16. Smith GA, Dietrich AM, Garcia CT, Shields BJ. Injuries to children related to shopping carts. *Pediatrics.* 1996;97:161–165

CHAPTER 15

Toy Safety

Toys and playing are important in growing up. They spark creativity and give children an opportunity to experiment, develop new skills, and experience a sense of accomplishment, and they offer an outlet for energy.

Nothing makes a child happier than receiving a toy or a game, and, ideally, parents, relatives, and friends will guide their selection and use. Unfortunately, toys that should enable harmless fun for children can pose hidden dangers that result in serious injury or even death.[1]

15.1 Deaths

Data from the Consumer Product Safety Commission (CPSC) show that between January 1, 1993, and September 30, 1994, 36 toy-related deaths were reported.[2] Table 15.1, p 304, shows the types of toys and hazards reported. The numbers represent a minimal estimate because reporting was still in progress for some data sources.

Choking continues to be associated with the largest number of toy-related fatalities and was reported to be involved in 22 of the previously mentioned 36 deaths. Nine children 7 months to 9 years of age choked on balloons and eight choked on various types of small balls; the ages for seven of these children ranged from 9 months to 4 years.

Ten deaths occurred in children riding on toys. Four children 3 and 4 years of age rode a toy vehicle into a swimming pool and drowned. The three victims between 4 and 6 years were struck by motor vehicles.

15.2 Injuries

Data from the National Electronic Injury Surveillance System showed that an estimated 165 400 persons were treated in US hospital emergency departments for toy-related injuries in 1993[2] (Table 15.2, p 305). Almost half of the injuries (80 300) were to children younger than

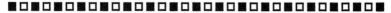
TABLE 15.1.
**Reported Toy-Related Deaths by Type of Toy and Date of Death,
January 1993 — September 1994***

Type of Toy	Total	1993	January-September 1994
Total	36	25	11
Tricycles, riding toys	10	5	5
Hit by motor vehicle	6	3	3
Rode into swimming pool	4	2	2
Balloons	11	8	3
Choked on balloon	9	6	3
Strangled on string of balloon	1	1	...
Suffocated by mylar balloon	1	1	...
Balls	8	6	2
Choked on ball	8	6	2
Toy Storage†	1	1	...
Suffocated in cedar chest	1	1	...
Other	6	5	1
Choked on toy dart	1	1	...
Choked on toy figure	1	1	...
Choked on piece from game	1	1	...
Choked on cap of water toy	1	...	1
Choked on detachable toy part	1	1	...
Strangled in small hammock	1	1	...

*Age range of victims is 6 months to 12 years. Source: Death Certificate, In-Depth Investigation, and Injury or Potential Injury Incident Files, 1993–1994, US Consumer Product Safety Commission.

†Although used to store toys, item was not manufactured for toy storage.

5 years, and almost 80% (130 300) were to children younger than 15 years. Most injuries were minor; an estimated 62% of the patients were treated for lacerations, contusions, and abrasions. Hospitalized victims accounted for 1.3% compared with a 4% overall hospitalization rate for all victims of product-related injuries. Almost two thirds of the victims were boys; there was little change in the data from previous years. Most of the injuries continued to be incidental to the toy (eg, tripping over a toy, bumping into a toy, or being hit by a thrown toy), rather than directly related to design of the toy.

Riding toys were associated with the largest group of injuries (38 500 or almost 25%), with most victims injured when they fell from the toy. Tricycles accounted for 9000 falls and children's wagons for 7300 of the falls from riding toys.

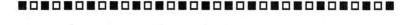
15.3 Toy-Related Safety Legislation

The federal government began regulating potentially hazardous products – including toys – to which children may be exposed under the Federal Hazardous Substances Labeling Act passed by Congress in 1960. The Child Protection Act of 1966, subsequently changed to The Federal Hazardous Substances Act (FHSA), added provisions banning toys consisting of or containing any of the hazardous substances defined. The Toy Protection and Toy Safety Act of 1969 authorized the issuance of rules banning toys or children's articles presenting an electrical, mechanical, or thermal hazard.

In 1972, The Consumer Product Safety Act established the CPSC, which was given authority to administer and enforce the FHSA. This legislation authorized the agency to issue safety standards for consumer products sold to or used in or around a household, a school, in recreation, or in similar places and activities; toys fell within this definition. The Toy Safety Act of 1984 improved the process by which the CPSC can ban and recall hazardous toys and products, allowing for greater expediency.

In 1994, The Child Safety Protection Act added provisions to the FHSA requiring labeling of balls, latex balloons, marbles, and certain toys and games (which include these small parts) that are intended for use by children 3 years of age and older. Certain balls intended for use by children 3 years of age and younger were banned. Manufacturers are also required to report to the CPSC information about choking incidents.

TABLE 15.2.
Toy-Related Injuries by Age of Victim, Calendar Year 1993

Age of Victim, y	No. of Estimated Injuries	Percentage
Total	165 400*	100
<5	80 300	49
5–14	50 000	30
15–24	12 000	7
25+	23 200	14

*Column detail does not add to total due to rounding. Source: National Electronic Injury Surveillance System, 1993, US Consumer Product Safety Commission.

While the CPSC has no authority to approve or endorse toys for safety under the FHSA, it has promulgated safety regulations for certain toys. Manufacturers must design and manufacture their products to meet these regulations so hazardous products are not sold. The effectiveness of CPSC regulations depends, in part, on resources made available to the agency for enforcement. At least 2.5 billion toys and games were sold in the United States in 1993. The CPSC recalled 108 hazardous toys and other children's products representing over 3.3 million units. Half a million units of hazardous toys were seized by US Customs. (For background on the CPSC, see Appendix G.)

Toy Manufacturers of America has developed a voluntary product standard (PS 72–76) that establishes safety requirements and tests. However, many manufacturers do not belong to the association, and more than 80 000 different toys are imported into the United States each year.

15.4 Hazards of Toys

15.4.1 Choking Dangers
(See also chapter 13.)

Toys and toy parts should be large enough that they cannot be swallowed. Toys intended for use by children younger than 3 years should not have accessible small parts that fit into a standard truncated cylinder with an inside diameter of $1\frac{1}{4}$ in and depth varying from 1 to $2\frac{1}{4}$ in. This standard cylinder (available at some juvenile products stores and through catalogs) can be used to test toy parts (Fig 13.1). Parents can also test toys using a toilet paper role, which has a diameter of approximately $1\frac{3}{4}$ in. If the widest part of any toy piece fits within the toilet paper role, the toy is too small for a child younger than 3 years because it represents a potential choking hazard.

Federal regulations require rattles to be large enough so they cannot become lodged in an infant's throat or be separated into small parts. A rattle test fixture with particular dimensions is specified. The device has an oval opening measuring approximately $1\frac{3}{8}$ by 2 in and is $1\frac{3}{16}$ in deep. Rattles should be larger than these dimensions because any part, such as the handle, that passes through this opening could enter a child's throat and become lodged in the back. Voluntary safety standards for teethers and squeeze toys require that they are large enough so they cannot enter an infant's throat and become lodged.

Previous toy labeling requirements have been believed to be inadequate.[3] To comply with labeling requirements of The Child Safety Protection Act of 1994, toys and games that contain small parts and are intended for use by children to 6 years of age must include the following cautionary statement:

> **! WARNING: Choking Hazards**
> **Small Parts. Not for children under 3 years.**

During childhood, latex balloons are a major cause of deaths from choking.[4] Young children also frequently choke on small rubber balls. Packaging, descriptive materials, bins, containers for retail display, and vending machines for balloons, small balls, and marbles intended for use by children 3 years of age or older must include specific cautionary statements. According to CPSC data, at least 121 children died by choking on balloons between 1973 and 1988.[5] The highest mortality occurred in infants; 30 (25%) of the deaths involved children aged 6 years or older. The following cautionary statements are required:

For latex balloons:

> **! WARNING: Choking Hazard**
> **Children under 8 years can choke or suffocate**
> **on uninflated or broken balloons. Adult supervision**
> **required. Keep uninflated balloons from children.**
> **Discard broken balloons at once.**

For balls:

> **! WARNING: Choking Hazard**
> **This toy is a small ball. Not for children under 3 years.**

For marbles:

> **! WARNING: Choking Hazard**
> **This toy is a marble. Not for children under 3 years.**

For toys and games containing small balls and marbles:

> ! WARNING: Choking Hazard – toy contains a marble
> or a small ball. Not for children under 3 years.

15.4.2 Electric Toys

Battery-operated toys are preferred over electric toys. Electric toys that are improperly constructed, wired, or used can shock or burn. These toys must meet requirements for maximum surface temperatures and electrical construction and must have prominent warning labels. Toys with heating elements are recommended only for children older than 8 years, and hobby items such as wood-burning kits are not recommended for children younger than 12 years. Adult supervision and instruction should be exercised. Despite a manufacturer's compliance with labeling requirements, burns and shocks may result from frayed cords or misuse.

15.4.3 Sharp Edges and Sharp Points

Exposed sharp edges, glass, or rigid plastic parts have caused a variety of injuries. New toys intended for use by children younger than 8 years must, by regulation, be free of sharp edges and dangerous points. With use, toys may break, exposing edges that may cause lacerations. Regulations established as technical guidelines provide manufacturers with test methods to ensure compliance.

15.4.4 Loud Noise

Noise above 100 dB can damage hearing. Toy caps and some noise-making guns and other toys can produce noise above this level. The law requires the following label on loud caps (138 to 158 dB):

> ! WARNING — Do not fire closer than one foot
> to the ear. Do not use indoors.

Caps producing noise likely to injure a child's hearing (above 158 dB) are banned.

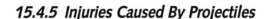
15.4.5 Injuries Caused By Projectiles

The most serious injuries by projectiles affect the eye. Children should never be permitted to play with lawn darts or other hobby or sporting equipment with sharp points. Lawn darts were banned from sale in the United States on December 19, 1988, because they were responsible for serious and fatal injuries to children. Adult supervision during use of projectile-type toys is essential. Arrows or darts used by children should have soft cork tips, rubber suction cups, or other protective tips. Dart guns or other toys capable of firing objects not intended for use in the toy, such as pencils or nails, should be avoided. Industry-promulgated voluntary safety standards require that projectiles fired from toys must not be "small parts" and those exceeding a specified energy level must have a resilient tip that is not detachable. The discharge mechanism of these toys must be designed to prevent discharge of improvised projectiles such as pencils or pebbles. The standards for projectile-type toy guns do not include specifications for projectile tip geometry, maximum velocity, impact force, or protective devices.[6] Currently, no federal, state, or local regulations exist for these devices.

15.4.6 Strangulation

Ropes or loops can strangle young children. Strings on pull toys should be less than 12-in long. Toys with long strings, cords, loops, or ribbons should never be hung in a crib or playpen. Crib gyms should be labeled to be removed from the crib when children can pull up on their hands and knees (at 4 to 5 months of age).

15.4.7 Art and Craft Materials

Art and craft materials, including large crayons used by toddlers and paints, clay, markers, chalk, and the many other materials used for creative play by older toddlers, preschoolers, and older school-age children, can present substantial hazards.

The Labeling of Hazardous Art Materials Act (PL 100-695), signed into law November 18, 1988, requires that art materials be reviewed to determine their potential for causing chronic hazards and that appropriate warning labels be put on hazardous materials. The law applies to many children's art and craft products such as crayons, chalk, paint sets, modeling clay, coloring books, pencils, and any other product used by children to produce a work of visual or graphic art.

Products that are hazardous are banned for distribution to young children, whether the hazard is based on chronic toxic effects, acute toxic effects, flammability, or other hazards identified by the FHSA.

Materials labeled as hazards should not be used by children. Other materials can be substituted for most hazardous materials, eg, water-based adhesives, nonleaded or nontoxic ceramic glazes. Safe art materials indicate on the label that they conform to "ASTM D-4236." No art material should be transferred from its original container to an unmarked container.

15.5 Choosing Safe Toys

Although the federal government has given the CPSC increasing authority to develop mandatory safety standards and ban toys if they present unreasonable risk of personal injury during normal use or when subjected to foreseeable damage or abuse, data about injuries show that continued efforts are necessary to keep potentially harmful products out of children's hands. This is particularly true in a political climate that favors reducing regulations and product liability of manufacturers. Choosing safe toys and supervising children at play continues to be the responsibility of parents, family, and other caregivers. Educating consumers to think of safety when purchasing toys is the pediatrician's challenge. Through an understanding of the threats and dangers that certain toys can pose and an appreciation of the developmental capabilities of young children, anticipatory guidance can be used to minimize injury.

Great strides have been made to impress on parents the need to consider maturity as well as chronological age when determining a child's ability to handle toys safely. The new toy labeling statements addressing the hazards of small parts contained in toys and games intended for older children address a gap that previously caused great concern.[3]

The American Academy of Pediatrics pamphlet, "Toy Safety Guidelines for Parents," describes how children are injured, how to prevent injuries from toys, tips for purchasing toys, and age-appropriate toys.[7] Table 15.3, pp 325–326, includes some of this information.

TABLE 15.3.
Age-Appropriate Toys*

Age Group and Developmental Considerations	Suggested Toys
Newborn to 1-year-old Choose eye-catching toys that appeal to your baby's sight, hearing, and touch.	• Large blocks of wood or plastic • Pots and pans • Rattles • Soft, washable animals, dolls, or balls • Bright, movable objects that are out of baby's reach • Busy boards • Floating bath toys • Squeeze toys
1- to 2-year-old toddler Toys for this age group should be safe and able to withstand a toddler's curious nature.	• Cloth or plastic books with large pictures • Sturdy dolls • Kiddy cars • Musical tops • Nesting blocks • Push or pull toys, but without long strings • Stacking toys • Toy telephone, but without long cords
2- to 5-year-old preschooler Toys for this age group are usually experimental and should imitate the activities of parents and older children.	• Books (short stories or action stories) • Chalkboard and chalk • Building blocks • Crayons, nontoxic finger paints, clay • Hammer and bench • Housekeeping toys • Outdoor toys (eg, sandbox with lid, slide, swing, playhouse) • Transportation toys (eg, tricycles, cars, or wagons) • Tape or record player • Simple puzzles with large pieces • Dress-up clothes • Tea party utensils
5- to 9-year-old child Toys for this age group should help a child promote skill development and creativity.	• Blunt scissors or sewing sets • Card games • Doctor and nurse kits • Hand puppets • Balls • Bicycles • Crafts • Electric trains • Paper dolls • Jump ropes • Roller skates • Sports equipment • Table games

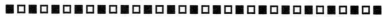
TABLE 15.3. Age-Appropriate Toys, continued	
Age Group and Developmental Considerations	**Suggested Toys**
10- to 14-year-old child Hobbies and scientific activities are ideal for this age group.	• Computer games • Sewing, knitting, or needlework • Microscopes or telescopes • Table and board games • Sports equipment • Hobby collections

*This list of age-appropriate toys is provided for consideration for specific age groups.[7] These suggestions may be useful when shopping for toys. Parents should watch for and avoid mislabeled toys and always provide proper supervision for younger children playing with toys.

The CPSC issued a consumer's guide for selecting suitable toys titled "Which Toy for Which Child — Ages Birth Through Five" and another guide for "Ages Six Through Twelve." These booklets are organized by abilities and interests of children and by categories of appropriate toy lists. In addition, a pamphlet titled "For Kid's Sake Think Toy Safety — by Knowing the Nine Toy Dangers" is also available. See the Resources section for contact information for the CPSC.

A CPSC toll-free hotline number, 800-638-CPSC, can be used to report unsafe products including toys. The hotline also offers recorded recall and safety information 24 hours a day, 7 days a week.

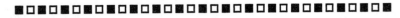

15.6 Resources

Consumer Product Safety Commission
Office of Information and Public Affairs
Washington, DC 20207
301-504-0580
800-638-CPSC (toll-free hotline)

Toy Safety Guidelines for Parents
American Academy of Pediatrics
Division of Publications
141 Northwest Point Blvd
PO Box 927
Elk Grove Village, IL 60009-0927

References

1. Baker MD. Toy safety. *Contemp Pediatr.* 1985;2:42–48

2. Cassidy S. Toy Related Deaths and Injuries, January 1, 1993–September 30, 1994. (Memorandum). Washington, DC: Consumer Product Safety Commission; 1994

3. Langlois JA, Wallen BA, Teret SP, Bailey LA, Hershey JH, Peeler MO. The impact of specific toy warning labels. *JAMA.* 1991;265:2848–2850

4. Ryan CA, Yacoub W, Paton T, Avard D. Childhood deaths from toy balloons. *Am J Dis Child.* 1990;144:1221–1224

5. Tinsworth DK. *Analysis of Choking-related Hazards Associated With Children's Products.* Washington, DC: Consumer Product Safety Commission, Directorate for Epidemiology Division of Hazard Analysis; 1989

6. American Academy of Pediatrics, Committee on Accident and Poison Prevention. Injuries related to "toy" firearms. *Pediatrics.* 1987;79:473–474

7. *Toy Safety Guidelines for Parents* (pamphlet). Elk Grove Village, IL: American Academy of Pediatrics; 1994

CHAPTER 16

Sports Safety

16.1 Introduction

Injuries that occur while playing sports are not only a cause of significant morbidity and occasional mortality, they are also expensive. In one study in Massachusetts, sports-related injuries ranked second to falls in per capita expenditures for treating injuries to children.[1] Compared with other areas of injury control, sports-related injuries present unique challenges for accuracy of reporting. Passive means of reporting such as reports developed from record reviews and emergency department logs do not accurately reflect injury rates associated with specific activities. The best epidemiologic studies of sports-related injuries use data collected by athletic trainers, school nurses, and team physicians covering practices and competitions. The severity of the injury is usually expressed in terms of time lost from participation in a sport. Most studies define an injury as a loss of at least one practice session or one competition. Injury rates are often expressed as number of injuries per 100 athletes per season, but are more meaningfully expressed as injuries per athlete per unit of exposure (eg, per hour of play, per game).

Sports injuries can be classified as *acute*, if caused by a one-time transfer of energy to vulnerable tissues, or as *chronic* (or *overuse*) if caused by repetitive microtrauma. Acute injuries are not necessarily related to the behavior of the injured athlete, whereas chronic injuries are usually directly related to the behavior of the host. Chronic injuries are often due to training errors such as a rapid increase in training duration or intensity, or a combination of both.

Some children become injured because they participate in too many activities during one season. During the child's health supervision visit before participation in sports, guidance about the level of participation and preparation required for the planned activity can help prevent chronic injuries. For example, participation in summer sports camps may result in chronic injury if the athlete does not undertake some sports-specific training for several weeks prior to attending camp.

Parents often ask pediatricians about their child's risk of injury in a particular sport, such as football. In general, the injury rates are low for all sports at the youth level. Prepubertal athletes do not generate enough force to cause a substantial number of injuries even in collision sports such as football and ice hockey. Injury rates climb considerably when participants reach puberty and are substantial in youth of high school age or older. Despite parents' best efforts, children choose their sports activities based on choices of their peers, their own talents, and their past success in a particular sport. Pediatricians should not impose their own values about sports on families, but they should inform parents of risks and benefits so children and parents can make more informed choices about sporting activities.

Parents often forget that all activities carry risk. Absence of activity also poses health risks. And some children are more likely to take additional risks no matter what activity they choose. Injury-prone athletes appear to have some of the same characteristics as their counterparts who are prone to injury outside the athletic setting.

Data are lacking about the relative risks of participation in recreational sports. For organized sports, comparison of injuries during various high school sports revealed a consistent pattern. Although data are limited, two studies performed 12 years apart in different areas of the United States obtained similar results[2,3] (Table 16.1, p 331). The sports with the highest number of injuries are football, gymnastics, wrestling, and ice hockey. Soccer and track and field produce significant injury rates with a greater proportion of chronic injuries.

Pediatricians and parents may be most concerned about severe neurologic injuries, and particularly the so-called catastrophic events. (A *catastrophic injury* results in permanent, severe neurologic disability. Serious injuries resulting in *transient* functional neurologic disability are noncatastrophic.) No accurate method exists to account for all of these relatively rare events. On the basis of data from the National Center for Catastrophic Sports Injury Research, Mueller and Cantu[4] reported the incidence of such injuries from 1982 to 1988 at the high school and collegiate levels. There is no reporting system for participants in grades below the high school level. The college and high school data showed that gymnastics, ice hockey, and football were the sports most closely

■□■□■□■□■□■□■□■□■□■□■□■□■□■□■□■□■□■

TABLE 16.1. Injury Rates for High School Sports*		
Sport	Garrick and Requa[2]	McLain and Reynolds[3]
Football	81	61
Gymnastics		
Boys	28	40
Girls	40	46
Wrestling	75	40
Basketball		
Boys	31	37
Girls	25	31
Volleyball	10	17
Baseball	18	15
Cross-country		
Boys	29	13
Girls	35	7
Soccer		
Boys	30	13
Girls	...	17
Softball	44	13
Track		
Boys	33	10
Girls	35	18
Badminton	6	7
Field Hockey		6
Tennis		
Boys	3	0
Girls	7	3
Swimming		
Boys	1	0
Girls	9	0

*Injuries are reported per 100 participants per year.

associated with risk of catastrophic injury per participant, with rates of 3.3, 3.7, and 4.5 catastrophic injuries per 100 000 participants per year, respectively. However, this system depends on voluntary reporting, and underreporting is likely, especially at the high school level.

Injury control measures should target these most severe injuries as well as the less serious injuries. Improvements in equipment have reduced injuries in many sports, but some of the most effective injury prevention measures have involved changing the rules of the games. For example, in football, severe cervical spine injuries were found to be associated with the practice of "spearing" — driving one's helmet into the body of another player at the initial contact. When a change was instituted and enforced to make this practice against the rules, a dramatic reduction of cervical spine injuries resulted.

A discussion of all sports activities is beyond the scope of this manual. The sports with the highest levels of youth participation are reviewed with a focus on the high-injury sports. The most important issues to be discussed in the pediatrician's office are emphasized. Additional information is available in the *Sports Medicine: Health Care for Young Athletes* manual published by the American Academy of Pediatrics (AAP).[5]

16.2 Football

In football, the most important reductions in injury have occurred in the area of the head and neck. Improvements in helmets have reduced the frequency and severity of head injuries. Face masks and mouth guards greatly reduce dental injuries. Mouth guards are mandatory in most football leagues.

Lawsuits have reduced the number of football helmet manufacturers to two. Helmets are produced under strict guidelines written by the National Operating Committee on Standards for Athletic Equipment. Football helmets often do not fit well, especially on the youngest and most inexperienced players. No studies have been conducted of the role of helmet fit in the pathogenesis of brain or cervical injury. Theoretically, a loose helmet is less protective than a snug helmet. A properly fitting helmet does not move about the head when it is rotated or rocked back and forth.

The popularity of prophylactic knee bracing at the professional and collegiate levels prompted families to ask physicians about its efficacy in high school sports. The best studies of knee braces found no evidence that they effectively prevented knee injuries. The AAP has issued a statement recommending that they "*not* be considered standard equipment" for football players.[6]

Lace-up ankle braces are receiving increasing attention and seem to be used more often in football and other sports. Unlike knee braces, however, evidence exists that they are effective at preventing ankle sprains and may be more effective than the traditional taping of ankles.[7] Although it is premature to recommend ankle braces as standard equipment, many teams that used protective taping of ankles in the past now use lace-up ankle braces because of reduced cost and equal or improved efficacy.

Other football pads prevent injuries. In general, the better the construction of the pads, the more protective the pads. For example, on the basis of anecdotal experience, thicker shoulder pads reduce the risk of acromioclavicular sprains.

16.3 Baseball

Baseball, long the most popular youth sport in the United States, has been only recently surpassed by soccer as having the most participants. Sliding into a base poses the highest risk of injury, often resulting in foot, ankle, and lower leg injuries. The breakaway base has been shown to reduce the number of injuries substantially in adults involved in recreational and collegiate programs, but its use in children's games has not been studied.[8] Helmets used by batters and runners on the bases help reduce head injuries and should be mandatory equipment in all baseball programs. Eye injuries occur in baseball and are entirely preventable by wearing safety goggles or a polycarbonate shield connected to the batting helmet. These devices also prevent the majority of facial injuries by a pitched ball and should also be worn while guarding bases. Eye protection during baseball should be strongly encouraged in children with normal vision and protective eyewear should be mandatory for functionally one-eyed athletes (a visual acuity <20/40 corrected in one eye).

Rarely, chest impact from a baseball results in sudden death in young baseball players. Sometimes called *commotio cordis*, this apparent concussion of the heart seems to cause immediate ventricular fibrillation or asystole.[9] According to the Consumer Product Safety Commission, 38 deaths occurred in baseball players 5 to 14 years old from 1973 to 1995 due to the impact of the ball to the chest. Although sudden death occurs infrequently, interest has increased about possible interventions to reduce this risk. It is suggested that Little League coaches should be instructed to teach children to turn away from the oncoming baseball. Methods to reduce the force of the impact on the chest include chest protectors and softer baseballs. To date, there are no data to support the contention that softer baseballs can reduce or eliminate sudden death from "cardiac concussion." There is evidence, however, to suggest that softer baseballs reduce the incidence and severity of head injuries.[10]

A 1994 policy statement of the AAP reviews protective strategies in baseball and softball for school-age children.[11]

16.4 Soccer

With the boom in soccer participation by youth, injury prevention issues are amplified. Shin guards help prevent tibial fractures, but data are lacking on their effectiveness. Children's soccer shoes, to make them affordable, are usually not as well constructed as running shoes, which contributes to some of the chronic injuries to the lower extremities such as calcaneal apophysitis (Sever disease) and shin splint syndrome. Improvements in the composition of shoes are expected because of the expanded market.

Soccer goal posts are a potential hazard for youth soccer players because they can tip over. The cross-bar can strike a player, causing severe injury and death. In a 1994 report from the Centers for Disease Control and Prevention, two deaths were reported — a 16-year-old boy and a 3-year-old boy.[12] Consumer Product Safety Commission data revealed that from 1979 to 1993, 27 persons were injured or killed by falling soccer goal posts.[13] The reports indicated that the injuries were associated with climbing, swinging, doing chin-ups, and lifting the posts. In 1992, goal post manufacturers adopted standards specifying the need to anchor or counterweight the goal posts using driving stakes, auger stakes, vertical pole sleeves, or sandbags. Additional information on anchoring is available from the Coalition to Promote Soccer Safety (800-527-7510).

16.5 Gymnastics

Gymnastics is associated with a high injury rate overall and has a large number of catastrophic injuries. Padding around landing areas is important, but the quality of the supervision and the number of supervisors are the most important factors in reducing injury. Spotting for difficult maneuvers is an important method of reducing the risk of injury. In addition, good coaches match the skill level of the gymnast with the appropriate move. Young gymnasts must learn that supervision is an important element of training and that new moves should always involve spotters in the gym.

Some gymnastic coaches (and diving coaches) incorporate workouts on trampolines to teach selected skills. The AAP has published a statement regarding the risks of trampolines and the associated high number of injuries resulting in quadriplegia.[13] Trampolines have no role in routine physical education or in competitive or recreational gymnastics. If trampolines are used in training, the activity must be closely supervised. To our knowledge, however, no evidence exists that skill, training, instruction, spotters, or safety harnesses can prevent catastrophic injury.[14]

16.6 Racquet Sports

Among child athletes, tennis, racquetball, and squash produce acute and chronic injuries by the time the athletes enter high school. Because of the forces on the upper extremities, chronic injuries often occur at the elbow and shoulder. If the muscle imbalances that develop in many players are detected early, more serious problems may be prevented.[15] Studies are in progress to determine the effect of conditioning and a specific strengthening program to prevent such injuries.

During racquet sports, eye injuries are likely to occur because of the size and speed of the ball. Protective eyewear should be worn at all times. The AAP and the American Academy of Ophthalmology have published a statement about the importance of protective eyewear in these sports, especially in functionally one-eyed athletes.[16]

16.7 Conclusion

Because of the frequency of sports injuries, their considerable morbidity, and their high cost, pediatricians should be knowledgeable about injury control measures in sports. Protective equipment has improved over the years and has reduced injuries in many sports. Parents should look for evidence of approval of equipment from the American Society for Testing Materials or the National Operating Committee on Standards for

Athletic Equipment. Among the most important pieces of equipment are helmets for use in football, ice hockey, baseball, equestrian activities, and cycling. Protective eyewear should be worn in sports with the highest risk of eye injuries such as racquet sports, handball, basketball, and baseball. Injury surveillance studies are needed to identify the highest need for intervention and to evaluate the impact of new equipment or rule changes in sports.

References

1. Malek M, Chang BH, Gallagher SS, Guyer B. The cost of medical care for injuries to children. *Ann Emerg Med.* 1991;20:997–1005

2. Garrick JG, Requa RK. Injuries in high school sports. *Pediatrics.* 1978;61:465–469

3. McLain LG, Reynolds S. Sports injuries in a high school. *Pediatrics.* 1989;84:446–450

4. Mueller FO, Cantu RC. Catastrophic injuries and fatalities in high school and college sports, fall 1982–spring 1988. *Med Sci Sports Exerc.* 1990;22:737–741

5. American Academy of Pediatrics, Committee on Sports Medicine and Fitness. *Sports Medicine: Health Care for Young Athletes,* 2nd ed. Elk Grove Village, IL: American Academy of Pediatrics; 1991

6. American Academy of Pediatrics, Committee on Sports Medicine. Knee brace use by athletes. *Pediatrics.* 1990;85:228

7. Bunch RP, Bednarski K, Holland D, Macinanti R. Ankle joint support: a comparison of reusable lace-on braces with taping and wrapping. *Phys Sportsmed.* 1985;13:59–62

8. Janda DH, Maguire R, Mackesy D, et al. Sliding injuries in college and professional baseball: a prospective study comparing standard and break-away bases. *Clin J Sports Med.* 1993;3:78–81

9. Maron BJ, Poliac LC, Kaplan JA, Mueller FO. Blunt impact to the chest leading to sudden death from cardiac arrest during sports activities. *N Engl J Med.* 1995;333:337–342

10. Kyle SB, Adler P, Monticone RC. Reducing youth baseball injuries with protective equipment. *Consumer Product Safety Review* (USCPSC). 1996;1:1–4

11. American Academy of Pediatrics, Committee on Sports Medicine and Fitness. Risk of injury from baseball and softball in children 5 to 14 years of age. *Pediatrics.* 1994;93:690–692

12. Centers for Disease Control. Injuries associated with soccer goalposts – United States, 1979–1993. *MMWR Morb Mortal Wkly Rep.* 1994;43:153–155

13. American Academy of Pediatrics, Committee on Accident and Poison Prevention and Committee on Pediatric Aspects of Physical Fitness, Recreation, and Sports. Trampolines II. *Pediatrics.* 1981;67:438

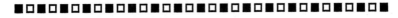

14. Torg JS, Das M. Trampoline-related quadriplegia: review of the literature and reflections on the American Academy of Pediatrics' position statement. *Pediatrics.* 1984;74:804–812

15. Kibler WB, Chandler TJ. Musculoskeletal adaptations and injuries associated with intense participation in youth sports. In: Cahill BR, Pearl AJ, eds. *Intensive Participation in Children's Sports.* Champaign, IL: Human Kinetics Publishers, 1993:203–217

16. American Academy of Pediatrics, Committee on Sports Medicine and Fitness; American Academy of Ophthalmology, Committee on Eye Safety and Sports Ophthalmology. Protective eyewear for young athletes. *Pediatrics.* 1996;98:311–313

CHAPTER 17

Recreational Activities and Vehicles

Year round, children and adolescents enjoy a variety of sports and recreational activities. In the United States, young people sustain between 3 and 5 million injuries each year from such leisure activity; this represents more than a third of injuries from all causes.[1] This chapter deals with recreational activities: on wheels, on snow, and on horseback. These activities commonly are loosely organized, engaged in by individuals or small groups, and informally supervised or undersupervised. All of these activities involve speeds that place children at risk of injury. This is particularly true for motorized recreational activities, during which heightened kinetic energy makes injury possible and likely. Table 17.1, p 340, shows the number of injuries from these recreational activities. Injury control in recreational activities requires an understanding of the basic epidemiology of each class of recreational injuries. For each activity, consider the human factors, the vehicle factors, and the environmental factors that either predispose to, or protect from, injury. For the selected activities listed in Table 17.1, there are more than three quarters of a million injuries treated in emergency departments annually; more than half of the injuries are attributable to bicycle riding. This chapter discusses how the majority of these injuries may be prevented and provides guidance for the pediatrician, who can be instrumental in educating children and parents, both in the office and as a catalyst for community-based prevention activities.

17.1 Bicycles

Bicycling is a popular recreational activity for Americans of all ages; there are approximately 100 million bicyclists in the United States. More bicycles are sold in the United States than automobiles, with more than 11 million sold annually.[2] While increased popularity in recent years is primarily due to the rapidly increasing numbers of adult riders, there

TABLE 17.1.
**Estimated 1994 Emergency Department (ED) Treated Injuries:
Selected Recreational Vehicles and Activities —
United States, Birth Through 19 Years of Age***

Product or Activity	Estimated 1994 ED Visits	Age Distribution, y			
	Birth-19	Birth-4	5-9	10-14	15-19
Small Wheels					
Roller skates	65 254	2090	22 731	33 247	7185
In-line skates	52 031	468	13 164	30 334	8065
Skateboards	22 188	1441	5497	8623	6628
Skates (unspecified)	10 557	264	3051	5205	2038
Winter					
Sledding	40 393	3353	11 472	18 944	6624
Snow skiing	34 981	665	4303	15 007	14 972
Snowboarding	13 614	0	259	4479	8876
Snowmobiles	5509	523	540	2540	1906
Motorized					
All-terrain vehicles	34 347	1750	4884	15 728	11 989
Minibikes and trail bikes	18 396	166	1876	7782	8573
Mopeds	5095	224	652	2303	1916
Other					
Horseback riding	25 235	1565	4315	10 245	9110
Bicycles	457 619	56 287	177 556	174 353	49 423

*Data from the National Electronic Injury Surveillance System, US Consumer Product Safety Commission, courtesy of Joel Freedman. Moped includes power-assisted, two-wheeled cycles. Horseback riding is limited to "product-related" injuries. Bicycle data are for 1993.

remain, according to industry estimates, about 44 million bicyclists younger than 16 years.[2]

Children (5 to 15 years old) ride bicycles at least twice as frequently as older adolescents or young adults, making about 800 000 trips per year.[3] Eight of ten children own bicycles and ride them at least occasionally.[4] More than half of children in all age groups ride more than 100 hours per year.[5] For children and adults, bicycling can be an important source of aerobic exercise as well as a nonpolluting form of recreation and transportation.

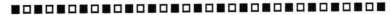
17.1.1 Scope of the Problem

Unfortunately, substantial morbidity and mortality are associated with bicycle riding. Each year, more than 900 bicyclists are killed, 20 000 are admitted to hospitals, and about half a million receive treatment in an emergency department.[3] While collisions with motor vehicles account for nine of ten bicycle-related deaths, at least 75% of nonfatal injuries are unrelated to motor vehicle crashes.[4]

Although most bicycle-related injuries for adults and children are minor and self-limited, central nervous system injuries represent the most significant cause of fatal and disabling injuries. Central nervous system trauma is a primary or contributing cause of three out of four deaths, two out of three hospitalizations, and a third of the emergency department visits.[4,6,7] Most mild and moderate head trauma to cyclists is unrelated to crashes with motor vehicles. Head trauma that is motor vehicle–related is more severe and, if survived, the outcomes are less satisfactory.[8]

Children between the ages of 5 and 15 years are disproportionately involved in crashes resulting in injury. While only four of ten cyclists are in this age group, they account for six of ten bicycle injuries treated in emergency departments.[2,3] Using Consumer Product Safety Commission (CPSC) emergency department data and data from the Federal Highway Administration's (FHA) 1990 Nationwide Personal Transportation Survey, Baker et al estimated that children in the 5- to 15-year-old age group are injured once every 2300 bike trips, that older teenagers are injured once every 3800 trips, and that adults in their 20s are injured only once every 6600 trips.[3,p64] Bicycle deaths per million trips are five times higher in 5- to 15-year-olds than in older teenagers and nearly twice as high as for cyclists in their 20s.

Children younger than 10 years ride primarily on sidewalks, playgrounds, and neighborhood streets. Their nontraffic injuries result from falling from the bike or colliding with fixed objects. As children get older, they venture more frequently into traffic, resulting in more crashes involving motor vehicles. Among elementary school children, nontraffic cycling injuries outnumber the traffic-related ones by 9 to 1. Among teenagers, the ratio is only 2.5 to 1.[9,10]

Despite the fact that head injuries are common and frequently severe, nationally less than 20% of bicycle riders wear a helmet all or most of the time.[4] This number may be higher in areas where there have been local campaigns to promote helmet usage or legislation or regulation has been enacted. Helmets are now lightweight, attractive, and relatively inexpensive compared with injury costs. They have been shown to reduce the risk of brain injury by about 85%, but they must be worn correctly to be beneficial.[7]

Younger children can be injured as passengers on bikes — typically in a rear-mounted carrier. These children are usually injured when the rider crashes, or occasionally when the bike tips over or the child falls from the seat,[11] resulting mainly in head and face injuries.[12]

17.1.2 Risk Factors

Age

Children in the 5- to 14-year-old age group are at maximal risk because of the quantity and the quality of their exposure. Hospital admissions (severe injuries), as well as fatalities, peak in the 10- to 14-year-old age group. A sharp peak in death rates occurs among males in this age group.[3]

Gender

As with most injuries, males have higher injury rates in all age groups. In the pediatric population, the rates increase with age. In 5- to 9-year-olds the male-female ratio is 1.6; in 10- to 14-year-olds, 2.6; and in 15- to 19-year-olds, four boys are injured for every girl.[3] The increased injury rate in boys is due largely, but not entirely, to their riding more.[5]

Riding environment

Children are at increased risk of severe injury and death riding in traffic. Nighttime poses additional risk because the cyclist is less visible to the motorist. Nearly half of bicycle fatalities occur at dusk, dawn, or in the dark.[3] One of three injured riders reports that road surface conditions (bumps, gravel) contributed to injury.[13] Ice on roads in winter is also a hazard.

Riding practices

Certain unsafe practices put children at increased risk of injury. Specifically, the literature suggests that stunt riding, riding double, riding too fast, and riding a borrowed bike may pose additional risk.[13,14] Ignorance of, or failure to follow, rules of the road is hazardous. Failure to ride on the right, with traffic, is confusing to motorists.[15] According to police reports, nearly four of ten cyclists killed in traffic either failed to yield the right-of-way or improperly crossed a roadway or intersection.[16,p132] Child cyclists who have collided with automobiles have overwhelmingly acted in a way that made them "probably responsible" for the collision. Among adult cyclists, it is more often the motorist who is "probably responsible" for the collision.[17]

Equipment

If a bicycle helmet is not used during riding, the relative risk of head injury is 6.6 and the relative risk of brain injury is 8.3.[7] A poorly maintained bicycle, with defects in steering and/or braking, can cause the cyclist to lose control and crash, but is an infrequent cause of injury.

17.1.3 Intervention Strategies

Following the Haddon model, intervention strategies may be divided into human factors, vehicle factors, and environmental factors.[3,18] Important human factors include the use of helmets and the education of parents and children about safe cycling practices. Vehicle factors include proper sizing and maintenance of the bicycle. The most important environmental factor involves efforts to physically separate bicycles from motor traffic.

Human factors: bicycle helmets

Properly fitted bicycle helmets are extremely effective in preventing injuries to the brain. Helmets owe their energy-absorbing qualities primarily to their compressible polystyrene liners. Currently in the United States, three organizations — American National Standards Institute (ANSI), Snell Memorial Foundation, and American Society for Testing and Materials (ASTM) — have published voluntary standards covering the protective capabilities of bicycle helmets, and federal standards for helmets are forthcoming from the CPSC.[4] All helmet standards define and measure impact protection by dropping a helmeted "headform" onto a metal anvil from a measured height and then measuring the amount of force transmitted to the headform. Current standards require that the headforms sustain no more than $300g$ deceleration, which is within a range considered concussive but not life-threatening.[19] In addition, helmets must pass a test of strength of the retaining straps and buckles. Currently, the Snell standard is more stringent than the ANSI standard, in part because the helmet is dropped from a greater height onto the anvil.[4] Additionally, Snell-certified helmets are independently tested by Snell laboratories and are certified by Snell to meet the standard. The other standards are "self-certifying," meaning that the manufacturer assures that the helmets are in compliance with the standard.

Cover materials on helmets vary widely. Those with hard plastic shells are more durable and puncture-resistant and therefore make a good choice for children.

Cyclists of all ages should use helmets that meet the ANSI, ASTM, or Snell standard (or a subsequent generally recognized standard) and are so labeled.[20] Directions should be carefully followed to assure a good fit and proper retention in the event of a crash. Interior fitting pads of the proper thickness assure that the helmet does not move around on the head. Many helmets are supplied with fitting pads of several *different* thicknesses to accommodate a growing child's head. The position of the helmet on the child's head is important. A properly positioned helmet sits horizontally on the head to protect the forehead — not pushed to the back of the head. Parents should not purchase helmets for children "to grow into."

Bicycle helmets differ from helmets used in team sports in that they are "single-impact" helmets. In the act of absorbing the impact forces of a crash, the helmet is partially destroyed, though damage to the polystyrene liner may not be readily visible. Bicycle helmets that are dented, cracked, or otherwise visibly damaged (inside or out) should be discarded and replaced. Those that have been in a crash but are not visibly damaged should either be discarded and replaced or returned to the manufacturer for inspection.[21]

Pediatricians can have the greatest impact on reducing serious injury by encouraging the use of helmets.[10,20] Physicians must address the currently recognized barriers to helmet use — lack of awareness, negative peer pressure, cost, comfort, and lack of physician counseling.[22–24] With this in mind, pediatricians' efforts need to extend beyond the office and into the community.[25]

To date, community campaigns to increase helmet use have had mixed success. Their success depends, in part, on the socioeconomic mix of the target community and the coexistence of helmet legislation. In Ontario, a school-based intervention was successful in increasing helmet use in middle-income families but not among those of more modest income, even when subsidies were provided to make helmets more affordable.[26,27] On the other hand, a broad-based community-wide effort in Seattle, Wash, has successfully raised helmet use among children, as measured by observation, from 5.5% to 40% during a 5-year period.[28] A helmet campaign combined with legislation in Howard County, Md, an economically more advantaged population, achieved a similar magnitude of increase in usage in only a 1-year period.[29] The American Academy of Pediatrics (AAP) has model state legislation available on this topic. Several organizations have sample campaign materials available (see Resources section).

Human factors: cycling practices

In addition to assuring that helmets are worn at all times by bicycle riders, there are a variety of other safety practices that lower the risk of injury to young cyclists. Physicians should give the following advice to parents and patients:

- Children must understand traffic rules and be able to demonstrate hand signals before riding in the street.
- Children should not be permitted to venture onto roadways until they have demonstrated competence in handling the bike on the sidewalk. Skills include braking, turning, and looking over one's shoulder while riding forward.
- When riding on the roadway, it is essential that children ride with traffic — not against traffic. In addition, they must respect all traffic signals such as stop signs and traffic lights.
- Children should not be permitted to ride at dusk or after dark.
- Children should wear bright light-colored clothes.
- Children should not ride double on a bike.
- Parents should wear helmets for protection and appropriate role modeling.

The age at which children should be allowed to ride bikes in the street is a question analogous to the question of when children should be allowed to cross the street unsupervised (see chapter 9.2). As with street crossing, it depends not solely on age but rather on the child (maturity and temperament) and on the street (volume and speed of traffic). Children must be able to control the bicycle, to understand and follow rules of the road, and to exercise good judgment. Child cyclists new to street riding should be allowed only on portions of roadway that are straight, with good visibility; slow, light traffic; and no challenging intersections. Only with practice and demonstrated competence should children be allowed to ride in more challenging traffic. While some 8- and 9-year-olds may be capable of riding safely on some streets, others may not. Parents should require a substantial period of adult-supervised street riding at first.

The rationale for riding on the right, with traffic, is not widely appreciated. It is the opposite of how pedestrians should walk in roadways without sidewalks. Bicycling against traffic confuses motorists at intersections. Motorists expect traffic to be entering the intersection from the opposite direction of the cyclist riding the wrong way and are not typically looking for traffic from that direction. Also, cyclists riding the wrong way are forced to cross paths with oncoming traffic at times of neither's choosing. An automobile can approach and wait to pass a cyclist traveling in the same direction at a time when it is safe. In contrast, a motorist approaching an oncoming "wrong-way" cyclist must pass him at a time that may be less than ideal — and at a time the motorist cannot choose. A cyclist traveling with traffic gives motor vehicles the opportunity to wait and pass at a safe opportunity.[15]

Vehicle factors: the bicycle

Bicycles that are not the appropriate size for the child's age are hard to control. The bicycle size should not be selected for the child to "grow into." The child, sitting on the seat with the hands on the handlebars, should be able to place the balls of both feet on the ground. When straddling the bar, the child should be able to stand flat-footed on the ground and reach the handle bars comfortably. There should be least a 1-in clearance between the child's crotch and the bar. Children younger than 8 years usually lack sufficient hand strength and coordination to operate hand brakes; therefore, bicycles for younger children should be equipped with coaster brakes.

Bicycles should be periodically inspected and maintained. This is a good joint responsibility and activity for parents and children who are mechanically inclined. Special attention should be paid to the steering mechanism, the brakes, the condition of the tires, and the chain guard. If parents are unable to routinely maintain their children's bikes, they should have a bike shop do the maintenance.

Vehicle factors: children as passengers on adult bikes

Children who ride as passengers on adult bikes make the bicycle less stable and increase the braking time. Parents should be advised of these problems and should ride with caution.[11,12] Children should only be carried in well-designed, rear-mounted seats and should wear helmets. Seats should be securely mounted over the rear wheel and have a spoke guard to prevent the child's hands and feet from being caught in the wheel. Seats should also have a high back and a shoulder harness and lap belt that will support a sleeping child. Children who lack back and neck support (those younger than 1 year) should not be passengers on bicycles. As children approach 4 years of age, their weight makes the bike increasingly unstable and difficult to handle. Children who cannot cooperate and sit still should not be passengers. Infant carriers such as backpacks and front packs are unsafe to transport infants on bicycles.

Parents riding bicycles with passengers should confine their bike riding to low-traffic areas and reasonable speeds. Children should never be left alone in a bike carrier.

Although data are unavailable, use of bike trailers to carry a young child as a passenger has at least two theoretic advantages over rear-mounted seats. They do not make the bike unstable from being top-heavy and they attach by a pivot joint so that the child is not thrown if the bike tips over. Trailers should not be used in the roadway as they are low and may not be seen by motorists. Passengers in trailers must wear helmets.

Environmental factors: separating bikes from traffic

With 90% of fatalities and large percentages of serious injuries related to traffic, there is good reason to try to separate young recreational cyclists from traffic. Bike paths provide a good alternative but are seldom available to the urban cyclist. The "Rails to Trails" initiatives in various states are an encouraging development and are particularly appropriate and appealing to the current generation of mountain bike and hybrid bike riders. Special bicycle lanes may seem like a good idea, but they may lead to a paradoxical increase in collisions with motor traffic at curves and intersections.[30]

17.1.4 Recommendations for Pediatricians

Because bicycle riding is an almost universal activity of childhood, pediatricians should become knowledgeable about bike safety and become involved with bicycle safety activities. Bicycling as a source of recreation and exercise should not be discouraged. Safety activities include advocating and promoting proper bicycle safety education in the schools; working with community agencies (fire and rescue teams, school personnel, police, Scouts) to promote bicycle helmet use through coupons, rebates, and giveaways; and studying the possibility of legislation to enforce helmet use.

Local regulation and legislation have ultimately been shown to produce the greatest increases in helmet usage and reduction of head injuries. Pediatricians should be aware of this and be prepared to advocate for legislation when it seems appropriate.[31]

17.2 In-line Skating, Roller Skating, and Skateboarding

Three modern sports, in-line skating, roller skating, and skateboarding, are attractive to children and adolescents, perhaps because they provide greater mobility, transportation, exercise, recreation, and competition, are readily affordable, and can be done in many environments. The epidemiology of injuries in these sports has recently been explored.[32] Estimates of injuries treated in emergency departments are shown in Table 17.1. Although the relative importance of sequestered paths or parks, protective equipment, lessons, and ability on preventing injuries has not been determined for all these sports, some consensus recommendations for prevention of injuries are given below.

17.2.1 In-line Skating

In-line skating has become the fastest growing recreational sport in the United States. In 1994, an estimated 19.5 million people participated in the sport, an increase of 57% over the previous year.[33] Half the participants skated more than 25 times annually. More than 100 models of skates are manufactured by more than 33 companies, and at least three publications and three national or international associations exist.

Most in-line skaters are young. In 1994, 77% were younger than 25 years, and 38% were younger than 12 years. The number of male and female participants is approximately equal. About one third of all American skaters live in the North Central states. About 37% of participants live in households with an annual income exceeding $50 000.[33]

Risk factors associated with injury and the likelihood of injury are presently under study. It seems that speed, obstacles, lack of protective gear, and the hard impact surface all contribute to the risk of injury. Cruising speeds of 10 to 17 mph are commonly reached,[34] and anecdotal reports cite speeds in excess of 70 mph, especially when skaters are "skitching," the undesirable practice of holding onto a fast-moving motor vehicle while skating.[35] Furthermore, when skating outdoors, participants must share the roadway with motor vehicles, bicyclists, pedestrians, and pets, as well as steer around pavement defects and road debris.

In the year ending July 1, 1993, about 31 000 injuries were reported for adults and children,[1] including 20 000 injuries in children and adolescents younger than 21 years. In 1994, about 53 000 injuries were reported in young persons, of which 63% involved males (NEISS, CPSC, unpublished data). The reason that more males are injured than females is unknown; possibly more males skate than females, their inexperience may place them at higher risk than females, or they may have a greater propensity to take risks. April, May, and September were the peak months for injury. The wrist area, including the lower arm, was the site most frequently injured (40%), followed by the knee, face, and elbow. The head was injured in about 5% of cases. About 41% of all injured children sustained a fracture. Less than 2% of this total required hospitalization. Many of those injured were first-time skaters who lost control and fell. Others were experienced skaters who were injured while performing a trick or traveling at excessive speed.

17.2.2 Roller Skating

Unlike in-line skating, roller skating is mainly an indoor activity. In 1994 in the United States, roller skating–related injuries resulted in an estimated 66 000 visits to emergency departments by children and adolescents annually (CPSC, NEISS, unpublished data). The wrist area was the most commonly injured site (43%), followed by the ankle, elbow, knee, finger, and hand. Thirty-nine percent of all injuries treated were fractures. Sixty-five percent of those injured were girls. The peak months of injuries were January through April, probably because of the nature of this sport as an indoor activity. In two other reports, surgery was frequently required for those hospitalized.[36,37] Loss of balance, irregular surfaces, and collision with other skaters have been cited as the main factors leading to injury.[36,37] Better rink discipline, instruction classes, and safety publicity were countermeasures recommended by some authors,[6] whereas others recommended use of protective gear and establishment of a separate skating area indoors for beginners.[38]

17.2.3 Skateboarding

The frequency of skateboard-related injuries peaked in 1977, resurged in the late 1980s, and has declined again.[39] In 1994, skateboard-related injuries resulted in an estimated 23 000 visits to emergency departments by children and adolescents in the United States (CPSC, NEISS, unpublished data). Eighty-four percent of the injuries involved males. The most frequently injured body site was the ankle (16%), followed by the face, wrist, and elbow. About 24% of the total group sustained a contusion or abrasion, 23% sustained a sprain or strain, and 21% sustained a fracture. Hospitalization is rarely required, but most often results from the occurrence of a head injury. The peak incidence of injuries occurred in May, August, and September.

Retsky et al[39] have suggested several possible risk factors for skateboard injury, including immature motor coordination and the disproportionately large head of young children (which may account for a greater proportion of head injuries in this age group); risk-taking behavior of older children; the high speed of travel (faster than 40 to 50 mph); skateboard design — some with high maneuverability features that adversely affect the individual's ability to balance and control the skateboard and therefore requiring considerable skill to ride; and the sensitivity of the small wheels to road obstacles or irregularities, which may lead to a crash.

The AAP recommends that children younger than 5 years not ride skateboards, citing as reasons their high center of gravity, immature neuromuscular system, poor judgment skills, and insufficient ability to protect themselves from injury (ie, knowing how to react to obstacles, knowing how to fall).[40] The AAP holds that skateboards should not be used near traffic, and their use should be prohibited on streets and highways — a controversial position not universally held.[41,42] The AAP encourages skateboarders to use protective gear (discussed in the next section). Furthermore, they recommend that pediatricians should discuss skateboard safety with parents and children. Some years ago, a request for a ban on the manufacture and/or sale of skateboards was denied by the CPSC. They noted that skateboard-associated injuries usually relate more to the misuse of the product, rather than an inherent flaw in the product itself.[43]

17.2.4 Recommendations

Protective gear

The International In-line Skating Association,[34] AAP,[40] and several authors[37] recommend that participants of all three sports use full protective gear — helmets, wristguards, and knee and elbow pads. The Roller Skating Association, a national industry trade association of roller rink owners, notes that protective gear is needed for indoor roller hockey but is optional for indoor skating.

For participants in all these sports, the wrist appears to be particularly vulnerable to injury, as might be expected when skaters fall and by reflex outstretch their arms with their wrists hyperextended. Wrist guards, which sandwich the wrist area between two stiff plastic or metal plates, protect against such sudden hyperextension. They also provide a barrier to direct contact of the wrist with hard surfaces.

Until recently, the relative degree of effectiveness of wrist guards in preventing wrist injuries was not known. Preliminary results in injured in-line skaters indicate, however, that wrist guards are virtually completely protective against lacerations, sprains, and strains, and that they reduce the overall odds of sustaining a wrist injury more than sixfold.[44] Elbow- and knee-pad protectors might also help prevent local injuries, but their degree of effectiveness is unknown. Further evaluation of the effectiveness of wrist, knee, and elbow pads in reducing or eliminating injuries is warranted.

The issue of protection against head injury is particularly important because of the potential for long-term disability. Although the percentage of injured participants in each sport who sustain a head injury appears low, each such event has the potential to cause enormous and lasting medical, social, and financial consequences. Approved bicycle helmets and multipurpose helmets are quite effective in reducing the incidence of serious head injuries to bicyclists,[7] and their use is recommended for these sports.

Special considerations for novice participants

Novices seem to be at particularly high risk of injury.[36,37] In a CPSC study, 24% of those injured on skateboards were first-time participants.[45] Besides wearing protective gear, novices should avoid roadways with traffic, uneven surfaces, hills (even small ones), and obstacles. They should avoid roadways shared by bicyclists and pedestrians until they are capable of steering themselves successfully. Skating instruction may reduce the likelihood of injury and safe skating practices are likely to improve skills, especially in the early phases of learning.[36] Special attention should be paid to learning to fall properly to help avoid injuries.

Trails, parks, and rinks

Although more experienced in-line skaters may be able to share the road with bicyclists and pedestrians safely, separate trails are advisable where possible. Trail designs have been published,[34] including recommendations for design speed, drainage, trail width, sight distances, and surface materials. Skate parks for skateboarders have been recommended by some[46,47] but refuted by others.[41]

General measures

Skates and skateboards, especially wheels, should be maintained in good condition. Skaters and skateboarders should skate on the right, pass on the left, and yield to pedestrians. On public roads, all traffic regulations must be observed, just as in bicycle riding. Skitching should be strongly discouraged. This practice potentially endangers the skater if the vehicle suddenly slows down, stops, or turns. During a fall, a skater's enhanced momentum results in a greater impact with the roadway (or another vehicle) and is likely to cause a more severe injury. Control, not speed, should be the principal skill emphasized for inexperienced participants. Children should not participate in these sports on wet surfaces or after dark.

What is the most appropriate age to allow children to begin participating in these sports? Assuming they have normal strength, coordination, and judgment, young elementary school children can participate. Roller skating should probably be the first sport attempted, because it is usually practiced indoors, where lighting is good, speed is monitored and controlled, horseplay is not allowed, and where the skating surface is flat and free from defects or debris. Also, roller skate wheels can be tightened to roll more slowly and afford greater control. Teachers are available at many indoor rinks, and some rinks have a separate area for beginners. Roller skates (and often in-line skates) can be rented, and are generally subject to regular maintenance. However, these safeguards cannot be expected to eliminate completely the possibility of an injury occurring, even indoors — the rink-specific injury incidence rate has been estimated at 1.2%.[36,48]

Once the basics of roller skating have been learned, in-line skating (if desired) may be attempted by children, preferably at an indoor rink, or at the very least, outdoors on a flat surface free of road debris and defects and protected from traffic. Skateboarding activities may follow once the child has sufficient skill, strength, and coordination to steer the board adequately. Overall, acquiring more experience in the early phases of learning to skate may lessen the possibility of injuries occurring later.

17.2.5 Conclusion

In-line skating, skateboarding, and roller skating are popular sports that provide excellent recreational outlets for children and adolescents. Although in the United States the frequency of bicycle-related injuries far exceeds that of injuries from any of these sports, more studies of exposure risk are needed to determine their relative safety. Subsequent studies should be conducted to assess the risk factors for injury, especially the relative importance of environmental and behavioral aspects. Certain groups of participants also warrant additional study, particularly those who may be exposed to greater risk because they spend more time participating in the sport than other persons, skate at higher speeds or at higher performance levels (such as speed skating and trick skating), or have greater exposure to bodily contact (eg, in-line hockey players). Pediatricians and parents should recognize that these sports are not without risk, even when full protective gear is worn and good technique is used.

17.3 Winter Recreation

Winter recreation usually involves frost, freezing temperatures, and snow. This can mean fun for children of all ages, but it also brings certain hazards. Cold weather brings the risk of cold injury (frostbite or hypothermia). Wind and wet clothing can make this problem worse. As a general rule children need all parts of their body covered (with gloves, hats that cover the ears, and waterproof boots). Wool is an excellent insulator, even when wet, but wet mittens and boots should be removed quickly to avoid chilling.

This section does not address all winter recreation, but considers and provides guidelines for control of injury for the most popular recreational activities specifically associated with cold weather and snow — sledding, skiing, snowboarding, and snowmobiling (skimobiling). In each case, the thrill, as well as the risk, is associated with speed, which sometimes exceeds 30 mph.[49] Together, sledding, skiing, snowboarding, and snowmobiling are responsible for more than 90 000 emergency department visits annually in the pediatric population (Table 17.1).

17.3.1 Sledding Injuries

Sledding is almost a universal outdoor activity wherever or whenever snow falls. Traditional wooden sleds have two metal runners and a steering bar that turn the sled. Now, most sledders use a plastic model without runners or a steering mechanism. The traditional wooden sleds with flexible steel runners are more easily steered by 6- to 12-year-olds than the snow disks that rely only on weight shifts and foot dragging to steer.[50] Snow disks are capable great speeds, and injuries are common.

Injury patterns and risk

Injuries cluster in the 5- to 14-year-old age group because this group has the greatest exposure. Most injuries are minor — lacerations, contusions, sprains, and strains — but the face and head may also be involved, accounting for about a third of injuries.[51] The younger the sledder, the more likely a head injury may occur. One third of injuries treated in an emergency department are serious: concussions, internal injuries, and fractures.[51] The chances of severe injury are increased by impact with a fixed object or motor vehicle or by hard-packed icy conditions. Parents are frequently injured while riding on sleds with their children, by twisting or breaking their legs in an attempt to steer or brake the sled.

Intervention strategies

Think about interventions in terms of the host (the child), the equipment (the sled), and the environment (the slope and surroundings).[49] Some interventions that may control the risk of injury are the following:

- *Host:* Educate children and parents about safe practices (see below). Gloves and boots should be worn to protect hands and feet. To lessen the risk of a head injury, sledding should not be done in the prone position (not head first).
- *Equipment:* Encourage the use of steerable sleds rather than snow disks or inner tubes. The steering mechanism should be well lubricated and the sled should be free of sharp edges, splinters, and structurally sound.
- *Environment:* Recreational sledding is safest when slopes are away from traffic, are free of fixed obstructions (fire hydrants or fences) or ice, and have a slope less than 30° and flat runoff; slopes should not be overcrowded, with younger sledders separated from adolescents and constant supervision provided by adults.

Recommendations for pediatricians

Pediatricians should provide appropriate advice about winter recreation to parents of children, particularly parents of 5- to 14-year-olds. Younger children should be supervised, and children of widely varying ages should be separated, as older children may place younger children at risk for injury. The most important preventive measure is to separate sledders from motor traffic. Head injuries may be avoided if children sled feet first or sitting up instead of the traditional head-first prone position.

Pediatricians can participate in community efforts to provide sledders with a safe, supervised environment.

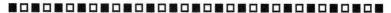
17.3.2 Skiing

Alpine, or downhill, skiing continues to grow in popularity, fueled by televised competitive events, improved equipment, and manufactured snow that makes conditions more predictable. Approximately 10% of the 5 to 10 million downhill skiers in the United States are younger than 16 years.[52] Despite improved equipment and better facilities, children and adolescents continue to suffer injuries and, rarely, fatalities. Most injuries occur as a result of falls or collisions, but hypothermia may also contribute to the associated morbidity. The 35 000 pediatric skiing injuries treated annually in emergency departments mainly involve children and adolescents 10 years old and older, but 4000 annual injuries occur in younger children. It is sometimes difficult to estimate the true incidence of skiing injuries because only persons with severe or perceived to be severe injuries are transported down the mountain.[53] Others who are less seriously injured may seek medical attention after returning home.

Injury patterns and risk

Although children constitute 10% of skiers, they sustain 20% of the injuries.[52] Children are particularly prone to lower extremity injuries, particularly tibial fractures.[52] Children also frequently suffer medial collateral ligament sprains and ankle sprains, as do adults.[54] Head injuries are not common, but are often severe. Large percentages of lower extremity injuries have been attributed to equipment, particularly failure of boot bindings to release, which may be associated with poor fit or maintenance.[55]

A number of known factors can combine to increase the risk of injury. The age and experience of the skier seem to have a direct correlation with injury. Less experienced skiers are injured more often, as are younger skiers.[53] As a group, young skiers are more prone to injury for a variety of reasons. They are more likely to be novices; they possess less skill and judgment than older skiers; their bones are more prone to fracture; and they more often use second-hand, poorly maintained, ill-fitting, or poorly adjusted equipment. Among children, those injured tend to be the less experienced and less skillful; they are often injured at the beginning of the season.[55]

In alpine skiing, fatigue is associated with incidence of injury. The last run of the day frequently has injuries. The type and function of the ski bindings also influence the severity of injuries. In three of four lower leg injuries, the bindings do not release.[56] Bindings need to be adjusted to the weight of the skier and to snow conditions; adjustment usually needs to be done by an experienced professional.

Crowding or obstacles on the slopes can contribute to injuries. Injuries typically result when a skier's speed is disproportionate to his or her skill, leading to loss of control.[53] Seventy-five percent of injuries result from collisions.[52]

Intervention strategies

- *Host:* Children are best taught how to ski by a trained instructor rather than their parents. Children should be taught in a ski school program designed for children.[52] With limitations in judgment, children require supervision on the slopes depending on individual maturity and skill.
- *Equipment:* Safety bindings prevent many long bone fractures. To be protective they must be adjusted at least every year and perhaps more often if snow conditions change significantly (icy to deep, soft snow). Equipment should be well-fitting, relying on guidance from ski shop personnel experienced in outfitting children. The role of helmets is controversial, but a warm, lightweight ski helmet can provide protection for the young skier.[52] Helmets are commonly used by child skiers in Europe. Head injuries are uncommon, but when they occur they may be severe or catastrophic. Most fatalities are related to head injuries from collisions with another skier or with a fixed object such as a lift tower or tree. Warm, dry clothing is necessary to prevent hypothermia or frostbite.
- *Environment:* Special ski programs and special slopes for children are the ideal. Skiers should stick to slopes appropriate to their experience and ability. Parents should not pressure children into the sport until they express interest and are ready.

Recommendations for pediatricians

Pediatricians who practice in areas where skiing is popular should advise and educate parents about injury prevention. Neophyte skiers should be encouraged to purchase safe, proper fitting equipment, which includes close-fitting boots, short, flexible skis, and well-chosen and properly adjusted safety bindings. Lessons by a qualified instructor should be encouraged that teach not only technique, but proper etiquette on the slopes.

17.3.3 Snowboarding

Snowboarding, which began in the 1970s, has become an extremely popular winter sport, competing in popularity with downhill skiing, particularly among young people and males. By the mid-1990s, snowboarders comprised 20% to 25% of participants at some downhill slopes.[57]

Snowboards resemble skateboards and measure between 140 and 190 cm in length. The boards are constructed similarly to skis with fiberglass bodies and plastic bases. Snowboarders ride snowboards much the way surfers ride surfboards, with the back foot positioned perpendicular to the long axis of the board and the forward foot at 45°. In contrast to alpine skiing, boot bindings are nonreleasable, and the participant does not use ski poles. Steering is accomplished by twisting and shifting of body weight. As in surfing and skateboarding, jumping to become airborne is a popular maneuver.[57] Snowboarders can achieve speed in excess of 40 mph.[58]

Injury patterns and risk

Several studies have looked at injury patterns among snowboarders.[57,59–61] When compared with alpine skiers, snowboarders have more upper extremity injuries than lower extremity injuries. The most common significant injury is to the wrist, often incurred from falling backward. Without ski poles, snowboarders instinctively use their arms to break a fall. (The thumb injuries often seen in skiers, presumably from the ski pole acting as a lever, do not occur frequently in snowboarding.) Lower extremity injuries occur as commonly to the ankle as the knee, in contrast to skiers who more commonly injure the knee. This is presumably the result of the twisting motions of the sport and the nonreleasable boot bindings. Among persons with severe injuries, head and abdominal injuries are more common among snowboarders than skiers.[60] In contrast to skiers, novices account for a significantly higher proportion of those treated for injury.[61] This may in part be an artifact of a rapidly growing sport in which there are many more new participants than seasoned ones and many who do not have the advantage of qualified instruction.

While skiing injuries occur with equal frequency in males and females, more than seven of ten injured snowboarders are male, likely reflecting the current demographics of the sport.[61]

Snowboard injuries are estimated to occur about twice as commonly as skiing injuries.[57] In one study, none of the injured participants wore protective equipment.[58]

Intervention strategies

- *Host:* Snowboarding is not recommended for children under 7 years of age. As with skiing, qualified instruction is important to instill safe technique and practice.
- *Equipment:* The snowboard should fit the child. It should stand no higher than the child's nose. Given the higher incidence of head injuries in snowboarding, an equal or stronger argument can be made for the use of helmets.[62] To help prevent distal radial fractures, gloves with built-in wrist guards should be worn.
- *Environment:* Snowboarders can probably safely share the same slopes as skiers.[61] However, the slope must fit the abilities and experience of the participants. Overcrowding should be avoided. Snowboarders should never snowboard alone.

Pediatricians who practice in areas where snowboarding is popular should be competent in advising and educating parents. Parents should be made aware of the risks to this emerging sport, particularly to new participants, those lacking protective equipment, and those who have not been instructed in safe practice.

17.3.4 Snowmobiles

Injury patterns and risk

Snowmobiles are motorized vehicles equipped with skis on the front and are capable of high speeds on the snow. Injuries occur from collisions with fixed objects, from immersion in water when they fall through icy surfaces, and from hypothermia when they break down in remote areas. Alcohol use is frequently involved in these crashes. Young adolescents are frequently involved as drivers and younger children are injured as passengers. Drowning is not uncommon when a snowmobile breaks through the ice. About 5000 injuries to the pediatric population are treated in emergency departments annually.

Intervention strategies

- *Host:* Individuals who are intoxicated, fatigued, or young should be discouraged or prohibited from operating snowmobiles. The vehicles are inappropriate for children (who lack skill and judgment) and young adolescents (who often lack judgment and take risks). Machines should be used only by those who have received safety instruction, and novices should be supervised by an experienced operator. Protective clothing (helmets, gloves, boots, goggles, or eye shields) gives some protection to riders.

- *Equipment:* Vehicles should have built-in protection in their design. The exhaust system should have protective cowlings to prevent burns to the extremities. Less powerful vehicles are inherently safer because they cannot attain the speeds of more powerful machines.

- *Environment:* Ponds and rivers should be avoided early in the season and again when spring thaws begin. This is the most common time for breaking through the ice, immersion injuries, or drownings.

Recommendations for pediatricians

Pediatricians should be aware of the hazards of snowmobiling and urge participants to receive proper instruction and follow safety guidelines. Parents should be made aware that snowmobiles are powerful motor vehicles not intended to be driven by children or young adolescents. The AAP recommends that snowmobiles only be operated by persons older than 16 years, and then only by persons who have had proper safety instruction.[63] Although in many rural areas snowmobiles are commonly operated by children, pediatricians should discourage this practice. Physicians should work with snowmobile clubs and other local groups to promote usage only by persons old enough to understand risks and to operate the vehicles safely.

17.4 Recreational Injuries: Motorized Recreational Vehicles

17.4.1 Definitions

Motorized recreational vehicles of various types are commonly used by adolescents for both recreation and transportation. Powered off-road use cycles include *minibikes* and *minicycles*, as well as *trail bikes*. *Minibikes* are small (weighing <45 kg) and have bicycle-style frames and lawn mower engines (with <4 horsepower).[64] *Minicycles* are constructed to resemble miniature motorcycles with suspension systems and transmissions, and they may have more horsepower. *Trail bikes* are larger than minicycles and have more power. They are specifically designed for use on rough terrain, and because they are intended for off-road use, neither the vehicles nor their riders are licensed. These cycles are particularly dangerous because of their design (small tires, short wheelbase, slow acceleration, and inadequate brakes) and because they are often used illegally on the roadway. *Snowmobiles* are considered off-road vehicles, and are discussed in the Winter Recreation section (see section 17.3).

Powered street-use cycles include *mopeds, scooters*, and *motorcycles*. *Mopeds* are bicycles with small, unenclosed assist motors, but they may obtain a top speed of about 30 mph. They are not intended to carry more than one person. Many states do not require licensing of mopeds and their drivers because they are classified as bicycles, although some states set a minimum age of 14 to 16 years for moped use, and helmet use is not generally required. Mopeds are often used in city traffic by adolescents with undeveloped driving skills, and the vehicles themselves have insufficient acceleration for mixing with city traffic. Scooters usually have an enclosed engine, automatic transmission, and small (10 to 12 in) wheels, with a larger engine (up to 250 cc). They may be designed to carry passengers, and top speed, determined by the available power, is usually enough to keep up with city traffic and occasionally enables freeway driving. *Motorcycles* can attain speeds greater than many passenger vehicles, but lack the stability and crash protection of cars. A state operator's license is required to drive motorcycles (see chapter 9.1).

All-terrain vehicles (ATVs) are motorized recreational vehicles with three or four large soft tires, a high center of gravity, a poor or absent suspension system, and no rear-wheel differential. They may attain speeds of 30 to 50 mph. Because these vehicles are not designed for on-road use, licensing is not required. In fact, ATVs are often promoted for use by young children, and many states do not set a minimum age limit for their operation.

17.4.2 Scope of the Problem

Specific injury rates for the various kinds of recreational two-wheeled vehicles are not available − data are combined in injury statistics.

Motorcycles (See section 9.1.6 also.)

More than 4 million motorcycles are registered in the United States, about 2% of all registered vehicles. However, they account for about 7% of occupant deaths in motor vehicle crashes. About 2200 deaths and 54 000 injuries occurred in 1994, with about 350 of the deaths and 10 000 of the injuries involving children and adolescents.[65] The mileage death rate (per 1 million miles traveled) is about 20 times higher than that for occupants of other motor vehicles.[16] About half of the motorcyclists involved in fatal crashes in 1994 collided with another vehicle, the other half were single-vehicle crashes, of which half involved drivers with very high blood alcohol levels.[66]

Scooters and mopeds

Scooters and mopeds are more likely to be involved in a collision with another vehicle, presumably because they are used more in urban areas.[67] More than half of the victims of scooter- and moped-related injuries are younger than 20 years; in one study, the average age was younger than 13 years.[68] Motorcycles overturn and hit stationary objects more often than do scooters and mopeds. Injuries related to all two-, three-, and four-wheeled vehicles overwhelmingly involve males.

More than 23 000 people younger than 20 years are treated in emergency departments each year for injuries associated with two-wheeled, motorized off-road vehicles, of which 13 000 are children younger than 14 (Table 17.1). The injuries occur most often from loss of control of the vehicle after it strikes rocks, bumps, or holes. A significant number of injuries occur with illegal on-road use.

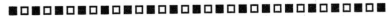
All-terrain vehicles

The CPSC estimates that 200 to 250 deaths each year are related to ATV use, and about 60 000 injuries from three- or four-wheeled ATVs are treated each year in emergency departments.[69] Children younger than 16 years experience four out of ten injuries; about 11% are younger than 10 years. There are about 2.5 million ATVs in use in the United States; the CPSC calculates a death rate of about one per 10 000 ATVs in use. For children, the death rate decreased from 1985 to 1987 and then remained stable through 1993. The number of ATV-associated injuries decreased more than 40% between 1987 and 1993. Since limitations were set on production of three-wheeled ATVs in 1987, an increasing percentage of the injuries are occurring on four-wheeled ATVs, up from 7% in 1984 to 64% in 1995.[69]

Head injuries account for most of the ATV-related deaths, and more than half of the deaths are instantaneous.[70] Serious nonfatal injuries include head trauma, spinal trauma, abdominal injuries, and multiple trauma.[71–73] Some studies, but not all, have suggested that children sustain more severe injuries. The severity of injury is the same for three- and four-wheeled off-road vehicles.[74]

There is an additional risk of burns on mopeds and minibikes when engines are not enclosed.[75]

17.4.3 Risk Factors

As previously indicated, important risk factors include the age and gender of the drivers; young males are much more likely to die or become injured from operating motorized recreational vehicles. Although risk ratios for young drivers of ATVs have decreased somewhat since the actions of the CPSC in 1987–1988, drivers younger than 16 years are at five times higher risk than older drivers. Males experience more than twice the risk of females. Also, driving experience reduces the risk of injury significantly.

The larger the engine on an ATV, the greater the likelihood of injury. Although the severity of injury is about the same regardless of the number of wheels, those riding three-wheeled vehicles are about 50% more likely to be injured; this difference has decreased since 1987. Those who use the ATVs for nonrecreational uses, eg, as a farm vehicle, are significantly less likely to be injured than those who use the vehicle primarily for recreation.

For street-use vehicles, in general, the larger the engine and thus the higher the top speed attainable, the more likely the driver is to be injured. Age, sex, and driving experience modify the risks for injury in the same fashion as for ATVs. Driving under the influence of alcohol is associated with a greater chance of injury and greater severity of injury.

17.4.4 Intervention Strategies

Education

It is probable that the most effective outcome of the 1988 consent decrees between the federal government and the ATV manufacturers (discussed later) was the attendant publicity. Widespread educational campaigns at the time of the decrees resulted in diminished use of ATVs by children and a decline in sales, even before the three-wheel ATV manufacturing ban could have had an effect or sufficiently "safer" vehicles were produced. It has also been postulated that these campaigns had an effect on the driving behavior of those operating the ATV. Education, both public and personal, may also have an effect in producing a public demand for regulation, eg, helmet laws.

Enforcement

Under pressure from the CPSC and numerous lawsuits, the ATV industry accepted consent decrees in early 1988. Under the decrees, the industry agreed to cease production and sale of new three-wheeled ATVs, to implement a rider's safety training program nationally, and to develop a voluntary standard to make ATVs safer.[76] Changes were made in the recommended age children could operate various sized ATVs. The adult size (>90-cc) engine is not recommended for children younger than 16 years; vehicles with the smaller (70- to 90-cc) engine are suggested for 12- to 15-year-olds, and, although the decrees did not prohibit the sales of ATVs with engines smaller than 70 cc originally promoted for children younger than 12 years, none have been made since 1986. The age recommendations are communicated by warnings on the vehicle as well as in the owner's manual and in advertisements. There have been problems with dealers specifically communicating the age restrictions to purchasers, although pressure and enforcement from the CPSC have improved this practice.

As younger children are at considerably greater risk, because of their age and lack of driving experience, legislation to prohibit use by children younger than 16 years and to require licensing of off-road vehicles and drivers has been proposed by the AAP and others.[77,78] Enforcement of existing legislation against on-road use of off-road vehicles and driving while intoxicated, even when not on public roads, could also lower the injury rate.

Equipment or design modification

Some requirements of the 1988 consent decrees related to modification of the vehicles to make them somewhat more stable and to improve the suspension systems, brakes, and switches, as well as speed limitations for the youth models. Because there are fewer three-wheeled ATVs, there should be some improvement in the risk of injury. Other modifications have been suggested, including the installation of seat belts, that would require that the vehicle also have a roll bar so the driver would not be crushed by the weight of the vehicle.[10] The addition of a sturdy leg guard could prevent injuries from sideswiping solid objects or being pinned to the ground. Headlights and flags may improve visibility; this strategy has been helpful for motorcycles. Other vehicle modification suggestions include throttle governors and a remote control device that would allow a child's caregiver to shut off the vehicle motor while the child is driving.

Helmet use has been proven to reduce deaths and serious head injuries for motorcyclists.[79,80] Studies of other recreational vehicles also suggest that helmet use is associated with fewer and less severe injuries. Motorcycle helmets, not bicycle helmets, should be used for all motorized vehicles. Protective clothing such as long-sleeved shirts, heavy pants, gloves, and boots can reduce trauma to the extremities.[78]

Many injuries are precipitated by encounters with rocks, bumps, and holes in the driving surface. Removal of these hazards by developing and maintaining trails for the use of off-road vehicles may help reduce the injury rates.

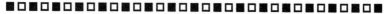
17.4.5 Recommendations for Pediatricians

Anticipatory guidance

Families should be asked, as part of routine counseling, about the kinds of recreational activities in which they engage. Just as those who have a swimming pool merit special counseling, so do families who engage in the use of off-road vehicles. Points to emphasize include:

- Off-road vehicles are particularly dangerous for children younger than 16 years. Children who do not know how to drive a car should not be allowed to operate off-road vehicles.
- Injuries frequently occur to passengers; riding double should not be permitted.
- Four-wheeled vehicles may be more stable than three-wheeled vehicles. Although three-wheeled models are no longer being manufactured, there is an active, although diminishing, market for used ones.
- All riders should wears helmets and protective clothing.
- Parents should never permit the street use of off-road vehicles.
- Flags and lights should be used to make vehicles more visible.
- Drivers of recreational vehicles should not drink alcohol.
- Young drivers should be discouraged from riding motorcycles because they are considerably more dangerous than passenger cars.

Advocacy

Pediatricians should lend support to public education programs, as well as efforts to regulate the use by children of off-road vehicles and to require helmet use. Many injuries occur in remote areas; improved prehospital care networks and emergency medical services could result in a decrease in the number of deaths.

17.5 Equestrian Injury

17.5.1 Scope of the Problem

There are more than 6 million horses in the United States, and 30 million Americans ride horses. The percentage of these riders who are children or adolescents is uncertain, but is thought to be large.[81] There were 240 000 young people involved in 4-H horse and pony programs in the United States in 1993.[82] About 25 000 injuries to pediatric-age horseback riders are treated in emergency departments each year. About three quarters of the injuries occur in children 10 years of age and older; the remaining one quarter are younger than 10 years. About half of all equestrian injuries occur during recreational use near home or on the farm; a smaller proportion occur specifically in sports and recreational settings.[83,84] Injuries most commonly result from falling off the horse and tend to be severe, as reflected by the facts that 20% to 30% of injured riders sustain head or neck injuries, about a third sustain fractures or dislocations, and at least 10% of the injured are hospitalized.[81,83] About 2000 children and adolescents are hospitalized each year for horse-related injuries. Injuries to horseback riders without helmets are comparable in severity to injuries sustained by pedestrians struck by automobiles.[85]

17.5.2 Risk Factors

Unlike many other classes of pediatric injury, horse-associated injuries are more common in girls, which may reflect frequency of exposure. Severity of injury is associated with the likelihood of a head injury; three quarters of deaths and the majority of hospitalizations are due to head injury.[81] Eight of ten head injuries are the result of falling from or being thrown from a horse.[85] Hospitalization and head injury are highly associated with not wearing a helmet.[86] Helmet use appears more common and more acceptable to participants in English-style riding than to those involved in Western-style riding.

Other risk factors have not been well-studied. The role of particular settings (eg, competitive riding), the breed of horse, the level of supervision, and the skill and experience of the rider are unknown.

17.5.3 Intervention Strategies

Despite the rather sparse epidemiologic knowledge of horseback riding injuries, a number of intervention strategies are considered reasonable. The AAP recommends the following[86]:

- All riders should wear helmets at all times while riding a horse. These should be hard shell helmets that meet the industry-wide ASTM standard (F1163-90) and are certified by the Safety Equipment Institute.

(Not all helmets available are so certified.) The United States Pony Club and other riding organizations require such helmets in all events, but this is not the case for all riding organizations.

- Riding activities should be supervised commensurate with the skill level of the rider.

- The horses that children ride should be appropriate for the capabilities of the young rider.

- All young riders should receive proper education and instruction that emphasize risk reduction and safety practices as well as riding skills.

Some evidence exists that nonuse of helmets is less related to lack of knowledge of their importance than to design characteristics that make them unappealing. Some riders find helmets uncomfortable, expensive, and inappropriate for some riding styles.[87]

17.5.4 Recommendations for Pediatricians

Pediatricians should inform parents and children about the risks of horseback riding, particularly emphasizing the importance of light, comfortable, certified helmets, qualified instruction, and adequate supervision. As in bicycle riding, helmets that have been in a crash, with or without visible damage, should be replaced. The physician may also emphasize the following additional important safety practices[88,89]:

- *Instruction and supervision:* Emphasize that riders receive training from competent instructors who teach safety. Children should be taught the proper techniques for mounting, dismounting, and controlling a horse. Those not competent in these skills should ride only with direct supervision. Children younger than 6 years should not ride alone. All children should be supervised around horses because they may be kicked, bitten, dragged, or trampled on. Children should never be tied to a horse or strapped to a saddle.

- *Clothing and footwear:* Avoid loose-fitting clothes that may snag on tree limbs or other objects while riding. All riders using stirrups should wear boots or shoes that have a heel and completely cover their ankles.

- *Equipment:* Inspect all equipment before riding. Make sure each piece of equipment is securely fastened.

Pediatricians can use their influence to help assure that all organized equestrian clubs or organizations, both local and national, require the use of certified helmets at all times.

17.6 The Role of a Multisport Helmet

A common theme in the epidemiology of recreational injuries is the central importance of head injuries in terms of frequency, severity, disability, and mortality. Sports and recreational activities account for about 20% of all brain injuries to children.[90] Head injuries account for disproportionately large percentages of hospital admissions. Hospital admissions are twice as common among patients with head injury as those with other injuries.[91] The majority of deaths from recreational injuries are caused by brain injury.

Helmets have been found to be highly protective in impacts sustained in recreational activities such as cycling and horseback riding. While bicycling is the major source of head trauma in school-age children, these children also experience considerable head trauma from skating, horseback riding, and playground activities. Younger children suffer head trauma from these causes as well as from children's vehicles such as wagons, scooters, and other riding toys.[91] It has been suggested that physicians and parents would be interested in an inexpensive multisport helmet that children could wear for a variety of impact-prone activities.[92] Any multisport helmet must balance the needs for comfort, protection, and affordability. For example, a helmet that is optimally protective for equestrian activities may not be optimal for skateboarding because it is too hot and heavy. For a helmet to be widely available, it may need to cost less than $20. It seems better to design a helmet that provides good protection and is widely accepted rather than design a helmet that provides excellent protection but is not accepted by parents and children. It has been suggested that the helmets be promoted for children between the ages of 5 and 14 years and for a limited set of activities that would include nonmotorized wheeled sports, ice skating, and playground activities.[92]

In 1994, the Snell Memorial Foundation issued a standard (N-94) for a multipurpose helmet for use in nonmotorized sports.[93] The standard addresses the four critical aspects of a sports helmet: impact management, helmet stability, the strap retention system, and the extent of protection. The N-94 standard differs from the bicycle helmet standard in two ways:

1. The standard requires more head coverage, especially in the back of the head because skaters are more likely to fall backward (and bicyclists forward).

2. The standard accounts for multiple impacts. Skaters are likely to experience a number of minor falls prior to a major fall. Therefore, the standard requires that the helmet retain its impact-absorbing properties after a number of small impacts.

Helmets meeting this standard are appropriate for wheeled sports (such as cycling and skateboarding) and playground activities, but not for skiing, team sports, or motorized recreational vehicles.

The concept of multisport helmets is new and evolving. As of late 1995, at least five manufacturers have brought to market multisport helmets. As such helmets become increasingly available, it remains to be seen how well they are accepted and how effective they are in controlling head injury in everyday recreational activities.

17.7 Resources

1. American Academy of Pediatrics
   141 Northwest Point Blvd
   PO Box 927
   Elk Grove Village, IL 60009-0927
   Publications Department: 847-228-5005

   TIPP materials on bicycle safety.

2. Bicycle Helmet Safety Institute
   4611 7th St
   Arlington, VA 22204-1419
   703-486-0100 (telephone and fax)

3. Consumer Product Safety Commission
National Injury Information Clearinghouse
US Consumer Product Safety Commission
Washington, DC 20207
301-504-0424
301-504-0124 (fax)

Statistics on emergency department–treated, product-related injuries.

4. CSN Rural Injury Prevention Resource Center
National Farm Medicine Center
100 North Oak Ave
Marshfield, WI 54449
715-389-4999
715-389-4950

Resource packets on all-terrain vehicles, equestrian injuries, and other injuries prevalent in rural areas. The center is supported by funding from the Maternal and Child Health Bureau.

5. Harborview Injury Prevention and Research Center
325 Ninth Ave, ZX-10
Seattle, WA 98104
206-521-1520
206-521-1562 (fax)

Harborview has produced a variety of educational materials, posters, brochures, and manuals used in their community-wide helmet promotion campaign.

6. Johns Hopkins Injury Prevention Center
The Johns Hopkins School of Hygiene and Public Health
624 North Broadway
Baltimore, MD 21205-1996

"Injuries to Bicyclists: A National Perspective" is a comprehensive monograph on the epidemiology of bicycle related injuries. The monograph is available from the CDC's National Center for Injury Prevention and Control.

7. National Center for Injury Prevention & Control
4770 Buford Highway, NE
Atlanta, GA 30341-3724
404-488-4400
404-488-4349 (fax)

For an epidemiologic review, ask for a copy of *Injuries to Bicyclists:
A National Perspective*, which was developed by the Johns Hopkins
Injury Prevention Research Center in cooperation with the Snell
Memorial Foundation. For bicycle helmet recommendations for
public health agencies ask for *Injury-Control Recommendations:
Bicycle Helmets*, a special issue of *MMWR*.

8. National SAFE KIDS Campaign
111 Michigan Avenue, NW
Washington, DC 20010
202-939-4993
301-650-8038 (fax)

The Safe Kids Campaign offers advice and materials for developing bicycle safety awareness and helmet use activities in community
campaigns.

9. Snell Memorial Foundation
PO Box 493
St. James, NY 11780
516-862-6440
516-862-6545 (fax)

Information on the Snell helmet standard and educational materials
regarding the importance of helmets.

10. Washington State 4-H Foundation
7612 Pioneer Way
Puyallup, WA 98371-4998
206-840-4570

The foundation has a video, *Every Time Every Ride*, on the value
and importance of helmets in equestrian sport and recreation.

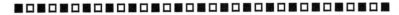
11. World Health Organization Helmet Initiative
Center for Injury Control
The Rollins School of Public Health
Emory University
1518 Clifton Rd, NE
Atlanta, GA 30322
404-727-9377
404-727-8744 (fax)

Information on helmet use initiatives internationally.

References

1. Bijur PE, Trumble A, Harel Y, Overpeck MD, Jones D, Scheidt PC. Sports and recreation injuries in US children and adolescents. *Arch Pediatr Adolesc Med.* 1995; 149:1009–1016

2. *The Bicycle Institute of America's Bicycling Reference Book,* 1993–1994. Washington, DC: The Bicycle Institute of America; 1993

3. Baker SP, Li G, Fowler C, Dannenberg AL. *Injuries to Bicyclists: A National Perspective.* Baltimore, MD: The Johns Hopkins Injury Prevention Center; 1993

4. Centers for Disease Control and Prevention. CDC surveillance summaries. Injury-control recommendations: bicycle helmets. *MMWR Morb Mortal Wkly Rep.* 1995; 44(RR-1):1–17

5. Hu X, Wesson DE, Chipman ML, Parkin PC. Bicycling exposure and severe injuries in school-age children: a population-based study. *Arch Pediatr Adolesc Med.* 1995; 149:437–441

6. Sacks JJ, Holmgreen P, Smith SM, Sosin DM. Bicycle-associated head injuries and deaths in the United States from 1984 through 1988: how many are preventable? *JAMA.* 1991;266:3016–3018

7. Thompson RS, Rivara FP, Thompson DC. A case-control study of the effectiveness of bicycle safety helmets. *N Engl J Med.* 1989;320:1361–1367

8. Kraus JF, Fife D, Conroy C. Incidence, severity, and outcome of brain injuries involving bicycles. *Am J Public Health.* 1987;77:76–78

9. Gallagher SS, Finison K, Guyer B, Goodenough S. The incidence of injuries among 87,000 Massachusetts children and adolescents: results of the 1980–81 statewide childhood injury prevention program surveillance system. *Am J Public Health.* 1984; 74:1340–1347

10. Widome MD. Pediatric injury prevention for the practitioner. *Curr Probl Pediatr.* 1991;21:428–468

11. Sargent JD, Peck MG, Weitzman M. Bicycle-mounted child seats: injury risk and prevention. *Am J Dis Child.* 1988;142:765–767

12. Tanz RR, Christoffel KK. Tykes on bikes: injuries associated with bicycle-mounted child seats. *Pediatr Emerg Care.* 1991;7:297–301

13. Selbst SM, Alexander D, Ruddy R. Bicycle-related injuries. *Am J Dis Child.* 1987; 141:140–144

14. Waller JA. Bicycle ownership, use, and injury patterns among elementary school children. *Pediatrics.* 1971;47:1042–1050

15. Schubert J. Why cyclists should ride with traffic: it's just madness for bicyclists to ride facing traffic. *Bicycling.* 1979;20:20–24

16. National Highway Traffic Safety Administration. *Traffic Safety Facts 1993.* Washington, DC: US Department of Transportation; 1994

17. Williams AF. Factors in the initiation of bicycle–motor vehicle collisions. *Am J Dis Child.* 1976;130:370–377

18. Haddon W Jr. Advances in the epidemiology of injuries as a basis for public policy. *Public Health Rep.* 1980;95:411–421

19. Burke ER. Safety standards for bicycle helmets. *Phys Sportsmed.* 1988;16:148–153

20. American Academy of Pediatrics, Committee on Injury and Poison Prevention. Bicycle helmets. *Pediatrics.* 1995;95:609–610

21. Snell Memorial Foundation. *1990 Standard for Protective Headgear for Use in Bicycling.* St James, NY: Snell Memorial Foundation, Inc; 1990

22. Weiss BD, Duncan B. Bicycle helmet use by children: knowledge and behavior of physicians. *Am J Public Health.* 1986;76:1022–1023

23. Howland J, Sargent J, Weitzman M, et al. Barriers to bicycle helmet use among children: results of focus groups with fourth, fifth, and sixth graders. *Am J Dis Child.* 1989; 143:741–744

24. DiGuiseppi CG, Rivara FP, Koepsell TD. Attitudes toward bicycle helmet ownership and use by school-age children. *Am J Dis Child.* 1990;144:83–86

25. Runyan CW, Runyan DK. How can physicians get kids to wear bicycle helmets? a prototypic challenge in injury prevention. *Am J Public Health.* 1991;81:972–973

26. Parkin PC, Spence LJ, Hu X, Kranz KE, Shortt LG, Wesson DE. Evaluation of a promotional strategy to increase bicycle helmet use by children. *Pediatrics.* 1993; 91:772–777

27. Parkin PC, Hu X, Spence LJ, Kranz KE, Shortt LG, Wesson DE. Evaluation of a subsidy program to increase bicycle helmet use by children of low income families. *Pediatrics.* 1995;96:283–287

28. Rivara FP, Thompson DC, Thompson RS, et al. The Seattle children's bicycle helmet campaign: changes in helmet use and head injury admissions. *Pediatrics.* 1994; 93:567–569

29. Coté TR, Sacks JJ, Lambert-Huber DA, Dannenberg AL, Kresnow MJ, Schmidt ER. Bicycle helmet use among Maryland children: effect of legislation and education. *Pediatrics.* 1992;89:1216–1220

30. Schubert J. Bike dangers. *Pediatrics.* 1993;92:882–883

31. Graitcer PL, Kellermann AL, Christoffel T. A review of educational and legislative strategies to promote bicycle helmets. *Inj Preven.* 1995;1:122–129

32. Schieber RA, Branche-Dorsey CM, Ryan GW. Comparison of in-line skating injuries with rollerskating and skateboarding injuries. *JAMA.* 1994;271:1856–1858

33. *American Sports Analysis: Summary Report.* Hartsdale, NY: American Sports Data, Inc; 1995

34. *Guidelines For Establishing In-Line Skate Trails in Parks and Recreation Areas.* Minneapolis, MN: International In-line Skating Association; 1992

35. Martin D. Skating by – at 72 mph. *The New York Times.* 1993; November 24:section B-1(col 1–2)

36. Shen WY, Chan KM, Leung PC. Roller skating – is it a dangerous sport? *Br J Sports Med.* 1987;21:125–126

37. Ferkel RD, Mai LL, Ullis KC, Fineman GA. An analysis of roller skating injuries. *Am J Sports Med.* 1981;10:24–30

38. Corcoran M. Survey of roller disco dance injuries. *Irish Med J.* 1980;73:238–239

39. Retsky J, Jaffe D, Christoffel K. Skateboarding injuries in children: a second wave. *Am J Dis Child.* 1991;145:188–192

40. American Academy of Pediatrics, Committee on Injury and Poison Prevention. Skateboard injuries. *Pediatrics.* 1995;95:611–612

41. Morgan WJ, Galloway DJ, Patel AR. Prevention of skateboard injuries. *Scottish Med J.* 1980;25:39–40

42. Illingworth CM, Jay A, Noble D, Collick M. 225 skateboard injuries in children. *Clin Pediatr (Phila).* 1978;17:781–789

43. No ban on skateboard manufacture. *JAMA.* 1979;242:1344

44. Schieber RA, Branche-Dorsey CM. In-line skating injuries: epidemiology and recommendations for prevention. *Sports Med.* 1995;19:427–432

45. Rutherford GW, Friedman J, Beale SP. *HIA Hazard Analysis Report–Skateboards.* Bethesda, MD: US Consumer Product Safety Commission; 1977

46. Fyfe IS, Guion AJ. Accident prevention in skateboarding. *J Sports Med Phys Fitness.* 1979;19:265–266

47. Hawkins RW, Lyne ED. Skateboarding fractures. *Am J Sports Med.* 1981;9:99–102

48. Esses S, Zaremba M, Langer F. Roller skating injuries. *Contemp Orthop.* 1982; 5:99–103

49. Larkin M. Sliding into sledding injuries. *Phys Sportsmed.* 1991;19:90–102

50. Ridenour MV. Children's snow sleds: age appropriateness and safety. *Percept Mot Skills.* 1989;68:883–890

51. Dershewitz R, Gallagher SS, Donahoe P. Sledding-related injuries in children. *Am J Dis Child.* 1990;144:1071–1073

52. Levy DJ, Buck J. Safety on the slopes. *Contemp Pediatr.* 1994 11:51–58

53. Johnson RJ. Skiing and snowboarding injuries: when schussing is a pain. *Postgrad Med.* 1990 88:36–51

54. Blitzer CM, Johnson RJ, Ettlinger CF, Aggeborn K. Downhill skiing injuries in children. *Am J Sports Med.* 1984;12:142–147

55. Ungerholm S, Gustavsson J. Skiing safety in children: a prospective study of downhill skiing injuries and their relation to the skier and his equipment. *Int J Sports Med.* 1985;6:353–358

56. Ungerholm S, Gierup J, Lindsjo U, Magnusson A. Skiing injuries in children: lower leg fractures. *Int J Sports Med.* 1985;6:292–297

57. Chow TK, Corbett SW, Farstad DJ. Spectrum of injuries from snowboarding. *J Trauma.* 1996;41:321–325

58. Callé SC, Evans JT. Snowboarding trauma. *J Pediatr Surg.* 1995;30:791–794

59. Pino EC, Colville MR. Snowboard injuries. *Am J Sports Med.* 1989;17:778–781

60. Prall JA, Winston KR, Brennan R. Severe snowboarding injuries. *Injury.* 1995; 26:539–542

61. Davidson TM, Laliotis AT. Snowboarding injuries: a four-year study with comparison with alpine ski injuries. *West J Med.* 1996;164:231–237

62. Brown JM, Ramsey LC, Weiss AL. Ski helmets: an idea whose time has come. *Contemp Pediatr.* 1997;14:115–125

63. American Academy of Pediatrics, Committee on Accident and Poison Prevention. Snowmobile statement. *Pediatrics.* 1988;82:798–799

64. Van Rooy CW. Minibikes. *Pediatrics.* 1981;67:154

65. Cerrelli EC. *1994 Traffic Crashes, Injuries, and Fatalities — Preliminary Report.* Washington, DC: National Highway Traffic Safety Administration; 1995

66. *Fatality Facts, 1995 Edition.* Arlington VA: Insurance Institute for Highway Safety; 1995

67. Salatka M, Arzemanian S, Kraus JF, Anderson CL. Fatal and severe injury: scooter and moped crashes in California, 1985. *Am J Public Health.* 1990;80:1122–1124

68. Westman JA, Morrow G III. Moped injuries in children. *Pediatrics.* 1984;74:820–822

69. *Update of All-Terrain Vehicle (ATV) Deaths and Injuries Using Data Available as of June 30, 1995.* Washington, DC: US Consumer Product Safety Commission; September 28, 1995 (memorandum); document 6003

70. Hargarten SW. All-terrain vehicle mortality in Wisconsin: a case study in injury control. *Am J Emerg Med.* 1991;9:149–52

71. Kriel RL, Sheehan M, Krach LE, Kriel HD, Rolewicz TF. Pediatric head injury resulting from all-terrain vehicle accidents. *Pediatrics.* 1986;78:933–935

72. Sneed RC, Stover SL, Fine PR. Spinal cord injury associated with all-terrain vehicle accidents. *Pediatrics.* 1986;77:271–274

73. Stevens WS, Rodgers BM, Newman BM. Pediatric trauma associated with all-terrain vehicles. *J Pediatr.* 1986;109:25–29

74. Dolan MA, Knapp JF, Andres J. Three-wheel and four-wheel all-terrain vehicle injuries in children. *Pediatrics.* 1989;84:694–698

75. Bantz E, Auerbach J. Leg burns from mopeds. *Pediatrics.* 1982;70:304–305

76. Final Consent Decree, United States of America v American Honda Motor Co. Inc. et al. US District Court for the District of Columbia, Civil Action No. 87–3525 GAG; 1988

77. Canadian Pediatric Society, Accident Prevention Committee. Two-, three- and four-wheeled unlicensed, off-road vehicles. *Can Med Assoc J.* 1987;136:119–120

78. American Academy of Pediatrics, Committee on Accident and Poison Prevention. All-terrain vehicles: two-, three-, and four-wheeled unlicensed motorized vehicles. *Pediatrics.* 1987;79:306–308

79. Rutledge R, Stutts J. The association of helmet use with the outcome of motorcycle crash injury when controlling for crash/injury severity. *Accid Anal Preven.* 1993; 25:347–353

80. Kraus JF, Peek C, McArthur DL, Williams A. The effect of the 1992 California motorcycle helmet use law on motorcycle crash fatalities and injuries. *JAMA.* 1994; 272:1506–1511

81. Nelson DE, Bixby-Hammett D. Equestrian injuries in children and young adults. *Am J Dis Child.* 1992:146:611–614

82. *Fact Sheet: Horse and Children.* Marshfield, WI: CSN Rural Injury Prevention Resource Center, National Farm Medicine Center; June 1995

83. Centers for Disease Control. Injuries associated with horseback riding – United States, 1987 and 1988. *MMWR Morb Mortal Wkly Rep.* 1990;39:329–332

84. Hamilton MG, Tranmer BI. Nervous system injuries in horseback-riding accidents. *J Trauma.* 1993;34:227–232

85. Bond GR, Christoph RA, Rodgers BM. Pediatric equestrian injuries: assessing the impact of helmet use. *Pediatrics.* 1995;95:487–489

86. American Academy of Pediatrics, Committee on Sports Medicine and Fitness. Horseback riding and head injuries. *Pediatrics.* 1992;82:512

87. Condie C, Rivara FP, Bergman AB. Strategies of a successful campaign to promote the use of equestrian helmets. *Public Health Rep.* 1993;108:121–126

88. Nelson DE, Rivara FP, Condie C. Helmets and horseback riders. *Am J Prev Med.* 1994; 10:15–19

89. Harborview Injury Prevention and Research Center. *Equestrian Safety: A Guide to Promotion of Helmet Use for Riding Clubs and Communities.* Pullman, WA: Washington State University Cooperative Extension; 1995

90. Rivara FP. Epidemiology and prevention of pediatric traumatic brain injury. *Pediatr Ann.* 1994;23:12–17

91. Baker SP, Fowler C, Li G, Warner M, Dannenberg AL. Head injuries incurred by children and young adults during informal recreation. *Am J Public Health.* 1994; 84:649–652

92. Rivara FP, ed. *Proceedings: Forum on Head Protection in Recreational Sports.* Seattle, WA: Harborview Injury Prevention and Research Center, University of Washington; 1994

93. *Standard for Protective Headgear for Use in Non-Motorized Sports.* St James, NY: Snell Memorial Foundation, Inc; 1994

CHAPTER 18

Injuries Caused by Animals

18.1 Introduction

Animal ownership is extremely popular worldwide. Animals provide companionship and assist in a variety of other functions in millions of households. Each year, many parents are faced with the responsibility of choosing appropriate pets to join their families. Although some may view these decisions as straightforward, parents of young children should view such decisions with great care. Parents should carefully consider the health and safety issues associated with pet ownership in addition to the pet's physical appearance and adult size. When animals are properly matched with families, family members can look forward to many years of rewarding interaction.

18.2 Safety Issues

Many human health problems are linked to exposure to animals. Most parents, however, when asked to identify the most common health issue related to pet ownership, correctly cite bite injuries. In the United States alone, between 2 and 4 million animal bites are reported each year.[1] In a survey of one pediatric practice, 20% of children had been bitten at least once by a dog.[2] It is estimated that 0.5% to 1.5% of all emergency department visits by children are due to injuries from animal bites.[3]

Fortunately, most injuries from animal bites are minor, although many severe injuries have been reported[4,5]; an estimated 10 to 20 deaths occur from dog bites each year in the United States.[6,7] As with nonfatal injuries from animal bites, deaths due to animal bites involve a disproportionately higher percentage of infants and young children. One report of 157 fatalities related to dog bites (which occurred over 10 years) indicated that 70% occurred among children who were younger than 10 years.[7] In this report, aggressive breeds of dogs (pit bulls, German shepherds, huskies, malamutes, Doberman pinschers, and rottweilers) were the most common offenders.

Children and young adults are most often the victims of nonfatal animal bites. The highest incidence occurs in school children, 5 to 14 years old, who may overexcite, mistreat, or unintentionally threaten an animal. Although this age group makes up only 20% of the US population, it accounts for almost half of all injuries from domestic animals.[1] Boys are bitten by dogs twice as frequently as girls, perhaps because they are more active and play more aggressively. Girls, however, are twice as likely to be bitten by cats.

Dog bites account for 90% of injuries caused by animals. Slightly less than 10% are caused by cats. Dogs that most often bite are not strays or wild, but are usually owned by the family or neighbors and are well known to the victim.[3] It is therefore imperative that parents give careful thought and use sound judgment when choosing a pet.

18.3 Behavioral Issues

Family pets should be well-trained and properly disciplined as they grow up, which includes careful monitoring of their interactions with children. Children are often responsible for the injuries that occur from pets. This is especially true in children younger than 5 years, who may not realize that playful actions can cause an angry or defensive reaction from an otherwise friendly pet. In this age group of children, more than two thirds of pet-related injuries are provoked by the child.[3] Children need to be advised that certain animal activities need to be recognized as "private times" for the animal. Mealtimes occupy the top of this list. Dogs can be very possessive and protective of their food and should not be disturbed while eating. In general, respect for animals should be engendered in all children.

18.4 Selecting a Pet

When a child expresses the desire for a pet, parents are often faced with a dilemma. The most popular animal requested is a dog. Dogs, however, are also involved in most animal-related injuries. The risk of dog bites can be lessened if parents use sound judgment in the timing of acquisition and choice of a pet. If a pet, but not necessarily a dog, is desired, a less-hazardous type of animal should be considered, particularly for a preschool child.

Having a dog as a pet is best deferred until children are old enough to be trusted to understand which interactions with the dog may be perceived by the animal as threatening. This ability is rare in children younger than 4 years and unusual in children younger than 6. Factors to be considered at any age are the maturity and disposition of the child and the animal.

Pets other than dogs include tropical or other fish, small birds (such as parakeets), and small rodents such as hamsters or gerbils. Cats make good pets. Kittens, however, tend to bite and scratch frequently during play and when they are frightened. These animals are also probably best avoided when there are young children (<4 years) in the family. Cats and kittens are also a poor choice of pet if a child has asthma. Raccoons, ferrets, and other wild animals are inappropriate as household pets.

Parents should observe some selection guidelines when choosing a dog as their family pet. Although little consensus exists about which breeds of dogs are most suitable for children, most authorities agree that dogs bred for their aggressive qualities are dangerous. More than half of all severe dog bites involve pit bulls, German shepherds, large mixed breeds, and, to a lesser extent, other large dogs such as rottweilers and Dobermans. However, many smaller dogs (eg, poodles, terriers, and mixed breeds) can also be aggressive. A list of dogs known for their gentle behavior is presented in Table 18.1, p 382.

18.5 Parenting Guidelines

A child's relationship with a pet can be a valuable part of growing up. However, along with pet exposure or ownership comes a number of health concerns. It is important to be a responsible pet owner by providing proper care for pets. Parents should be certain that pets receive veterinary care, particularly rabies immunization. Children should be taught never to bother animals that are eating or sleeping, never to approach an animal they do not know well, and never to tease an animal. Children who are too young to understand these guidelines are probably too young to have a pet. Tables 18.2, p 382, and 18.3, p 383, list other helpful hints for parents regarding their children's interactions with animals.

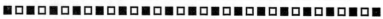
TABLE 18.1.
Recommended Pets That Are Generally Safe With Children

Large Dogs	Small Dogs
Bearded collie	Beagle
Border collie	Bichon frise
Boxer	Boston terrier
Collie	Cairn terrier
English springer spaniel	Jack Russell terrier
French bull dog (medium sized)	Norfolk terrier
Golden retriever	Norwich terrier
Greyhound	Poodle (toy)
Labrador retriever	Pug
Poodle (standard)	Sheltie
	Yorkshire terrier

Cats

Domestic short haired

Domestic long haired

Pure bred, eg, Siamese, tend to be less docile with small children

Others

Rabbits	Care and maintenance are very important.
Mice/guinea pigs/hamsters	Care and maintenance are very important.

TABLE 18.2.
What to Tell Children About Animals

- Avoid *all* strange animals, especially those that are wild or appear sick or injured. The same techniques employed in teaching children not to talk to strangers should be used to teach children not to approach strange animals.
- Never break up a fight between animals (even when his or her own pet is involved).
- Do not disturb an animal that is eating or sleeping. Always speak to an animal that is being approached to avoid startling the animal.
- Never tease an animal, pull an animal's tail, or take away an animal's food, bone, or toy.
- Never hold an animal close to your face.
- Respect animals; never intentionally hurt an animal (parents should set a good example by their own behavior).

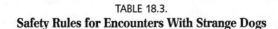

TABLE 18.3.
Safety Rules for Encounters With Strange Dogs

Remain calm! Stop, stand still, and speak softly.

Wait and see what the dog is going to do.

Look for the signs of an unsafe dog:
- Rigid body
- Still tail at "half mast"
- Shrill, hysterical bark
- Crouching position, head lowered, nose close to ground
- Staring expression
- An attempt to circle behind you

Pivot slowly if the dog tries to circle behind you. Wait until the dog stops moving, then move away slowly.

Never turn your back on a dog moving toward you.

Never touch a strange dog.

Never strike, kick, or make any other threatening gesture during the encounter.

Do not hand a person a package or shake hands when the persons' dog is nearby; this may be interpreted as a threat by a dog.

Do not make the first overture of friendship with a dog. Allow the dog to initiate friendship by smelling you.

18.6 Management of Injuries From Animal Bites

Wounds from animal bites should be managed in the same way as non-bite wounds. The primary focus should be directed toward thorough cleansing of the wound, which is the most effective means of preventing secondary infection. Infection occurs in approximately 5% of wounds from dog bites and in up to 50% of wounds from cat bites.

The higher rate of infection in cat bite wounds is thought to be due to the mechanical nature of the injury. Cats have sharp, small-caliber teeth that inflict deep puncture wounds that may be difficult to cleanse, whereas the teeth of dogs rip the skin and cause larger (more open) punctures and lacerations that tend to be easier to cleanse and, therefore, less prone to develop infection.

Wounds should be cleansed as soon as possible after the injury. Parents should be advised to clean smaller wounds at home with mild soap and plenty of water. Seek medical attention for larger wounds; if they require repair, they should be properly anesthetized and irrigated with copious amounts of sterile fluid (100 cc of normal saline per 1 cm of laceration). Crushed, devitalized tissue should be judiciously debrided.

Antibiotics should be administered to children whose wounds appear infected. In addition, high-risk injuries, including the following, may require prophylactic antibiotics:

- Injury from any cat bite
- Deep puncture wounds from a dog bite
- Deep (hard to cleanse) lacerations from a dog bite
- Any nonsuperficial animal bite on the hand

The use of prophylactic antibiotics remains controversial for two types of injuries from animal bites — wounds to the face and wounds requiring sutures. Because facial wounds have a relatively low incidence of secondary infection, most patients do not benefit from administration of prophylactic antibiotics. With cat bites or other deep wounds, antibiotics should be administered. Although it is difficult to predict which wounds requiring sutures will become infected, the majority will not. Nevertheless, most "experts" tend to use prophylactic antibiotics when sutured wounds are more than superficial and not easily cleansed.

Wounds from cat and dog bites can become infected with a variety of organisms, including *Pasteurella multocida* (in up to 50% of cat bite wounds and up to 25% of dog bite wounds), *Staphylococcus aureus, Streptococcus* species, and other enteric and anaerobic pathogens. Often, more than one organism is isolated from an infected wound. Therefore, a broad-spectrum antibiotic should be used for treatment. The most widely used treatment is amoxicillin/clavulanic acid (Augmentin). Infection in children allergic to penicillin can be managed with erythromycin.

Tetanus and rabies are other possible infections from animal bites that should always be considered. Tetanus prophylaxis should be given in accordance with the recommendations given in the *Red Book* (Report of the Committee on Infectious Diseases, American Academy of Pediatrics).[8] Rabies immunization should be given for treatment of bites by an unobservable carnivore in a rabies-endemic area. In many areas of the United States, bites by stray or otherwise unobservable dogs or cats are considered to be prone to have rabies. Rabies prophylaxis consists of administration of rabies immune globulin (20 IU/kg) at the time of initial wound management and human diploid cell vaccine, which is given in a 1-cc dose (for all patients) on days 0 (the day the wound is inflicted, if possible), 3, 7, 14, and 28. Consult the *Red Book* for further details. Local or state public health authorities should be consulted whenever there are questions about the appropriateness of rabies prophylaxis.

References

1. Baker MD. Bites and scratches: when pets fight back. *Contemp Pediatr.* 1989;6:76–84

2. Lauer EA, White WC, Lauer BA. Dog bites: a neglected problem in accident prevention. *Am J Dis Child.* 1982;136:202–204

3. Avner JR, Baker MD. Dog bites in urban children. *Pediatrics.* 1991;88:55–57

4. Wright JC. Severe attacks by dogs: characteristics of the dogs, the victims, and attack settings. *Public Health Rep.* 1985;100:55–61

5. Brogan TV, Bratton SL, Dowd MD, Hegenbarth MA. Severe dog bites in children. *Pediatrics.* 1995;96:947–950

6. Pinckney LE, Kennedy LA. Traumatic deaths from dog attacks in the United States. *Pediatrics.* 1982;69:193–196

7. Sacks JJ, Sattin RW, Bonzo SE. Dog bite-related fatalities from 1979 through 1988. *JAMA.* 1989;262:1489–1492

8. American Academy of Pediatrics. Peter G, ed. *1997 Red Book: Report of the Committee on Infectious Diseases.* 24th ed. Elk Grove Village, IL: American Academy of Pediatrics; 1997

Injury Death Rates

Injury Deaths and Death Rates Among Children and Teenagers: United States, 1995

	Birth-19 y		Under 1 y		1-4 y		5-9 y		10-14 y		15-19 y	
	Deaths	Rate	Deaths	Rate	Deaths	Rate	Deaths	Rate	Deaths	Rate	Deaths	Rate
All Injury	20 269	26.7	1129	29.3	2746	17.4	1773	9.2	2686	14.2	11 935	66.1
MOTOR VEHICLE												
TRAFFIC, ALL (a)	7940	10.5	172	4.5	703	4.5	854	4.4	1104	5.8	5107	28.3
Unintentional (b)	7925	10.5	172	4.5	703	4.5	854	4.4	1102	5.8	5094	28.2
Occupant	4680	8.3	126	4.2	361	2.9	369	2.4	513	3.6	3311	25.2
Motorcyclist	156	0.3	0	*	0	*	3	*	25	0.2	128	1.0
Pedal cyclist	292	0.4	0	*	8	*	96	0.5	126	0.7	62	0.3
Pedestrian	1100	1.5	10	*	235	1.5	285	1.5	262	1.4	308	1.7
Unspecified	1690	$	36	$	97	$	101	$	175	$	1281	$
FIREARM	5285	7.0	8	*	97	0.6	107	0.6	641	3.4	4432	24.5
Unintentional	440	0.6	0	*	20	0.1	32	0.2	129	0.7	259	1.4
Suicide	1450	1.9	na	na	na	na	1	*	183	1.0	1266	7.0
Homicide	3249	4.3	8	*	74	0.5	70	0.4	310	1.6	2787	15.4
Undetermined	115	0.2	0	*	3	*	4	*	18	*	90	0.5
Other	31								1		30	0.2
POISONING (c)	480	0.6	19	*	47	0.3	21	0.1	45	0.2	348	1.9
Unintentional	258	0.3	7	*	31	0.2	14	*	28	0.1	178	1.0
Suicide	151	0.2	na	na	na	na	2	*	14	*	135	0.7
Undetermined	55	0.1	8	*	10	*	1	*	2	*	34	0.2
FALL (d)	271	0.4	20	0.5	42	0.3	28	0.1	36	0.2	145	0.8
Unintentional	218	0.3	20	0.5	41	0.3	27	0.1	33	0.2	97	0.5
Suicide	42	0.1	na	na	na	na			1	*	41	0.2

	Birth-19 y		Under 1 y		1-4 y		5-9 y		10-14 y		15-19 y	
	Deaths	Rate	Deaths	Rate	Deaths	Rate	Deaths	Rate	Deaths	Rate	Deaths	Rate
SUFFOCATION	1438	1.9	424	11.0	200	1.3	91	0.5	211	1.1	512	2.8
Unintentional	739	1.0	376	9.8	162	1.0	74	0.4	60	0.3	67	0.4
Suicide	497	0.7	na	na	na	na	3	*	123	0.7	371	2.1
Homicide	169	0.2	31	0.8	34	0.2	13	*	18	*	73	0.4
Undetermined	33	0.0	17	*	4	*	1	*	10	*	1	*
DROWNING (e)	1567	2.1	74	1.9	557	3.5	229	1.2	246	1.3	461	2.6
Unintentional	1502	2.0	59	1.5	537	3.4	222	1.2	242	1.3	442	2.4
FIRE/HOT OBJECT/ SUBSTANCE (f)	1014	1.3	78	2.0	488	3.1	249	1.3	115	0.6	84	0.5
Unintentional	913	1.2	66	1.7	455	2.9	225	1.2	99	0.5	68	0.4
Homicide	82	0.1	7	*	26	0.2	24	0.1	15	*	10	*
CUT/PIERCE (g)	323	0.4	4	*	18	*	7	*	38	0.2	256	1.4
Homicide	303	0.4	4	*	15	*	6	*	33	0.2	245	1.4
STRUCK BY/ AGAINST	166	0.2	7	*	54	0.3	20	0.1	26	0.1	59	0.3
Unintentional	127	0.2	4	*	48	0.3	19	*	20	0.1	36	0.2
Homicide	39	0.1	3	*	6	*	1	*	6	*	23	0.1
MACHINERY	74	0.1	1	*	14	*	19	*	10	*	30	0.2
PEDAL CYCLE, OTHER	32	0.0	0	*	3	*	10	*	11	*	8	*
PEDESTRIAN, OTHER	233	0.3	5	*	109	0.7	24	0.1	29	0.2	66	0.4
TRANSP, OTHER	235	0.3	3	*	22	0.1	44	0.2	66	0.3	100	0.6

Injury Deaths and Death Rates Among Children and Teenagers: United States, 1995, continued

Injury Deaths and Death Rates Among Children and Teenagers: United States, 1995, continued

	Birth-19 y		Under 1 y		1-4 y		5-9 y		10-14 y		15-19 y	
	Deaths	Rate	Deaths	Rate	Deaths	Rate	Deaths	Rate	Deaths	Rate	Deaths	Rate
NATURAL/ENVIRONMENTAL (h)	116	0.2	19	*	38	0.2	8	*	19	*	32	0.2
Unintentional	115	0.2	19	*	38	0.2	8	*	19	*	31	0.2
OVEREXERTION	2	*	0	*					1	*	1	*
OTHER SPECIFIED	481	0.6	146	3.8	154	1.0	32	0.2	49	0.3	100	0.6
NOT ELSEWHERE CLASSIFIED	159	0.2	15	*	46	0.3	8	*	11	*	79	0.4
NOT SPECIFIED	453	0.6	134	3.5	154	1.0	22	0.1	28	0.1	115	0.6
All injury												
Unintentional	13 122	17.3	761	19.8	2249	14.3	1598	8.3	1916	10.1	6598	36.5
Suicide	2227	2.9	na	na	na	na	7	*	330	1.7	1890	10.5
Homicide	4586	6.1	311	8.1	452	2.9	157	0.8	404	2.1	3262	18.1
Undetermined	302	0.4	57	1.5	45	0.3	11	*	35	0.2	154	0.9
Other	32	0.0	0	*	0	*	0	*	1	*	31	0.2
Adverse events (i)	112	0.1	26	0.7	31	0.2	14	*	16	*	25	0.1
All causes of death	59 661	78.7	29 583	768.8	6393	40.6	3780	19.7	4816	25.5	15 089	83.5
Population	75 790 153		3 848 106		15 743 042		19 219 956		18 914 532		18 064 517	

Source: National Center for Health Statistics. Data computed by the Office of Analysis, Epidemiology and Health Promotion from data compiled by the Division of Vital Statistics; US Bureau of Census population file RESD0795.

In addition, see the following table, "Proposed Matrix for External Cause of Injury Mortality and Morbidity Data," for E codes.

Rates are deaths per 100 000 population.

* Rates based on fewer than 20 deaths are unstable.

$ In the rate calculations, the 4th digit .9 codes were proportionately distributed according to the known distribution of occupant and motorcyclist deaths in each age group.

0.0 rate is greater than 0 but less than 0.5.

a) Includes mvt suicide and undetermined.
b) Includes 4th digits .4,.5,.8 not shown separately.
c) Includes homicide.
d) Includes homicide and undetermined.
e) Includes suicide, homicide and undetermined.
f) Includes suicide and undetermined.
g) Includes unintentional, suicide and undetermined.
h) Includes suicide.
i) Not considered injury, but part of all external causes.

Proposed Matrix for External Cause of Injury Mortality and Morbidity Data

Mechanism or Cause	Unintentional	Manner or Intent			
		Suicide/ Self-inflicted	Homicide/ Assault	Undetermined	Other
Cut/pierce	E920.0–.9	E956	E966	E986	E974
Drowning/submersion	E830.0–.9, 832.0–.9, 910.0–.9	E954	E964	E984	...
Fall	E880.0–886.9, 888	E957.0–.9	E968.1	E987.0–.9	...
Fire/hot object or substance[1]	E890.0–899, 924.0–.9	E958.1,.2,.7	E961, 968.0,.3	E988.1,.2,.7	...
Fire/fame	E890.0–899	E958.1	E968.0	E988.1	...
Hot object/scald	E924.0–.9	E958.2,.7	E961, 968.3	E988.2,.7	...
Firearm	E922.0–.9	E955.0–.4	E965.0–.4	E985.0–.4	E970
Machinery	E919.0–.9	...	...	...	...
Motor vehicle traffic	E810–819 (.0–.9)	E958.5	E968.5	E988.5	...
Occupant	E810–819 (.0, .1)	...	...		...
Motorcyclist	E810–819 (.2, .3)	...	...		...
Pedal cyclist	E810–819 (.6)	...	...		...
Pedestrian	E810–819 (.7)	...	...		...
Unspecified	E810–819 (.9)	...	...		...
Pedal cyclist, other	E800–807 (.3), E820–825 (.6), E826 (1,.9), 827–829 (.1)	...	...	...	...
Pedestrian, other	E800–807 (.2), E820–825 (.7), E826–829 (.0)	...	...	...	...

■□■□■□■□■□■□■□■□■□■□■□■□■□■□■□■□■□■□■□■

Proposed Matrix for External Cause of Injury Mortality and Morbidity Data, continued

Mechanism or Cause	Unintentional	Manner or Intent			
		Suicide/Self-inflicted	Homicide/Assault	Undetermined	Other
Transport, other	E800–807 (.0–.1, .8–.9), E820–825 (.0–.5,.8–.9), E826 (.2–8), 827–829, (.2–.9) E831.0–9, 833.0–845.9	E958.6	...	E988.6	...
Natural/environmental factors	E900.0–909, 928.0–.2	E958.3	...	E988.3	...
Bites and stings	E905.0–.6, .9, 906.0–.4, .5, .9	...	...	...	...
Overexertion	E927				
Poisoning	E850.0–869.9	E950.0–952.9	E962.0–9	E980.0–982.9	E972
Struck by, against	E916–917.9	...	E960.0, 968.2	...	E973, 975
Suffocation	E911–913.9	E953.0–9	E963	E983.0–9	...
Other specified and classifiable	E846–848, 914–915, 918, E921.0–9, 923.0–9, E925.0–926.9, 929.0–5	E955.5, .9, 958.0, .4	E960.1, 965.5–9, E967.0–9, 968.4	E985.5, 988.0, .4	E971, 978 E990–994, 996, E997.0–2
Other specified, NEC[2]	E928.8, 929.8	E958.8, 959	E968.8, 989	E988.9, 989	E995, 997.8, 977, E998–999
Unspecified	E887, 928.9, 929.9	E958.9	E968.9	E988.9	E976, 997.9
All injury[3]	E800–869, 880–929	E950–959	E960–969	E980–989	E970–978 E990–999

[1]In the text of the chartbook, this category name is simplified to "fire/burn."
[2]Not elsewhere classifiable.
[3]Excludes fatal and nonfatal events caused by adverse events (E-codes E870–E879 and E930–E949).
NOTE: E968.5 and E906.5 are the only codes that are singled out that are in ICD-9-CM but not in ICD-9. All of the other codes that are in CM only are folded into larger groupings in the matrix.

■□■□■□■□■□■□■□■□■□■□■□■□■□■□■□■

Child Advocacy and Partnerships With Government

Most of the important work to control injuries must take place beyond the walls of the physician's office. Pediatricians have a long history of working on behalf of children as advocates on a community level and in concert with governments: local, state, and national. This tradition of advocacy extends back to the founding of pediatrics as a specialty. Abraham Jacobi, in his presidential address at the founding of the American Pediatric Society in 1889 said, "Every physician is by destiny a 'political being'...with many rights and great responsibilities." This discussion is meant to serve as an introduction and encouragement to those who wish to take their concern for the safety of children beyond office practice, where the frustrations are many, but so are the rewards.

B.1 The Need for "Champions"

Good ideas need a "champion." Champions are the people who tenaciously embrace a good idea to solve an unmet need and refuse to let go until the need is met. Their role is to take the idea to those who are affected by the problem, those with authority, those with expertise, and pass it around to generate support and enthusiasm for its implementation. Champions can be most effective if they have access to legislators, political leaders, and power brokers in the legislature, and/or state administration. Pediatricians make great champions. They have knowledge and credibility at the state and local levels.

A champion builds support for his or her idea one person at a time. Champions know that they have a good idea, and they look for opportunities to talk to anyone and everyone to mobilize grassroots support. These discussions, in good faith, give new perspective to the need and proposed solution. Through this process, the project is reshaped and molded to fit local community conditions.

B.2 Child Advocacy: Examples

The following examples demonstrate that energetic and persistent pediatricians — champions — can make a difference in the lives of thousands of children.

B.2.1 Flammable Fabrics

Although the problem of flammable clothing was one of the first issues highlighted by the American Academy of Pediatrics (AAP) Accident Prevention Committee in 1955, early legislation of fabric flammability was weak and poorly enforced. Over the next 2 decades, however, the law was considerably strengthened. Much of the credit for this goes to the efforts of Seattle pediatrician Abe Bergman, who worked with Washington Senator Warren Magnuson to realize the eventual passage of the federal Flammable Fabrics Act of 1977.[1] Dr Bergman further helped assure that a reluctant apparel industry comply with the law by helping to produce a television documentary, *The Burned Child*, which dramatized the problem of clothing ignition to the government and public.

B.2.2 Child Passenger Protection

In 1972, Edward Casey of the Tennessee Department of Public Health recommended the formation of a statewide multidisciplinary Task Force on Accidents. That group included individuals representing government, law enforcement, medicine, education, and public health. Although a universal seat belt usage law was originally proposed, the focus was eventually narrowed to the concept of a child passenger protection bill. Dr Robert Sanders, a pediatrician and county public health officer, soon became keenly aware of the possibilities inherent in such a legislative and public health measure. In his early and innovative advocacy for a state child passenger protection law, Dr Sanders gathered available supporting data and obtained the endorsement of his state AAP chapter, the state medical society, and other medical groups. He recruited like-minded medical colleagues across the state to lobby state lawmakers, and particularly called upon the pediatricians of the lawmakers' children to serve as advocates and lobbyists.

Dr Sanders' first legislative initiatives died in committee. Not discouraged, Sanders and his colleagues regrouped and developed an improved strategy for the subsequent legislative session. They attracted expanded media coverage for the issue and generated wider support and visibility throughout the state. They enlisted endorsements from the governor, the director of the state police, and other influential individuals. A child passenger protection bill finally passed the Tennessee legislature in 1977, making Tennessee the first state to have such a law.[2] Despite the weaknesses in Tennessee's early law (since amended), Dr Sanders' example influenced pediatricians across the country to similarly lobby for child safety seat legislation in their own states. Thus, by 1985 child passenger protection legislation was passed in every state.

B.2.3 Tap Water Scald Burns

Scalds can be less severe if hot tap water is less hot. Wisconsin pediatrician Murray Katcher, MD, PhD, became interested in this simple fact after listening to a presentation of pioneering work in this area by Seattle pediatrician Kenneth Feldman, MD.[3] Dr Katcher collected local data on tap water scald burns and began a community education project in cooperation with the local power company, water company, department of public health, and even senior citizen groups, whose constituency shares with children a disproportionate number of injuries from scalds. He later developed a multimedia campaign to encourage families to turn down water heater temperatures in their homes. Working with the Wisconsin Electric Power Company, he arranged to have pamphlets about the problem sent to all of the utility's subscribers. Newspaper, television, and radio ads, along with posters and pamphlets in physicians' offices, were also used to educate the public. Inexpensive thermometers were distributed to allow parents to check the water temperature at the tap.

This program was rigorously evaluated and the results were published.[4] Encouraged by initial efforts, Dr Katcher began an initiative to encourage the passage of legislation in Wisconsin to require safe water temperatures on all new water heaters sold in the state. The gathering of supporters, the answering to detractors, and persistence in the face of obstacles very much mirrored the early efforts of advocates of child passenger protection legislation. After many delays, disappointments, and frustrations, a bill finally passed in Wisconsin a decade after Dr Katcher had first heard Dr Feldman's presentation.

Dr Katcher then took his idea beyond the state level. He worked with the water heater trade association to ask that all new home water heaters sold in the United States were factory set at a safer temperature and included appropriate warnings to installers and to families to keep the water at a reasonable temperature. In that effort, Dr Katcher worked closely with the Washington DC office of the AAP, the Consumer Federation of America, and the National Safety Council.[5] Through persistence and focus, Dr Katcher succeeded in assuring that factory setting of water heaters at a safer temperature was at last a national industry standard.

B.3 Partnership With Government: Examples

A key to successful advocacy efforts is often in facilitating the establishment of effective partnerships between the private and public sectors. Public/private partnerships can effectively assess local and statewide need, advocate for change, and participate in the implementation of laws, regulations, and programs. Several examples of successful programs in the areas of *regulation, legislation,* and *education* that have been facilitated by pediatricians under the auspices of one state AAP chapter are given below.

B.3.1 Partnerships in Regulation

Public Law 99-457 was passed in 1989 to enable children with disabilities full access to a number of services offered through their school district if they are older than 3 years, or through the department of public welfare if they are younger than 3 years. This entitlement opened doors for children with disabilities; however, minimal in-service training effort was expended on some key school personnel who had the difficult task of caring for children with severe medical problems. The following illustration demonstrates the value of linking the public and private sectors to solve highly technical problems related to a specific group of high-risk children.

Transportation as a related service is often overlooked when a child with special health care needs has his or her individual education plan (IEP) meeting. The IEP meeting is the most significant planning tool for children with special needs. Once information is included in the IEP document and approved by the school district and guardian, it is a binding legal contract. The IEP is the key to safe transportation to and from school for the child with special health care and transportation needs. School transportation directors, while expected to provide safe transportation for children with involved medical histories, often have inadequate information about the child and the special requirements necessary.

In October 1993, several school transportation directors, a pediatrician, and two highway safety professionals met in Pennsylvania to develop a standardized "transportation medical certificate" for children with special needs. The project's champion was a transportation director whose daily life was complicated by the problems of transporting children with special needs. The transportation medical certificate provides transportation staff with a functional assessment of the child and a suggested list of the necessary equipment to transport the child safely. This form was developed for use by participants at the IEP meeting, and subsequently by the transportation department. By July 1994, the committee was expanded to include additional representatives from the public and private sectors, including individuals from state agencies, private insurance companies, an early childhood education expert, and additional pediatricians. Without the champion, the project would not have gone forward. As of 1995, the Special Needs Child Transportation Medical Certificate was being pilot tested in five states.

B.3.2 Partnerships in Legislation

Legislation alone does not assure adoption of healthy behaviors. While legislation is often critical, it must be combined with effective enforcement and education to change behavior and attitudes. In 1983, the Pennsylvania legislature passed Act 53: The Child Passenger Safety Act. Effective, coordinated, and consistent advocacy by a broad coalition of community and professional groups resulted in this legislative action. As often is the case, an initial law is imperfect due to political compromise. In Pennsylvania, although Act 53 mandated extensive public education, advocates were concerned about the enforcement difficulties associated with some elements of the law. Child safety advocates began efforts to educate the public about the key points of the law. Planning started immediately to modify the law at a future time.

To educate the public about the law, the Pennsylvania Chapter of the AAP submitted an unsolicited proposal to the Department of Transportation. The objective of the proposal was to increase public awareness about the law and to provide specific training and consultation to law enforcement agencies, hospitals, and other health care institutions on effective implementation of Act 53 provisions. The project, the Pennsylvania Traffic Injury Prevention Project, is now in its second decade. The original law has been modified, providing for improved enforceability. The credibility of a professional association of physicians as a legislative champion, combined with advocacy efforts of other organizations, facilitated incremental change in the law resulting in more effective enforcement and public acceptance.

B.3.3 Partnerships in Education

Education as a component of behavior change is crucial. Education, backed by legislation and enforcement, presents a strong, unified image that evokes confidence in the public. A pertinent example is the annual Youth Driving Challenge in York, Pa. This initiative combines the resources of the local police and a local insurance company with school district and highway safety personnel funded by the state Department of Transportation. Students compete for scholarship assistance with tests of driving skills competency, essays, and written examination on the law. The goal of the competition is to have students recognize their limitations while driving. The combined efforts of private sector participants and donors with public agency support make the effort highly visible, contributing to its success.

B.4 Identifying Community Resources

Successful local advocacy requires that injury prevention is identified in the community. Some communities have a variety of resources, others have few. Some resources are organized, others are waiting for someone to organize them. Pediatricians interested in community advocacy should develop links with community groups with interest in pertinent issues such as gun control, violence prevention, bicycle safety, and automobile safety. Local chapters of national organizations such as MADD (Mothers Against Drunk Driving), SADD (Students Against Driving Drunk), Boys and Girls Clubs, Scouts, the local hospital, religious groups, and PTA groups are often involved in activities related to injury control. Many communities have developed task forces on violence prevention and other injury issues. Such task forces may have broad cross-sectional representation from community leaders but be without the benefit of a pediatrician's contributions.

In the absence of organized resources, there are logical allies in the community with whom pediatricians can forge bonds. These may include teachers, coaches, lawyers, law enforcement officers, school nurses, and fire fighters, among others. Many national organizations (see B.7) can provide valuable information, material, and assistance in efforts to organize local efforts. The National Safe Kids Campaign is one such organization,[6] which has nearly 200 state and local coalitions. Safe Kids attempts to build awareness among adults about the magnitude of the childhood injury problem, and it works to create grassroots efforts to implement childhood injury control strategies. If there is not a Safe Kids Coalition in the area, pediatricians may consider helping to start one.

B.5 Working With Government

Interaction with government may occur in the context of individuals or organizations persuading, petitioning, or lobbying for passage, enforcement, or application of laws or regulations for the protection of children. In other cases, this interaction may take the form of a partnership in which private individuals and organizations assist the government — sometimes under contract or grant — to fulfill its objectives or obligations. In either case, the underlying premise is that government has an obligation to act to improve the public health and welfare. Furthermore, this obligation is particularly pressing for child health, for which the state has a special duty to protect children.

In the first case, pediatricians need to have some knowledge of legislative and administrative process; in the latter, pediatricians need to know how to develop a working relationship with appropriate government agencies.

Resources are available for pediatricians who seek organized training in advocacy and legislative processes. The AAP sponsors an annual legislative conference at which individuals have the opportunity to go to Washington, DC, learn about specific legislative issues, and learn how to influence decision makers in government. The AAP and other professional organizations also often include sessions on governmental affairs during continuing medical education meetings and conventions. The *Government Affairs Handbook*,[7] published by the AAP, is an excellent resource and includes sections on lobbying, coalition building, working with the media, and knowing the opposition. The book includes the addresses of a number of national and state advocacy organizations. Additionally, individuals can develop legislative and advocacy skills by volunteering to serve on the government affairs committee of their AAP chapter or the public affairs committee of another child advocacy organization.

To develop a working relationship with a government agency, the first step is to define the issues and goals in terms of meeting an unmet public need. Then the state governmental agency that may have a legal obligation to meet that goal needs to be identified. Is it the department of public welfare (to get Medicaid funds for child safety seats for children with special needs), the department of health (to initiate an emergency services for children project), or the department of transportation (to support child safety seat loan programs)? Once the target is identified, efforts can be focused.

Pediatricians need to contact the appropriate state agency to express their interest in helping the agency achieve their goal. Public funding may also be available. An RFP (request for proposal) is often listed in statewide publications to alert organizations and individuals that money has been allocated to study and/or address a problem. A telephone call to the appropriate state agency will allow pediatricians to obtain specific information about the RFP process and will indicate what RFPs are currently available.

Government agencies are usually interested in working with the local, nonprofit, community entities that are most qualified to meet their objectives. Pediatricians should find a sponsoring local entity (AAP state chapter, community group, hospital) and assist in writing proposals to satisfy the RFP requirements. The response to the RFP will usually consist of problem identification, goals/objectives, an action plan, a budget, and budget justification. Many RFPs are in the range of $25 000 to $50 000 a year, which makes them attractive to local voluntary groups and organizations. The keys to success include persistence and organization.

B.6 Conclusion: Elements of Successful Advocacy

The program elements common to successful advocacy efforts include[8,9]:
- The presence of a champion
- Availability of pertinent, convincing data
- Development of early, effective public education
- Development of a legislative initiative where appropriate
- Early acquisition of broad-based community support
- The passage of the necessary time for ideas to percolate, for objection to be countered, and for acceptance to develop

Pediatricians wishing to become involved in child advocacy efforts in injury control (or other areas of child and adolescent health) are encouraged to be in contact with officers of their AAP chapter.

B.7 Representative Advocacy Organizations and Resources

General

Association of Junior Leagues, International
660 1st Ave
New York, NY 10016
212-683-1515

Big Brothers/Big Sisters of America
230 N 13th St
Philadelphia, PA 19107
212-567-7000

Children's Defense Fund
25 E St, NW
Washington, DC 20001
202-628-8787
800-CDF-1200

Boy Scouts of America
1325 W Walnut Hill Ln
PO Box 152079
Irving, TX 75015
214-580-2000

Girl Scouts of America
420 5th Ave
New York, NY 10018-2702
212-852-8000

National Safety Council
1121 Spring Lake Dr
Itasca, IL 60143-3201
847-285-1121

National Safe Kids Campaign
1301 Pennsylvania Ave, NW
Suite 1000
Washington, DC 20004-1707
212-662-0600

National PTA-National Congress of Parents and Teachers
330 N Wabash St, #2100
Chicago, IL 60611-3604
312-670-6782

YMCA-USA
101 N Wacker Dr
Chicago, IL 60606
312-977-0031

YWCA-USA
766 Broadway
New York, NY 10003
212-614-2700

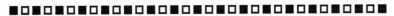
Abuse

Child Welfare League of America
440 1st St, NW, #310
Washington, DC 20001
202-638-2952

International Society for Prevention of Child Abuse and Neglect
1205 Oneida St
Denver, CO 80220
303-321-3963

Gun Control

Coalition to Stop Gun Violence
100 Maryland Ave, NW
Washington, DC 20002
202-544-7190

Education Fund to End Handgun Violence
110 Maryland Ave, NW
Washington, DC 20002
202-544-7227

Handgun Control Inc.
1225 Eye St, NW
Washington, DC 20005
202-898-0792

The HELP Network — Handgun Epidemic Lowering Plan
The Children's Memorial Medical Center
2300 Children's Plaza, #88
Chicago, IL 60614
312-880-3826

Motor Vehicle

Mothers Against Drunk Driving — MADD
511 E John Carpenter Freeway, #700
Irving, TX 75062
214-744-6233
800-GET-MADD

Advocates for Highway & Auto Safety
777 N Capital St, NE, #410
Washington, DC 20001
202-408-1711

This list is not all-inclusive. It is meant to give the provider some leads on organizations that may be contacted at a national or local level. Listing of a particular organization does not represent endorsement of its particular activity. See Appendix G of the *Government Affairs Handbook*[7] for a detailed list of addresses and telephone numbers of state affiliates or chapters of many of these organizations.

References

1. Baranowski J. His prescription for kids: a dose of 'political medicine.' *Contemp Pediatr.* 1989;6:44–54

2. Price SC. Robert Sanders: a lifelong advocate for children. *Childhood Injury Prevention Quarterly (National Safe Kids Campaign).* 1992;4(1):14–17

3. Feldman KW, Schaller RT, Feldman JA, McMillon M. Tap water scald burns in children. *Pediatrics.* 1978;62:1–7

4. Katcher ML. Prevention of tap water scald burns: evaluation of a multi-media injury control program. *Am J Public Health.* 1987;77:1195–1197

5. Wilson M. A lesson in child advocacy. *Newsletter of the Ambulatory Pediatric Association.* 1988;24:1,7–9

6. Mickalide A. The National SAFE KIDS Campaign (USA). *Inj Prev.* 1995;1:119–121

7. American Academy of Pediatrics. *Government Affairs Handbook.* Elk Grove Village, IL: American Academy of Pediatrics; 1992

8. Erdmann TC, Feldman KW, Rivara FP, Heimbach DM, Wall HA. Tap water burn prevention: the effect of legislation. *Pediatrics.* 1991;88:572–577

9. Scheidt PC, Wilson MH, Stern MS. Bicycle helmet law for children: a case study of activism in injury control. *Pediatrics.* 1992;89:1248–1250

AAP Policy Statements Related to Injury Prevention Issues

Following is a list of policy statements relating to injury prevention issues published by the American Academy of Pediatrics (AAP). These statements represent a consensus of the Academy and leading pediatric experts.

To order the complete text of individual policy statements listed below, call the AAP Department of Marketing and Publications at 847-228-5005, or mail your order to: AAP Publications, 141 Northwest Point Blvd, PO Box 927, Elk Grove Village, IL 60009-0927. All reprints are $1.95 each — prepaid orders only. No shipping or handling charge on reprint orders less than $10.

Committee on Adolescence

RE9233　Firearms and Adolescents, 4/92
RE9433　Sexual Assault and the Adolescent, 11/94
RE8108　Suicide and Suicide Attempts in Adolescents and Young Adults, 2/88, reaffirmed 4/92

Committee on Child Abuse and Neglect

RE9423　Distinguishing Sudden Infant Death From Child Abuse Fatalities, 7/94
RE9202　Guidelines for the Evaluation of Sexual Abuse of Children, 2/91, reaffirmed 6/94
RE9336　Investigation and Review of Unexpected Infant and Child Deaths, 11/93
RE9337　Shaken Baby Syndrome: Inflicted Cerebral Trauma, 12/93

Committee on Communications

RE9144   Impact of Rock Lyrics and Music Videos on Children and Youth, 2/89

RE9526   Media Violence, 6/95

Committee on Early Childhood, Adoption, and Dependent Care

RE9417   The Application of Health and Safety Guidelines to Out-of-Home Child Care Programs, 6/94

RE6068   Oral and Dental Aspects of Child Abuse and Neglect, 9/86, reaffirmed 2/90

Committee on Environmental Health

RE9509   Hazards of Child Labor, 2/95

RE9307   Lead Poisoning: From Screening to Primary Prevention, 7/93

Committee on Hospital Care

RE7077   Medical Necessity for the Hospitalization of the Abused and Neglected Child, 2/87, reaffirmed 4/91

Committee on Injury and Poison Prevention

RE9176   All-Terrain Vehicles, 2/87, reaffirmed 2/90

RE9176   Bicycle Helmets, 4/95

RE9218   Children and Fireworks, 9/91, reaffirmed 5/94

RE9216   Children in Pickup Trucks, 8/91, reaffirmed 5/94

RE9319   Drowning in Infants, Children and Adolescents, 8/93

RE9619   Efforts to Reduce the Toll of Injuries in Childhood Require Expanded Research, 5/96

RE9228   55 Miles Per Hour Maximum Speed Limit, 9/91, reaffirmed 5/94

RE9234   Firearm Injuries Affecting the Pediatric Population, 4/92

RE9248   Hospital Discharge Data on Injury: The Need for E Codes, 3/92

RE9520   Injuries Associated With Infant Walkers, 5/95

RE7085	Injuries Related to Toy Firearms, 3/87, reaffirmed 4/93
RE9164	Office-Based Counseling for Injury Prevention, 10/94
RE2408	Reducing the Toll of Injuries in Childhood Requires Support for a Focused Effort, 11/83
RE9181	Ride-On Mower Injuries in Children, 7/90, reaffirmed 5/93
RE8113	Rural Injuries, 6/88, reaffirmed 4/93
RE9190	Safe Transportation of Newborns Discharged From the Hospital, 9/90, reaffirmed 4/93
RE9188	Safe Transportation of Premature Infants, 1/91
RE9617	Safe Transportation of Premature and Low Birth Weight Infants, 5/96
RE9401	School Bus Transportation of Children With Special Needs, 1/94
RE9616	School Transportation Safety, 5/96
RE9618	Selecting and Using the Most Appropriate Car Safety Seats for Growing Children: Guidelines for Counseling Parents, 5/96
RE9157	Skateboard Injuries, 4/95
RE8129	Snowmobile Statement, 11/88, reaffirmed 4/93
RE2214	Trampolines II, 3/81, reaffirmed 2/90
REX031	Transporting Children With Special Needs, 1/93

Committee on Pediatric Emergency Medicine

RE9260	Access to Emergency Medical Care, 10/92
RE9309	Consent for Medical Services for Children and Adolescents, 8/93
RE9413	Death of a Child in the Emergency Department, 5/94
RE9323	First Aid for the Choking Child, 9/93
RE9247	Intraosseous Infusion, 3/92
RE9420	Pediatrician's Role in Advocating Life Support Courses for Parents, 7/94
RE8115	Pediatrician's Role in Emergency Medical Services for Children, 5/88, reaffirmed 1/92

Committee on School Health

RE9616   School Transportation Safety, 5/96

Committee on Sports Medicine

RE9245   Horseback Riding and Head Injuries, 3/92

RE8132   Infant Exercise Programs, 11/88, reaffirmed 11/94

RE5045   Infant Swimming Programs 9/85, reaffirmed 2/90

RE2219   Participation in Boxing Among Children and Young Adults, 8/84, reaffirmed 2/90

RE9630   Protective Eyewear for Young Athletes, 8/96

RE9409   Risk of Injury From Baseball and Softball in Children 5 to 14 Years of Age, 4/94

RE9192   Risks in Distance Running for Children, 11/90, reaffirmed 1/94

RE9196   Strength Training, Weight and Power Lifting, and Body Building by Children and Adolescents, 11/90, reaffirmed 1/94

RE2214   Trampolines II, 3/81, reaffirmed 2/90

RE9635   Triathlon Participation by Children and Adolescents, 9/96

■□■□■□■□■□■□■□■□■□■□■□■□■□■□■□■□■□■

AAP Professional and Patient Education Materials Related to Injury Prevention Issues

Following is a list of American Academy of Pediatrics (AAP) professional and patient education materials relating to injury prevention issues. To obtain pricing information or to order the materials, contact the AAP Department of Marketing and Publications at 847-228-5005.

MA0056	The Visual Diagnosis of Child Physical Abuse
CD0006	Focus on Child Abuse: Resources for Prevention, Recognition, and Treatment
HE0199S	Portraits of Promise — Preventing Shaken Baby Syndrome
MA0061	A Guide to References and Resources in Child Abuse and Neglect
MA0019	Handbook of Common Poisonings in Children, 3rd ed
MA0018	Sports Medicine: Health Care for Young Athletes, 2nd Edition
CD007	KidSTAT Plus: The AAP Pediatric Emergency Medicine Resource
MA0052	Emergency Medical Services for Children: The Role of the Primary Care Provider
MA0039	APLS: The Pediatric Emergency Medicine Course Manual
MA0055	Guidelines for Air and Ground Transport of Neonatal and Pediatric Patients
M10045	Caring for Our Children: National Health and Safety Performance Standards for Out-of-Home Child Care Programs
MA0073	Caring for Our Children: Video Series
MA0032	Health in Day Care: A Manual for Health Professionals
MA0031	School Health: Policy and Practice, 5th ed

Ambulatory Care Quality Improvement Program

AC0037   Injury Prevention Counseling
AC0035   Office Emergency Procedures

State Legislation Packets

CH0009   Firearms and Children
CH0010   Impaired Driving and Adolescents
CH0011   Children and Pickup Trucks
CH0013   Swimming Pool Enclosures
CH0014   Bicycle Helmets
CH0015   Child Death Investigation and Review
CH0016   Emergency Medical Services for Children

For Your Patients

HE0160   Safe Baby Tags
HE0008   First Aid Chart
HE0139   Rx For Good Health Growth Chart

TIPP®—The Injury Prevention Program

TIPP® Age–Related Safety Sheets

HE0021-A   Birth to 6 months
HE0021-B   6 to 12 months
HE0021-C   1 to 2 years
HE0021-D   2 to 4 years

Bicycle TIPP® Safety Sheets

HE0075   About Bicycle Helmets
HE0076   Bicycle Safety: Myths and Facts
HE0079   Tips for Getting Your Kids to Wear Helmets
HE0080   Choosing the Right Size Bicycle for Your Child
HE0081   Safe Bicycling Starts Early
HE0082   The Child as Passenger on an Adult's Bicycle

TIPP® Safety Sheets

HE0022-A   The First Year of Life From 1 to 4 Years, Part 1
HE0022-C   The First Year of Life From 1 to 4 Years, Part 2
HE0067-A   From 5 to 9 Years
HE0067-B   From 10 to 12 Years

Child Safety Slips

HE0030   Infant Furniture: Cribs
HE0031   Baby-sitting Reminders
HE0032   Safety Tips for Home Playground Equipment
HE0033   Protect Your Child...Prevent Poisoning
HE0038   Safe Driving...A Parental Responsibility
HE0039   Protect Your Home Against Fire...Planning Saves Lives
HE0129   Water Safety for Your School-age Child
HE0130   Lawn Mower Safety
HE0131   Home Water Hazards for Young Children
HE0132   Pool Safety for Children
HE0133   Life Jackets and Life Preserves

Patient Education Brochures/Materials

HE0163   Keep Your Family Safe From Firearm Injury
ER6005   One-Minute Car Seat Safety Check-up
ER6006   Family Guide to Car Seats
HE0149   Toy Safety
HE0110   Playground Safety
HE0212   Emergency Medical Services for Children Fact Sheet
HE0198   A Parent's Guide to Water Safety
HE0066   Choking Prevention and First Aid for Infants and Children
HE0181   Fun in the Sun: Keep Your Baby Safe
HE0184   Raising Children to Resist Violence: What You Can Do
HE0029   Child Sexual Abuse: What It Is and How to Prevent It
HE0026   The Teen Driver

Other Resources

Special Delivery: Safe Transportation of Premature and
Small Infants

TIPP Materials

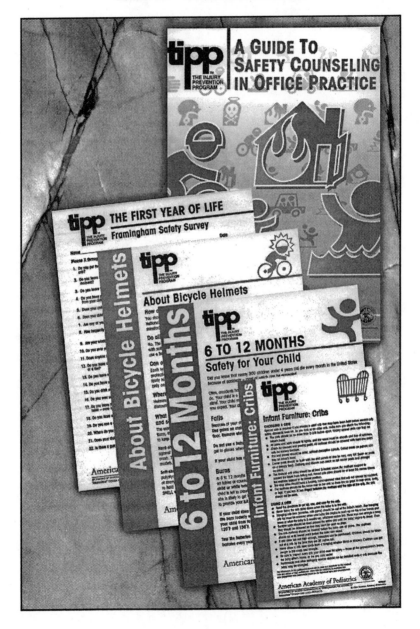

The AAP Committee on Injury and Poison Prevention and the Section on Injury and Poison Prevention

Committee on Injury and Poison Prevention

The seeds of an injury prevention program were sown by Dr George M. Wheatley in an editorial published in *Pediatrics* in September 1948 entitled "Child Accident Reduction: A Challenge to the Pediatrician."[1] This editorial announced the launching of a national campaign for child safety in which the American Academy of Pediatrics (AAP) was one of the leading participants. He also pointed out that even in 1948 "accidents" were the leading cause of deaths of children beyond infancy.

Shortly thereafter (October 1950), the Executive Board of the AAP created the Committee on Accident Prevention, appointing Dr Wheatley as its chairperson. This committee was different from other Academy committees in that it formed partnerships with nonmedical organizations, namely the National Safety Council and the Metropolitan Life Insurance Company. For the first time, the committee utilized the media to educate the public about injuries and their prevention. The committee also worked closely with government agencies to promote injury prevention through regulations. These themes still exist today.

Early efforts of the committee are best summarized from a roundtable discussion at the Annual Meeting in October 1951. At that time Dr Wheatley articulated the three cornerstones of injury prevention —

education, engineering, and enforcement, thereby laying the ground-work for subsequent efforts of the committee. Education involved making the public aware of existing hazards and potential countermeasures. Engineering dealt with the reduction of hazards through specific design modifications. In the area of enforcement, Dr Wheatley anticipated even in 1951 the role of government regulation in protecting the public from injuries.

Poisoning was an early concern of the committee, as were injuries attributable to flammable clothing and strangulation.[2] An early survey of injuries seen by pediatricians produced 2781 case reports, of which 50% were attributable to poisoning. Another 30% involved burns, half of which were caused by flammable clothing. There were 40 reported fatalities from the entire 2781 case reports.

The committee directed much of its early effort to unintentional poisonings and the lack of information to deal with these emergencies. In a move that foreshadowed the development of poison control centers, Dr Wheatley secured the help of the New York City Health Department and the New York Academy of Medicine to provide telephone responses to physicians' inquiries about childhood poisonings. In 1953, Dr Ed Press, a member of the committee, created the first organized poison control center in Chicago.[3] In this effort, he enlisted the help of the Chicago Board of Health, the Illinois State Toxicological Laboratory, and six Chicago hospitals.[4] The center soon expanded to include 20 hospitals covering the greater Chicago area. The recognition of the importance of this activity led to the creation of a Subcommittee on Poisoning in 1954, with Dr Press as chairperson. In 1955 this subcommittee published the manual, "Accidental Poisoning in Childhood," which was well received and widely acclaimed.[5] In 1976 this publication was succeeded by a second committee publication, "Handbook of Common Poisonings in Children," which was published by the Food and Drug Administration. Second and third editions were published by the AAP in 1982 and 1994, respectively.[6]

One of the early successes of the committee dealt with the issue of lead poisoning. In 1955, committee members, working with governmental agencies and paint manufacturers, set a voluntary standard of 1% lead for children's furniture, toys, and indoor areas. The committee continued to press for change, which resulted in 1970 federal legislation prohibiting the use of lead in household paint.[4]

Public education was a prominent activity of the committee, and many publications from the 1950s are still updated and published today. In 1959 the first aid chart developed by Dr Edward Wakeman was first published. Since then, it has undergone numerous revisions to reflect changes in practice and epidemiology. Also, in that same year, anticipatory guidance slips developed for the greater New Bedford Accident Prevention Program directed by Dr George Starbuck were published by the AAP. These safety slips were the forerunners of the safety slips published with TIPP materials. Drs Starbuck and Press succeeded Dr Wheatley as chairs of the committee.

During the 1960s, groundwork was laid for future legislation. Research on burns, begun shortly after the inception of the committee, culminated in the passage of the Flammable Fabrics Act of 1970. This was amended in 1971 at the urging of the committee to require that children's sleepwear through size 6x be flame retardant; in 1975 this legislation was extended to include sizes up to size 14. Continuing concern with unintentional poisoning in children led to the 1970 Poison Prevention Packaging Act.

In 1969, the Subcommittee on Accidental Poisoning rejoined the Committee on Accident Prevention and has since functioned as a single committee.

On the educational front, the committee was also very active. In June 1968, the committee sponsored the Second Annual National Childhood Injury Symposium in Richmond, Va. The proceedings were published as a supplement to *Pediatrics* in November 1969.[7] Experts from universities, government officials, and physicians presented papers on many common hazards, including falls, poisonings, drowning, motor vehicle injuries, and burns. There was no mention of injuries from firearm use, however. Dr Merritt Low, chairperson of the committee and future AAP president, presided.

Throughout the 1970s the committee continued its involvement with reducing the number of childhood poisonings. New agents were gradually added to the Poison Prevention Packaging Act, beginning with aspirin in 1972, furniture polish later that year, and finally acetaminophen in 1980. In September 1974 a symposium on poisoning was published in *Pediatrics* by the committee and others that dealt with treatment of common serious childhood poisonings. In his summation, Chairperson Dr Robert Scherz pointed out that prevention was by far the most effective treatment.[8]

Choking was another area of interest for the committee in the 1970s. The committee worked with the Consumer Product Safety Commission to develop the Child Protection and Toy Safety Act, which included a small parts standard for toys for children younger than 3 years. In addition the committee worked with toy manufacturers, specifically Mattel, to make plastic toy parts radiopaque by the addition of small amounts of barium, which facilitates identification and retrieval of aspirated small parts.

In 1981 the committee published the controversial statement, "First Aid For the Choking Child."[9-11] The statement advocated back blows and chest thrusts (sternal compressions) for choking infants and children and was based, in part, on a 1979 "expert opinion" consensus conference.[12] At the time the Heimlich maneuver — abdominal thrusts — was being advocated for adults. In 1985 another consensus conference concluded that back blows and sternal compressions should be reserved only for choking *infants*.[13] The AAP policy was revised to conform with these new national standards. Subsequent revisions of AAP policy (most recently by the Committee on Pediatric Emergency Medicine) have assured continued uniformity with recommendations of national organizations.[14-16] During this period of controversy, deaths from choking declined dramatically; whether this was due to new techniques or an increased awareness of the hazard is unclear. Efforts to resolve the best first aid measures for choking infants and children were spearheaded by Drs Howard Mofenson and Joseph Greensher, both leaders in the field of pediatric injury control and in committee activities.

In 1980 the committee chairperson, Dr James Holroyd, launched the "First Ride Safe Ride" program at the AAP Annual Meeting in Detroit. This program promoted the use of child safety seats for infants on the ride home from the hospital. With promotional literature and minigrants to AAP chapters to encourage safety seat use, this program became a model injury prevention program that motivated and trained a small core of pediatricians. These pediatricians then went back to their chapters to teach and encourage other practitioners to counsel on injury prevention activities. The program was later expanded to

"Every Ride a Safe Ride"; through program efforts, pediatricians helped assure that child passenger safety legislation was enacted in all 50 states.

In April 1983, the committee launched TIPP at the AAP spring meeting in Philadelphia.[17] Dr C. Everett Koop, Surgeon General and former committee member, pointed out "Accidents, poisonings, and injuries have emerged as one of the greatest threats to our children's health." TIPP had its origins in three Title V programs funded by the Bureau of Maternal and Child Health in California, Massachusetts, and Virginia and consisted of a policy statement on injury prevention from the committee, a counseling schedule appropriate to the development of the child, and a packet of materials (safety sheets, surveys, and anticipatory guidance materials). Original materials were designed for children from birth through age 4 years. These materials were expanded in 1988 to cover the child up to 12 years of age, and the entire package was revised in 1994 to cover from birth to 12 years. The program has been very successful and has helped to validate the value of anticipatory guidance in injury prevention in office practice.[18]

Over the years the agenda of the committee changed to meet the evolving epidemiology of injuries and the engineering advances that could combat them. In the late 1970s industry developed strong, lightweight plastics. With this technology, attractive, durable bicycle helmets were produced. Encouraged by colleagues at the Harborview Injury Prevention Center in Seattle, Wash, the AAP and the committee launched a bicycle helmet campaign in 1989. Following the format of "Safe Ride," there were minigrants to 25 chapters to promote helmet usage, and educational materials were developed. Helmets were distributed and legislation requiring helmets was passed in some communities. Thousands of new helmets were distributed as part of a promotional effort, and bicycle safety is now part of injury prevention counseling in most pediatric offices.

In the late 1980s, the committee became involved in another controversial issue with industry. In 1983 all-terrain vehicles (ATVs) were on the market, originally as an inexpensive toy for the whole family. Shortly thereafter, pediatricians began noting a surge of injuries attributed to these "toys." By 1987 more than 300 000 injuries and 900 deaths were attributed to ATV use, and nearly half of the injuries were to children younger than 16 years. The three-wheel version of ATV was inherently unstable and tipped over frequently and unpredictably. The committee worked with other organizations to bring about a ban on three-wheeled vehicle sales in 1988, but was unsuccessful in recalling previous purchases.[19] They were also unsuccessful in limiting sales or use of four-wheeled vehicles. Recent data would indicate that four-wheeled ATVs continue to cause an unacceptably high rate of injuries.

In September 1989, the AAP and the Henry J. Kaiser Family Foundation jointly sponsored a "Forum on Firearms and Children" in Chicago. The recommendations of this forum again reflected the three Es of injury prevention: Educating families, physicians, and the media of the hazards of firearms; Engineering firearm and bullet design modifications; and the Enforcement of an ultimate ban on certain types of firearms. As an outgrowth of this forum, the committee published a statement " Firearm Injuries Affecting the Pediatric Population" in April 1992, which stated that firearms should be removed from the environments where children live and play.[20] The statement also recognized a change in the ecology of firearm injuries. By 1991, firearms had become the leading cause of injury death in a number of states, exceeding deaths from motor vehicle injuries for the first time.[21]

In 1990 the name of the committee was changed to the Committee on *Injury* and Poison Prevention (COIPP). Thus injuries could be intentional or unintentional, but never truly chance or unpredictable events or *accidents*. Violence as a cause of injuries to children could no longer be ignored.

The committee has undertaken two other initiatives in the area of handguns and violence. In 1992, in conjunction with the Center to Prevent Handgun Violence, the education packet "Steps to Prevent (STOP) Firearm Injury" for pediatricians was developed. The packet contains counseling guidelines, a poster and audio tape, and promotional materials and attempts to encourage pediatricians to discuss firearms as a public health issue. Also in 1992, the committee sponsored a roundtable discussion on adolescent victims of violence, which noted that most teenagers who were assaulted and hospitalized were usually treated as adults, and many of their developmental/psychosocial adolescent needs were not addressed. As a result a task force has developed a policy statement and model protocol that addresses these needs.

Thus, over the years the committee has reflected the prevailing problems of injury as they affect the youth of America. The long delays between the description of the hazard and the institution of effective interventions are sometimes discouraging. Burns associated with sleepwear were described at the first committee meeting, but legislation to correct the problem took 20 years to enact. Infant walkers were reported to be a hazard in 1982, and finally in 1994 there was a voluntary cessation of production by some manufacturers. Progress has been made, in part, because pediatricians have been dedicated and persistent. The principles articulated by Dr George Wheatley a half century ago — to educate, to engineer, and to enforce — remain relevant in committee work to this day.

Section on Injury and Poison Prevention

The section on Injury and Poison Prevention was founded in 1990 and is dedicated to providing a forum to help educate pediatricians in all aspects of childhood injury and poison prevention and to vigorously work for the implementation of injury and poison prevention programs on local, state, and national levels. The section also encourages research in, and the teaching of, injury and poison prevention strategies.

While the section's membership is largely comprised of AAP members with an interest in injury and poison prevention and specifically general pediatricians who provide office-based counseling on injury prevention, it also includes emergency medicine and critical care specialists. In 1996, there were nearly 120 members.

In its short history, the section has established or participated in a number of successful special activities:

- The section presents two awards each year to honor significant achievement in injury prevention, one to an AAP fellow and one to a resident.
- The section's semiannual newsletter includes updates on section and committee activities, state legislation reports, meeting announcements, literature reviews, and abstracts.
- Members of the section worked closely with the COIPP on The Injury Prevention Program (TIPP) as it underwent extensive revision in 1993–1994.

- The section's Resident Education Subcommittee is developing a slide and speaker kit for program directors to educate residents on injury and poison prevention. A survey of pediatric training programs revealed a substantial need for such a kit.
- The section has consulted on and provided background for numerous resolutions considered at the annual Chapter Forum.
- The section has collaborated on activities and projects with the Committee on Native American Child Health, the AAP Department of Government Liaison, the Division of State Government and Chapter Affairs, and the Department of Communications. In addition, the section works closely with the COIPP through liaison representation.

The section holds two executive committee meetings annually, one at each AAP national meeting. The executive committee has relied on its own members to plan and implement the educational programs at the national meetings. A regular offering has been a successful session of abstracts, posters, and a review of the best articles of the year, presented at the Spring Meeting. With the growth of the section and its potential activities, the executive committee has also begun to utilize its members-at-large, who now serve as newsletter editors as well as on the subcommittees involved with awards, resident education, nominations, outcomes, membership assistance and resources, and minority access to care.

The leadership of the section keeps in contact with its members through its newsletter, which is published twice each year. The newsletter, which is typically 8 to 12 pages per issue, features commentaries, literature reviews, announcements of resources and programs, summaries of section and COIPP activities, legislative updates, and reports from educational sessions. In addition, the section surveys its members periodically in order to set program priorities. Members receive the annual call for nominations for the section's awards, the call for abstracts for the section's spring meetings, and the pocket program from the section's abstract session. The section's annual business meeting and its reception at AAP spring sessions present additional opportunities for interaction with section members. Finally, the section recently created a membership resources and assistance group to assist members with inquiries.

Looking to the future, the section will work on increasing its membership and continuing to involve its membership in more activities. There

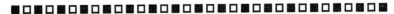
is great potential for expanding our member participation through our resources and assistance subcommittee. This group will also benefit the AAP as it seeks input from the section regarding issues of technical or programmatic importance. Another new endeavor of the section is the development of a group dedicated to monitoring outcomes research as it relates to injury prevention. Because injuries are the leading cause of death in childhood, this will likely be a resource of great value to the AAP in the years to come.

References

1. Wheatley GM. Child accident reduction: a challenge to the pediatrician. *Pediatrics.* 1948;2:367–368

2. Hughes JG. *American Academy of Pediatrics: The First 50 Years.* Evanston, IL: American Academy of Pediatrics; 1980

3. Scherz RG, Robertson WO. The history of poison control centers in the United States. *Clin Toxicol.* 1978;12:291–296

4. Wheatley GM. Accidents and poison prevention: a look back. Presented as part of the roundtable: *Forty Years of Injury Prevention* at the Annual Meeting, American Academy of Pediatrics. Boston, MA: October 9 1990

5. American Academy of Pediatrics, Committee on Accident Prevention. *Accidental Poisoning in Childhood.* Springfield, IL: Charles C. Thomas; 1955

6. American Academy of Pediatrics, Committee on Injury and Poison Prevention. *Handbook of Common Poisonings in Children.* 3rd ed. Elk Grove Village, IL: American Academy of Pediatrics; 1994

7. Childhood injuries: approaches and perspectives: a report of the Second National Childhood Injury Symposium, June 28–30, 1968, Charlottesville, Virginia. *Pediatrics.* 1969;44(5 Nov suppl):791–896

8. Scherz RG. The management of accidental childhood poisoning. *Pediatrics.* 1974; 54:323–324

9. American Academy of Pediatrics, Committee on Accident and Poison Prevention. First aid for the choking child. *Pediatrics.* 1981;67:744

10. Greensher J, Mofenson HC. Emergency treatment of the choking child. *Pediatrics.* 1982;70:110–112

11. Heimlich HJ. First aid for choking children: back blows and chest thrusts cause complications and death. *Pediatrics.* 1982;70:120–125

12. Standards and guidelines for cardiopulmonary resuscitation (CPR) and emergency cardiac care (ECC). *JAMA.* 1980;244:453–509

13. Standards for cardiopulmonary resuscitation (CPR) and emergency cardiac care (ECC), part IV: pediatric basic life support. *JAMA.* 1986;255:2954–2960

14. American Academy of Pediatrics, Committee on Accident and Poison Prevention. Revised first aid for the choking child. *Pediatrics*. 1986;78:177–178

15. American Academy of Pediatrics, Committee on Accident and Poison Prevention. First aid for the choking child, 1988. *Pediatrics*. 1988;81:740–742

16. American Academy of Pediatrics, Committee on Pediatric Emergency Medicine. First aid for the choking child. *Pediatrics*. 1993;92:477–479

17. Bass J. TIPP — the first ten years. *Pediatrics*. 1995;95:274–275

18. Miller TR, Galbraith M. Injury prevention counseling by pediatricians: a benefit-cost comparison. *Pediatrics*. 1995;96:1–4

19. Widome MD. Protecting children from all-terrain vehicles: a need to update legislation. *State Health Legislation Report*. 1988;16:1–5

20. American Academy of Pediatrics, Committee on Injury and Poison Prevention. Firearm injuries affecting the pediatric population. *Pediatrics*. 1992;89:788–790

21. Centers for Disease Control and Prevention. Deaths resulting from firearm- and motor-vehicle–related injuries: United States, 1968–1991. *MMWR Morb Mortal Wkly Rep*. 1994;43:37–42

Federal Agencies and Programs

G.1 Centers for Disease Control and Prevention (CDC)

G.1.1 Organizational Structure

The Centers for Disease Control and Prevention (CDC) is an agency of the US Public Health Service (PHS) within the Department of Health and Human Services. The CDC's mission is to promote health and quality of life by preventing and controlling disease, injury, and disability. What distinguishes the CDC from other health-related agencies is its strong emphasis on prevention rather than treatment and its focus on populations rather than individual patients.

The National Center for Injury Prevention and Control (NCIPC) in Atlanta, Ga, is the newest center of the CDC. Its activities were first established at the CDC in 1988 as the Division of Injury Control within the Center for Environmental Health and Injury Control, in response to recommendations made by the Institute of Medicine in a landmark monograph, *Injury in America.*[1] Three years later, a national consensus called for the establishment of a separate center for injury control within the CDC to "emphasize the importance of injuries as a public health issue and to lead a national program of effective action to address the problem."[2] Accordingly, NCIPC was established the following year, with its three main divisions — the Division of Unintentional Injury Prevention, the Division of Violence Prevention, and the Division of Acute Care, Rehabilitation Research, and Disability Prevention.

Other centers within the CDC also contribute to the scientific base for injury control, including the National Institute for Occupational Safety and Health (NIOSH), which is responsible for workplace-related injuries;

the National Center for Health Statistics (NCHS), which provides injury morbidity and mortality statistics; the Division of Adolescent and School Health (DASH) of the National Center for Chronic Disease Prevention and Health Promotion, which focuses on injuries in the context of comprehensive school health; and the Disabilities Prevention Program (DPP) of the National Center for Environmental Health, which addresses post-injury disabilities, especially the physical, psychological, and behavioral sequelae of traumatic brain and spinal cord injuries.

G.1.2 Unique Role of the NCIPC

The NCIPC differs from other federal, advocacy, and nonprofit organizations involved in injury prevention and control in that it is responsible for establishing and cultivating the science of this emerging field, as well as coordinating injury prevention activities among federal agencies. Included in the staff's diverse academic backgrounds is expertise in medicine (including pediatrics, internal medicine, family practice, emergency medicine, occupational medicine, general surgery, orthopedics, and preventive medicine), epidemiology, sociology, psychology, economics, education, demography, criminology, veterinary medicine, engineering, biostatistics, medical anthropology, and public health. The professional staff conducts intramural research, recommends topics for and subsequently reviews grant proposals, provides technical assistance to state and local health departments, and interacts substantially with other constituents — university research scientists, other federal agencies and nonprofit groups, the media, and the public.

G.1.3 NCIPC Objectives, Programs, and Functions

NCIPC goals and activities are consistent with targets established by *Healthy People 2000*, a consensus document that defines the nation's highest-priority objectives for health promotion and disease prevention, with target goals for the year 2000.[3] The NCIPC is the lead federal agency for the *Healthy People 2000* objectives related to unintentional injuries and violent and abusive behavior. NCIPC helps develop specific injury reduction goals and tracks progress towards their attainment. Within this framework, a more detailed national plan for injury control was established through collaboration with over 800 people in 1991, and was documented in a monograph endorsed by the American Academy of Pediatrics.[2]

■□■□■□■□■□■□■□■□■□■□■□■□■□■□■□■□■

Research and public programs are conducted by NCIPC through their intramural, extramural, and state programs. Work is conducted in five main areas of injury prevention and control: epidemiology, prevention, biomechanics, acute care, and rehabilitation. The traditional public health model depicted in the figure provides the structure for such research — defining the major problems (epidemiology), identifying their causes (risk factor analysis), determining what works (program development and its evaluation), and delivering effective programs to communities (technical and programmatic assistance to states, coordination among other agencies, and collaborative relationships with other groups). The overall goal of such research is to advance scientific knowledge and provide programs of proven effectiveness to state and local groups — including health departments and other public safety officials, schools, and community-based organizations.

Accordingly, the nearly 200 extramural projects funded by the Center are more likely to be applied research rather than basic science laboratory research, which is sponsored or conducted by other federal agencies. In the first half of the 1990s, funding was used to build state-level injury prevention capacity at state health departments to begin or enhance injury surveillance or intervention programs.

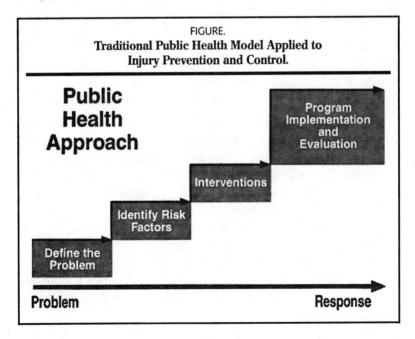

FIGURE.
Traditional Public Health Model Applied to Injury Prevention and Control.

Public Health Approach

Program Implementation and Evaluation

Interventions

Identify Risk Factors

Define the Problem

Problem → Response

Presently, state funding is used to promote the science of injury prevention by developing and evaluating intervention programs evaluating injury outcomes. In fiscal year 1995, with a total budget of about $45 million, NCIPC funded projects in 32 states, 40 academic institutions, and five nonprofit organizations.

G.1.4 Pediatric Injury Prevention at the CDC

The childhood and adolescent injury prevention program at the NCIPC has focused attention on subjects of major public health importance to children, as determined by (1) their leading rank in causing mortality, morbidity, disability, and/or excessive years of premature life lost, and (2) the known effectiveness of available countermeasures. Major target areas are motor vehicle occupant injuries, pedestrian and bicycle injuries, drowning, poisoning, burns, homicide, suicide, and family and intimate violence. Objectives include: (1) raising public and professional awareness and understanding of injury prevention in infants, children, and adolescents; (2) supporting a coordinated, national, science-based approach to injury prevention and control; (3) funding research concerning the major countermeasures, including child safety seats, drowning prevention programs, smoke detectors, bicycle helmets, parent education, and programs to reduce child abuse, teenage suicide, youth violence, family and intimate violence, and careless or hasty use of firearms; (4) establishing and/or improving injury surveillance systems of a national scope, including firearms injuries and unintentional childhood injuries; and (5) increasing the use of effective prevention strategies in all communities, particularly among the underserved.

Childhood injury prevention research is conducted in dozens of topics. A few examples include (1) studying risk factors for drowning among minorities; (2) studying risk factors associated with fatal and non-fatal residential fires; (3) evaluating the role of alcohol in fatal crashes; (4) evaluating the effectiveness of state bicycle helmet laws; (5) analyzing risk factors for injuries associated with in-line skating; (6) conducting surveillance on the magnitude, characteristics, and costs of injuries and disabilities caused by firearms, and on the types of firearms that inflict these injuries; (7) studying potentially modifiable causes of serious attempted suicide among adolescents; and (8) conducting a multistate surveillance system for traumatic brain and spinal cord injuries

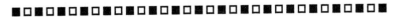
G.1.5 Other Activities

The NCIPC has several other key activities. It publishes recommendations for injury prevention, such as the recent recommendations for bicycle helmet use[4] and traumatic brain and spinal cord injury prevention.[5] It provides extramural grant funds and technical support to states and communities to support their efforts to develop state injury intervention programs, including the development, implementation, and evaluation of multifaceted injury prevention and surveillance programs. It tests the prevention effectiveness and cost-effectiveness of various model programs. It conducts primary surveillance to demonstrate the degree of national progress towards its goals. Such surveillance systems include its Injury Control and Risk Factor Survey, Firearm Injury Surveillance System (in collaboration with the US Consumer Product Safety Commission), national surveillance of traumatic brain and spinal cord injuries, and surveillance of special at-risk populations, including American Indians and Alaskan Natives, Hispanic children, and rural residents. And lastly, it provides liaison staff to other federal agencies, professional organizations, and nonprofit organizations, including the Committee on Injury and Poison Prevention and the Committee on Child Abuse and Neglect of the American Academy of Pediatrics.

G.2 Consumer Product Safety Commission

G.2.1 Background

The US Consumer Product Safety Commission (CPSC) is an independent federal regulatory agency created by Congress in 1972 under the Consumer Product Safety Act. The Agency's mission is to protect the public against unreasonable risks of injury and death associated with consumer products. The CPSC addresses product safety and health hazards for over 15 000 consumer products.

The Commission is a unique public asset because it is the only Federal agency that identifies and acts on this range of product safety hazards. The agency operates unique hazard identification systems, such as the National Electronic Injury Surveillance System (NEISS), a probability sample of US hospital emergency rooms; the Death Certificate Project;

the Medical Examiners and Coroners Alert Project (MECAP); and a toll-free hotline. The Commission utilizes a wide range of tools to reduce the risk of injuries and deaths, including mandatory or voluntary safety standards, product recalls, safety-related product modifications, and consumer information campaigns.

There are about 21 400 deaths and 29 million injuries each year related to consumer products under Commission jurisdiction. The deaths, injuries, and property damage associated with consumer products cost the nation about $200 billion annually. The Commission's actions have resulted in immediate reductions in the nation's health care costs and contributed substantially to the 20% decrease in the annual death and injury rate related to consumer products in the last decade. Past agency work in just four areas (electrocutions, children's poisonings, power mowers, and fire safety) save the nation about $2.5 billion each year. The recently issued Commission rule on child-resistant cigarette lighters is projected to save almost $300 million in societal costs each year.

The CPSC administers the Consumer Product Safety Act,[6] The Federal Hazardous Substances Act,[7] the Flammable Fabrics Act,[8] the Poison Prevention Packaging Act,[9] the Refrigerator Safety Act,[10] and the Child Safety Protection Act.[11] Hazards to children are specifically addressed by regulations for such products as cigarette lighters, lawn darts, refuse bins, garage door openers, lead-containing paints, toys, cribs, rattles, pacifiers, bicycles, children's sleepwear, certain medicines and household substances, and refrigerators.

G.2.2 Hazard Identification

The outcome of virtually every project undertaken by the CPSC depends on the availability of reliable data. First, data are used for surveillance to identify hazards. Later, data are used to assess the scope of the problem, to understand hazard patterns, and to evaluate the need for hazard reduction actions.

The foundation for Commission surveillance efforts to collect information on product-related injuries is the National Electronic Injury Surveillance System (NEISS). From this nationally representative sample of 100 US hospital emergency rooms, the CPSC annually collects over 330 000 injury and death reports. The current NEISS provides for four levels of data: timely surveillance of emergency room injuries; special information collected in the emergency department; follow-up telephone interviews with the injured person or parent; and more comprehensive on-site investigations with the injured person and other witnesses. In recent years, the NEISS has been invaluable in studying hazards associated with such children's products as baby walkers and other nursery equipment, bicycles, bunk beds, playground equipment, in-line skates, and toys.

A major source of product-related mortality data is the CPSC's Death Certificate Project. Through this activity, approximately 8700 death certificates are received each year from all 50 states, the District of Columbia, and Puerto Rico. Certificates purchased by the CPSC are those from "cause of death" categories that have a high probability of consumer product involvement. Additional information is often collected from police reports and other local records on fatal incidents for which there may be a specific Commission interest.

From the CPSC's Medical Examiners and Coroners Alert Project (MECAP), approximately 2400 reports are received each year from medical examiners and coroners throughout the country. The MECAP has proven to be very successful, alerting CPSC to product-related deaths much more quickly than is possible through the Death Certificate Project. While the number of reports received through MECAP is relatively small, the reports are especially useful to the CPSC because they have been determined by professionals in the field to be noteworthy. The CPSC was first alerted to major hazards associated with 5-gallon buckets, infant pillows, portable cribs, and other products by MECAP participants.

G.2.3 Involvement of Health Care Professionals

Hoping to build on the success of MECAP, the CPSC is encouraging the participation of other groups, such as pediatricians and other health care professionals, in reporting product-related injuries and deaths in a timely manner. The CPSC is interested in any incident in which a consumer product used in or around the home, school, or in recreation played a significant role in the resultant injury.* Cases involv-

---

* Certain products are under the jurisdiction of other government agencies and are therefore excluded from CPSC's jurisdiction: tobacco products, licensed motor vehicles, pesticides, licensed boats, licensed aircraft, drugs, medical devices, cosmetics, and food.

ing product defects and new hazards are of particular interest. A toll-free fax line (1-800-809-0924) provides a convenient way to file reports with the CPSC. Reports may also be made by toll-free telephone (1-800-638-8095), through the Internet (amcdonal@cpsc.gov), or by mail (Consumer Product Safety Commission, Division of Hazard and Injury Data Systems/EHDS, Washington, DC 20207).

Health care professionals should also encourage their patients to report unsafe products or product-related injuries through the CPSC's Hotline (1-800-638-2772; TTY number for the speech- or hearing-impaired, 1-800-638-8270; Internet address, info@cpsc.gov). In addition, the Hotline is an invaluable resource for obtaining information about product recalls or consumer alerts and ordering CPSC safety publications (For a list of CPSC publications, send a postcard to Publications List, CPSC, Washington, DC 20207. To obtain product recall information through Internet, gopher to cpsc.gov.)

Incidents reported to the CPSC from these and other sources are entered into computer databases, which are searchable by various topics. Data in these files are routinely used by Commission staff and also made available to the public and industry through CPSC's National Injury Information Clearinghouse.* In past years, data collected by the CPSC have been used extensively by other government agencies, standards-setting organizations, manufacturers/trade groups, and others having an interest in product safety.

G.2.4 Addressing Product Hazards

Data collected through all sources is continually reviewed by CPSC epidemiologists, health scientists, engineers, human factors specialists, and compliance officers. As hazards are identified, a variety of remedial actions are considered. For all aspects of product safety, however, the CPSC has the important task of informing and educating consumers of safety hazards through the media, state and local governments, and private organizations, and by responding to consumer inquiries. Future Commission efforts to reduce the annual toll of injuries to children will be greatly enhanced by the participation of pediatricians and other

---

* The computer record does not include data which would identify the victim or the reporter. Identifying information on the actual report is protected under Section 25(c) of the Consumer Product Safety Act and will not be released without consent.

health care professionals in identifying and reporting hazards to the CPSC and by participation in the dissemination of safety information.

G.3 Maternal and Child Health Bureau

G.3.1 Mission, Plan, and Activities

The Maternal and Child Health Bureau (MCHB) is the only Federal agency that focuses exclusively on improving the health and well-being of the nation's mothers and children. In general, the MCHB provides support to help build service systems that emphasize primary care and prevention and that encourage the reduction of risk behaviors and the prevention of disease, injury, and disability. The Bureau has long had an injury prevention focus in recognition of the seriousness of the impact of injury on child health.

Injury prevention activities of the MCHB have included demonstration grants to test specific interventions to prevent child and adolescent injury, grants to provide incentive funding to state public health programs to develop injury prevention activities, knowledge dissemination to inform and persuade a variety of audiences about the need for greater attention to injury, and technical assistance to help in the development of an injury prevention "infrastructure" at the state level.

In 1991, the MCHB developed a 10-year plan to address child and adolescent injury prevention. The plan identified several generic problems in the injury prevention field:

- Public perception. The general public still fails to appreciate the significance of injury. Education is needed to demonstrate that injuries can be prevented.

- Unapplied knowledge. There is a need to more fully apply proven injury control strategies. In many cases, the technology to prevent injuries is available, but there are obstacles to putting it into practice.

- Personnel training. There is a critical lack of trained personnel to develop injury prevention programs. Program implementation is difficult when personnel lack knowledge.

- Research and program evaluation. The continuing need for research and for better evaluation of pediatric injury control programs.

To address these problems, the 1991 plan included mechanisms for policy development, technical assistance, data analyses and publications, training opportunities, and enhanced program evaluation.

G.3.2 Children's Safety Network

A primary MCHB mechanism for carrying out many of the plan's objectives is the Children's Safety Network (CSN), funded to provide information and technical assistance to state and local maternal and child health agencies and other public and voluntary organizations. The CSN staff assist these organizations to collect and analyze data and to design and evaluate programs. The CSN also provides policy-relevant documents for use by states and communities in regulatory and legislative arenas and helps to identify ways in which injury prevention can be effectively integrated into MCHB programs, such as infant mortality reduction, home visiting and school health. Finally, the CSN develops and distributes publications, organizes conferences, and conducts training.* Many of the products developed by the CSN are useful to pediatricians, especially those working to promote policies and programs to prevent injury.

The CSN site at the Education Development Center in Massachusetts has identified a set of key activities, or core functions, in injury prevention that serve as markers for assessing the extent to which state MCH programs are addressing injury prevention in their states (see Table). The CSN uses the key activities to evaluate change over time.

G.3.3 Impact

In an effort to determine the impact of some of MCHB's incentive grants in injury prevention, the Bureau commissioned a study to examine the legacy of small grants awarded in the years 1987–88 for 3-year periods. The state agencies were assessed in terms of "key activities," before, during and after the grant. The evaluation found that the recipients of MCH grants exhibited a considerable increase in injury prevention capacity. Some 3 to 4 years after funding ceased, all seven states

---

* CSN is actually a group of six organizations, two of which are designated as the core sites and have the responsibility of addressing all aspects of injury and violence prevention. The other four sites are issue-specific. They cover the topics of rural injury prevention, economics and insurance issues, adolescent violence prevention, and injury data.

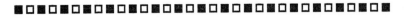

TABLE.
Key Activities for a Comprehensive
MCH Injury Prevention Program

MCH Injury Prevention Coordinator

Designation of an injury prevention coordinator within MCH, with broad-based training in concepts of injury prevention and program development.

Funding

Dedication of MCH funds to injury prevention efforts.

Advocacy

Advocacy within state government and among the public for injury prevention efforts aimed at children and adolescents.

Needs Assessment

Assessment of program needs based on analysis and dissemination of state and local data on:
- injury mortality and morbidity rates
- high-risk behaviors
- available services

Data Improvement

Participation in efforts to improve data sources and availability.

Intervention Plan

Development of an injury prevention service plan that
- targets key injuries, including those noted in *Healthy People 2000*, and targets high-risk groups
- uses proven strategies that incorporate education/behavior change, legislation/regulations, and engineering/technology
- integrates injury prevention into existing MCH and other programs

Support and Guidance for Local Programs

Support and guidance for effective local programs by providing direct funding and/or
- locally specific data reports
- information and materials on the injury problem and prevention strategies
- training and technical assistance

Evaluation

Requiring that programs have process and outcome evaluations.

Collaboration

Collaboration with other relevant government and private agencies and academic institutions to address injury from a multidisciplinary perspective.

studied increased their dedicated injury prevention staff, and six have maintained or increased that level of staffing. Funding for injury prevention also increased over this period. Most of the states greatly increased their capacity to collect and utilize injury morbidity and mortality data, although in most states, data analysis has still not been fully incorporated into the process of planning injury prevention programs. Advocacy for injury prevention increased over the time period in the states studied, and most importantly, injury prevention activities were supported at the local level to a much greater degree than prior to the period of funding. These findings support the concept of relatively small incentive grants as a mechanism for increasing attention and support for state and local injury prevention programming.

G.3.4 EMSC

While its main concern is to ensure that injury prevention is fully integrated into MCH programs at the state and local levels, MCHB also strives to incorporate injury prevention into other programs under its administrative responsibility, such as Emergency Medical Services for Children (EMSC). The EMSC program works with state Emergency Medical Services (EMS) agencies and others to ensure that EMS systems can meet the particular needs of children in emergency situations. Program activities include specialized training of providers, identification of hospitals with the resources to adequately care for ill and injured children, triage and transport guidelines, and other aspects of pediatric emergency care. Injury prevention is an integral component of EMSC; it is better to prevent injuries and entry of children into the EMS system than to treat an injured child.

Four years into MCHB's 10-year plan, much has been accomplished. The state MCH programs are addressing injury prevention and devoting more resources to it, and CSN is able to assist them in a variety of ways. EMSC grantees are also focusing increased attention on injury prevention. state and local MCH agencies have the ability to provide leadership and program funding for child and adolescent injury prevention. However, these agencies continue to be confronted with a myriad set of problems in child health, and these are occurring in an environment in which child poverty continues to increase while state, local, and federal budgets are being cut. It remains to be seen whether the successes

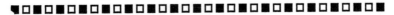
to date in developing the infrastructure for child and adolescent injury prevention at the state level can be sustained.

G.4 National Highway Traffic Safety Administration

G.4.1 Mission

The National Highway Traffic Safety Administration (NHTSA) was established by the Highway Safety Act of 1970 to carry out safety programs under the National Traffic and Motor Vehicle Safety Act of 1966 and the Highway Safety Act of 1966. It also implements consumer programs established by the Motor Vehicle Information and Cost Savings Act, enacted in 1972.

NHTSA's mission is the reduction of deaths, injuries and economic losses resulting from motor vehicle crashes. This is accomplished by establishing and enforcing safety performance standards for motor vehicles and motor vehicle equipment, and through grants to state and local governments and national organizations to implement effective local highway safety programs.

G.4.2 Programs

NHTSA investigates safety defects in motor vehicles, provides leadership to the public and private sector in planning and implementing highway safety programs, helps states and local communities reduce the threat of impaired drivers, promotes the use of safety belts, child safety seats and airbags, promotes the use of bicycle helmets and safe pedestrian behaviors, and provides consumer information on motor vehicle safety topics. NHTSA also conducts research on driver behavior and traffic safety to develop the most efficient and effective means of facilitating safety improvements.

The Agency program is implemented through a staff in Washington, DC, and ten regional offices. The "Section 403" (Highway Safety Research and Development Program) money funds research and development activities, demonstration projects, outreach to national organizations, materials development, training, and public information.

Implementation of state and community activities is conducted under the Highway Safety Act of 1966, which resulted in the establishment of a State Highway Safety Office. The state office is responsible for planning, implementing and evaluating the "Section 402" State and Community Highway Safety Grant program in each state.

G.4.3 Priority Areas

National traffic safety program priorities are established through a rule-making process that identifies those program areas found to be most effective in reducing highway fatalities, injuries, and economic losses. The process examines the extent of the problem and the available countermeasure strategies before assigning priority status to a program area. Currently there are nine priority program areas: alcohol and other drugs, occupant protection, traffic records, police traffic services, emergency medical services, motorcycle safety, pedestrian/bicycle safety, speed control, and roadway safety (a Federal Highway Administration program area). State-level problem identification serves to further define problems at the state and local level and inform decision makers where to invest limited highway safety resources.

G.4.4 Young People

Because motor vehicle injuries are the leading cause of death for young people, NHTSA's mission is clearly one of injury prevention. A variety of strategies are used to reduce motor vehicle injuries including effective legislation and law enforcement, sustained public information and education efforts, expanded partnerships with voluntary organizations, and engineering interventions. A combination of these approaches has been found to be most effective in reducing youth related fatal crashes.

In childhood and adolescent injury prevention, NHTSA's focus is in the areas of occupant protection, child passenger safety, pedestrian safety, bicycle safety, and alcohol programs. The goals of the programs include:

- increasing the correct use of child restraint systems and safety belts;
- increasing the use of bicycle helmets;
- decreasing pedestrian injuries by increasing the awareness of rights and responsibilities of pedestrians and motorists;
- decreasing the incidence of impaired driving and drinking among youth; and

- facilitating the development of community infrastructure to support motor vehicle injury prevention activities.

NHTSA has long worked with national organizations to carry out these goals. For example, NHTSA and the American Academy of Pediatrics have implemented the "Safe Ride" program to ensure that all children are transported safely in vehicles.

A new program in fiscal year 1996, "Patterns for Life," is designed to increase the safety of young children whether they are riding in a motor vehicle, walking down the street, or riding on a bicycle. It centers on increasing the effective use of child safety seats, bicycle helmets, and retroreflective clothing markers. Educational programs also teach parents and other caregivers about the correct use of these devices and provide other appropriate safety messages. The program focuses on building the infrastructure for the delivery of traffic safety services to young children, their parents, and other caregivers across the country. NHTSA's efforts will focus on the development, marketing, and distribution of training and educational materials that are usable by a widely diverse audience.

Training programs in the area of occupant protection and child passenger safety are designed to develop technical and advocacy skills for law enforcement, fire and rescue, public health/medical, child care providers, and other advocate groups.

Pedestrian and bicycle education focuses on the individual. These programs teach specific behaviors and skills needed to successfully interact in simple and complex traffic situations. Pedestrian programs focus on the young, old and impaired; bicycle programs promote helmet usage among all age groups.

In the impaired driving program, NHTSA focuses attention on two aspects of the problem; drinking and impaired driving. In both areas, the primary strategies revolve around prevention, enforcement, and legislation. Prevention emphasizes safe and healthy lifestyles, conveyed by messages and programs through organizations serving youth (such as PTA or SADD). Enforcement focuses on criminal justice system activities that will increase fear of apprehension for violating the law and reduce recurrence for those who are apprehended (eg, enforcement campaigns targeting underage drinking drivers). Legislation focuses on promoting laws directly related to teenage drinking or impaired driving. For instance, zero tolerance laws make it illegal for anyone under the age of 21 to drive after drinking *any* alcohol.

G.4.5 Available Resources

In all these program areas, NHTSA has a wealth of materials available for use by practitioners. Materials include brochures, fact sheets, resource guides, posters, stickers, and public service announcements. NHTSA also provides technical assistance, training, and data. For additional information, call 202-366-2683. In addition, NHTSA operates an Auto Safety Hotline that provides recall information and receives motor vehicle safety complaints. The Hotline operates from 8 am to 4 pm Eastern time, Monday through Friday. The toll-free number is 800-424-9393.

G.5 National Institute of Child Health and Human Development

The Human Learning and Behavior Branch, Center for Research on Mothers and Children, National Institute of Child Health and Human Development (NICHHD) supports research in the area of primary prevention of unintentional injury in children and adolescents.

Past research in injury prevention in children and youth has emphasized the epidemiologic and biomechanical approaches. While these approaches have been extremely useful, a better understanding of the behavioral aspects of injury causation is needed to supplement current understanding about how to most effectively reduce injury morbidity and mortality (see chapter 1.3).

Most injury prevention research in the past has not been based on theories or models of child and adolescent behavior and development — nor on the behavioral development of parents. While research has taken into consideration the natural and man made environments in which families live, there has been little attention paid to the child's *personal* environment (family members, peers, teachers). Primary prevention strategies based on engineering (environmental and product modification and enforcement (laws and regulations) have been effective in

■□■□■□■□■□■□■□■□■□■□■□■□■□■□■□■□■

reducing injury rates, yet injury remains the leading cause of mortality and morbidity in children and youth older than 1 year.

Injury prevention research in which active behavioral change is planned may be essential to further reduce injury rates. Current theory suggests that behavioral and developmental factors in both children and their parents should be considered when planning research. Interventions for prepubertal children are not the same as for adolescents because their physical, cognitive, social, and emotional development are different. Similarly, interventions aimed at changing parents' behaviors are not the same for teenage parents as for parents in their 30s because of the cognitive, social, and emotional differences between these two developmental groups.

The NICHD injury research primary prevention plan has an agenda that emphasizes the design and implementation of strategies that take into account developmental and behavioral factors in both children and their parents, as well as epidemiologic and biomechanical approaches.

Applicants may use a variety of funding mechanisms such as research projects, research career programs, fellowship programs, small business innovative research and others to apply for support. The following guidelines should be considered when applying for funding from the NIH:

- Understand the importance of a *developmental and behavioral* approach to primary injury prevention
- Utilize *theoretical and conceptual* approaches to research in primary injury prevention
- Choose the most appropriate *methods* for studying primary injury prevention — including evaluation research
- Choose the most appropriate *interventions* for primary injury prevention
- Consider the role of the *environment and context* in primary injury prevention

Pediatricians and others should contact the Human Learning and Behavior Branch (301-496-6591) for more detailed information about research submissions to the NIH involving primary injury prevention.

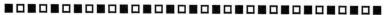
References

1. Committee on Trauma Research, Commission on Life Sciences, National Research Council, and the Institute of Medicine. *Injury in America: A Continuing Public Health Problem.* Washington, DC: National Academy Press; 1985

2. Centers for Disease Control and Prevention. *Injury Control in the 1990s: A National Plan for Action.* Washington, DC: US Public Health Service, Department of Health and Human Services; May 1993

3. *Healthy People 2000: National Health Promotion and Disease Prevention Objectives.* Washington, DC: Public Health Service; 1990. US Department of Health and Human Services publication PHS 90-50212

4. Centers for Disease Control and Prevention. Injury-control recommendations: bicycle helmets. *MMWR Morb Mortal Wkly Rep.* 1995;44:1-17

5. Thurman DJ, Sniezek JE, Johnson D, Greenspan A, Smith SM. Guidelines for Surveillance of Central Nervous System Injury. Atlanta, GA: Centers for Disease Control and Prevention, US Public Health Service, Department of Health and Human Services; 1995

6. Consumer Product Safety Act. 1972;15 USC §2051 et seq

7. Federal Hazardous Substances Act. 1960;15 USC §1261 et seq

8. Flammable Fabrics Act. 1953;15 USC §1191 et seq

9. Poison Prevention Packaging Act of 1970. 1970;15 USC §1471 et seq

10. The Refrigerator Safety Act. 1956;15 USC §1211-1214

11. Child Safety Protection Act. *xxUSC §xxx.* 1994

Index

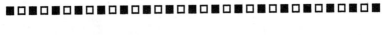

M

R

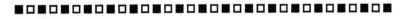